AF682879

Gerontological Nursing Certification Review Guide for the Generalist, Clinical Specialist, and Nurse Practitioner

Editor

Catharine A. Kopac, Ph.D., RN,CS
Gerontological Nurse Practitioner
Assistant Professor
School of Nursing
The Catholic University of America
Washington, D. C.

Associate Editor

Virginia Layng Millonig Ph.D., RN
Potomac, Maryland

Health Leadership Associates
Potomac, Maryland

Health Leadership Associates

Manuscript Editor: John O'Donnell
Production Manager: Martha M. Pounsberry

Copyright © 1993 by Health Leadership Associates, Inc.

All rights reserved. No part of this publication may be reproduced in any form or by any means, electronic, mechanical, photocopying, recording, or otherwise without prior permission in writing from the publisher.

Printed in the United States of America

Health Leadership Associates, Inc. • P. O. Box 59153 • Potomac, Maryland 20859

Library of Congress Cataloging-in-Publication Data

Gerontological nursing certification review guide for the generalist, clinical specialist, and nurse practitioner / editor, Catharine Kopac.
p. cm.
Includes bibliographical references and index.
ISBN 1-878028-08-1 : 38.95
1. Geriatric nursing—Outlines, syllabi, etc. 2. Geriatric nursing—Examinations, questions, etc. I. Kopac, Catharine.
[DNLM: 1. GeriatricNursing—examination questions.
2. Certification—examination questions. WY 18 G3765 1993]
RC954.G474 1993
610.73'65'076—dc20
DNLM/DLC
for Library of Congress 93-16823
CIP

NOTICE The editors, authors and publisher of this book have taken care that the information and recommendations contained herein are accurate and compatible with standards generally accepted at the time of publication. However, the editors, authors and publisher cannot accept responsibility for errors or omissions or for the consequences from application of the information in this book and make no warranty, express or implied with respect to the contents of the book.

To my children,
Michael and Jennifer for their love and support,

and

in loving memory of the late Mary Ellen Pomorski Watson,
a friend, a colleague, a nurse

Contributors

Pamela Z. Cacchione, M.S.N., RN,CS
Gerontological Nurse Practitioner
Doctoral Student
St Louis University
St. Louis, Missouri

Helene M. Clark, Ph.D., RN,C
Assistant Professor
Coordinator Adult Health Nursing
School of Nursing
The Catholic University of America
Washington, D. C.

Marguerite A. English, M.S.N., RN,CS
Gerontological Nurse Practitioner
Same Day Surgery Department
National Hospital for Orthopaedics and Rehabilitation
Arlington, Virginia

Deborah C. Francis, M.S., RN,CS
Gerontological Clinical Nurse Specialist
Hospital Clinical Education
University of California Davis Medical Center
Sacramento, California

Nancy Dickenson-Hazard, M.S.N., F.A.A.N.
Executive Director
National Certification
Board of Pediatric Nurse Practitioners & Nurses
Rockville, Maryland

Karen Cassidy King, M.S.N., RN,CS
Gerontological Nurse Practitioner
Assistant Professor
University of Louisville
School of Nursing
Louisville, Kentucky

Debbie G. Kramer, MS., RN, CS
Gerontological Nurse Practitioner
Adult Nurse Practitioner
BLSA Nurse Unit Manager
Baltimore Longitudinal Study of Aging
National Institutes on Aging
Francis Scott Key Medical Center
Baltimore, Maryland

Maren Stewart Mayhew, M.S.N., RN,CS
Gerontological Nurse Practitioner
Adult Nurse Practitioner
Instructor
School of Nursing
University of Maryland
Baltimore, Maryland

M. Eletta Morse, M.S.N., RN,CS
Gerontological Nurse Practitioner
Alexandria Hospital
Alexandria, Virginia

Anne S. Rosenberg, M.S.N., RN,CS
Family Nurse Practitioner
Baltimore Longitudinal Study of Aging
National Institutes on Aging
Francis Scott Key Medical Center
Baltimore, Maryland

Lois S. Walker, D.N.Sc., RN,CS
Clinical Nurse Specialist
Private Practice in Psychotherapy
Fairfax and Arlington, Virginia

Reviewers

Lynn C. Barnhart, M.S.N., RN,C
Department Chairperson
Department of Nursing
Cameron University
Lawton, Oklahoma

Paula A. Loftis, M.S., RN,CS
Director and Clinical Nurse Specialist
Department of Geriatrics
Parkland Memorial Hospital
Clinical Nurse Specialist
Zale-Lipshy University Hospital
The University of Texas Southwestern Medical Center
Dallas, Texas

Carol L. Panicucci, Ph.D., RN,C
Associate Professor and Chair
Community Health & Family Nursing
College of Nursing
University of Tennessee
Memphis, Tennessee

Preface

The Gerontological Nurse Certification Review Guide has been developed especially for nurses who are preparing to take Certification Examinations offered by the American Nurses Credentialing Center (ANCC). The Guide is inclusive in that it contains both basic and advanced content so that nurses seeking certification as generalists as well as nurses seeking certification as clinical specialists or nurse practitioners will find the guide useful for review. Basic content has been highlighted in shaded blocks throughout the text except for the chapters addressing test taking strategies, demography, and ethical and legal issues. The content in the test taking strategies chapter is essential information for all nurses who are taking certification examinations, the information provided in the chapters on demography and ethical and legal issues is foundational to gerontological nursing practice.

The purpose of the book is twofold. First, the material was designed to enhance the instruction provided in the Certification Review Courses offered by Health Leadership Associates, Inc. Secondly, this book will assist individuals engaged in self study preparation for Certification Examinations. Additionally, the book may be used as a brief reference guide in the practice setting.

Many nurses preparing for certification examinations find that reviewing an extensive body of scientific knowledge requires a very difficult search of many sources that must be synthesized to provide a review base for the examination. The purpose of this publication is to provide a succinct, yet comprehensive review of the core material.

The book has been organized to provide the reader with test taking strategies first. This is followed by the chapters on demographics and health assessment. A feature of the health assessment chapter is that it provides the reviewer with a summary of normal age changes that occur throughout the body and includes a chart on laboratory values that change with age. The next ten chapters address common disorders and provide succinct summaries of definitions, etiology, signs and symptoms, physical findings, differential diagnoses, management/treatment, and nursing considerations. Psychosocial problems are covered separately and include bereavement, depression, delirium, dementia, delusional disorders, and alcoholism. This is followed by the chapter on drug therapy which gives an overview of drug use in the elderly, provides a summary of pharmacokinetics and general principles of prescribing, and gives a good review of some of the major drug classifications that are frequently used with older adults. The final two chapters of the book focus on ethical/legal and the health policy and professional issues that confront gerontological nurses.

Following each chapter are test questions, which are intended to serve as an introduction to the testing arena. In addition a bibliography is included for those who need a more in depth discussion of the subject matter in each chapter. These references can serve as additional instructional material for the reader.

The editor and contributing authors are certified nurses who are respected experts in the field of gerontological nursing. They have designed this book to assist potential examinees to prepare for success in the certification examination process.

It is assumed that the reader of this review guide has completed a course of study in gerontological nursing. The Gerontological Nurse Certification Review Guide is not intended to be a basic learning tool.

Certification is a process that is gaining recognition both within and outside the profession. For the professional it is a means of gaining special recognition as a certified gerontological nurse which not only demonstrates a level of competency, but may also enhance professional opportunities and advancement. For the consumer, it means that a certified nurse has met certain predetermined standards set by the profession.

Acknowledgments

Special acknowledgements go to the authors and reviewers of this book; these individuals, all of whom are practicing professionals, gave unselfishly of their time to meet deadlines and provide exemplary work. Special thanks are given to the staff at Health Leadership Associates, Inc.; these people were always available to answer questions and provide support in preparing the manuscript. A special note of gratitude is offered to Chris Brush, who, as my secretary, provided moral support and edited manuscripts ''above and beyond the call of duty.''

CONTENTS

Test Taking Strategies and Techniques

Nancy A. Dickenson-Hazard

We all respond to testing situations in different ways. What separates the successful test taker from the unsuccessful one is knowing how to prepare for and take a test. Preparing yourself to be a successful test taker is as important as studying for the test. Each person needs to assess and develop their own test taking strategies and skills. The primary goal of this chapter is to assist potential examinees in knowing how to study for and take a test.

STRATEGY #1 Know Yourself

When faced with an examination, do you feel threatened, experience butterflies or sweaty palms, have trouble keeping your mind focused on studying or on the test question? These common symptoms of test anxiety plague many of us, but can be used advantageously if understood and handled correctly (Divine & Kylen, 1979). Over the years of test taking, each of us has developed certain testing behaviors, some of which are beneficial, while others present obstacles to successful test taking. You can take control of the test taking situation by identifying the undesirable behaviors, maintaining the desirable ones and developing skills to improve test performance.

Technique #1 From the following descriptions of test taking personalities, find yourself (Table 1). Write down those characteristics which describe you even if they are from different personality types. Carefully review the problem list associated with your test taking personality characteristics. Write down the problems which are most troublesome. Then make a list of how you can remedy these problems from the improvement strategies list. Be sure to use these strategies as you prepare for and take examinations.

STRATEGY #2 Develop Your Thinking Skills

Understanding Thought Processes: In order to improve your thinking skills and subsequent test performance, it is best to understand the types of thinking as well as the techniques to enhance the thought process.

Everyone has their own learning style, but we all must proceed through the same process to think.

Thinking occurs on two levels—the lower level of memory and comprehension and the higher level of application and analysis (ABP, 1989). Memory is the ability to recall facts. Without adequate retrieval of facts, progression through the higher levels of thinking can not occur easily. Comprehension is the ability to understand memorized facts. To be effective, comprehension skills must allow the person to translate recalled information from one context to another. Application, or the process of using information to know why it occurs, is a higher form of learning. Effective application relies on the use of understood memorized facts to verify intended action. Analysis is the ability to use abstract or logical forms of thought to show relationships and to distinguish the cause and effect between the variables in a situation.

Table 1

Test Taker Profile

Type	*Characteristics*	*Pitfalls*	*Improvement Strategies*
The Rusher	• Rushes to complete the test before the studied facts are forgotten	• Unable to read question and situation completely	• Practice progressive relaxation techniques
	• Arrives at test site early and waits anxiously	• At high risk for misreading, misinterpreting and mistakes	• Develop a study plan with sufficient time to review important content
	• Mumbles studied facts	• Difficult items heighten anxiety	• Avoid cramming and last minute studying
	• Tense body posture	• Likely to make quick, not well-thought-out guesses	• Take practice tests focusing on slowing down and reading and answering each option carefully
	• Accelerated pulse, respiration and neuromuscular excitement		• Read instructions and questions slowly
	• Answers questions rapidly and is generally one of the first to complete		
	• Experiences exhaustion once test is over		
The Turtle	• Moves slowly, methodically, deliberately through each question	• Last to finish; often does not complete the exam	• Take practice tests focusing on time spent per item
	• Repeated re-reading, underlining and checking	• Has to quickly complete questions in last part of exam, increasing errors	• Place watch in front of examination paper to keep track of time
	• Takes 60 to 90 seconds per question versus an average of 45 to 60 seconds	• Has difficulty completing timed examinations	• Mark answer sheet for where one should be halfway through exam based on total number of questions and total amount of time for exam
			• Study concepts not details
			• Attempt to answer each question as you progress through the exam

Type	*Characteristics*	*Pitfalls*	*Improvement Strategies*
The Personalizer	• Mature person who has personal knowledge and insight from life experiences	• Runs risk in relying on what has been learned through observation and experience since one may develop false understandings and stereotypes	• Focus on principles and standards that support nursing practice
		• Personal beliefs and experiences are frequently not the norm or standard tested	• Avoid making connections between patients in exam clinical situations and personal clinical experience
		• Has difficulty identifying expected standards measured by standardized examination	• Focus on generalities not experiences
The Squisher	• View exams as threat, rather than an expected event in education	• Procrastinates studying for exams	• Establish a plan of progressive, disciplined study
	• Preoccupied with grades and personal accomplishment	• Unable to study effectively since waits until last minute	• Use defined time frames for studying content and taking practice exams
	• Attempts to avoid responsibility and accountability associated with testing in order to reduce anxiety	• Increased anxiety over test since procrastinating in the study effort impairs ability to learn and perform	• Use relaxation techniques • Return to difficult items • Read carefully
The Philosopher	• Academically successful person who is well disciplined and structured in study habits	• Over analysis causes loss of sight of actual intent of question	• Focus on questions as they are written
	• Displays great intensity and concentration during exam	• Reads information into questions answering with own added information rather than answering the actual intent of question	• Work on self confidence and not on question. Initial response is usually correct
	• Searches questions for hidden or unintended meaning • Experiences anxiety over not knowing everything		• Avoid multiple re-readings of questions • Avoid adding own information and unintended meanings • Practice, practice, practice with sample tests
The Second Guesser	• Answers questions twice, first as an examinee, second as an examiner	• Altering an initial response frequently results in an incorrect answer	• Re-read only the few items of which one is unsure. Avoid changing initial responses

Type	*Characteristics*	*Pitfalls*	*Improvement Strategies*
	• Believes second look will allow one to find and correct errors	• Frequently changes answers because the pattern of response appears incorrect (i.e. too many "true" or too many "correct" responses)	• Take exam carefully and progressively first time, allowing little or no time for re-reading • Study facts • Avoid reading into questions
	• Frequently changes initial responses (i.e. grades own test)		
The Lawyer	• Attempts to place words or ideas into the question (leads the witness)	• Veers from the obvious answer and provides response from own point of view	• Focus on distinguishing what patient is saying in question and not on what is read into question
	• Occurs most frequently with psychosocial or communication questions which ask for the most appropriate response	• Reads a question, jumps to a conclusion then finds a response that leads to a predetermined conclusion	• Avoid formulating responses aimed at obtaining certain information • Choose responses that allow patient to express feelings which encourage hope, not catastrophe; those which are intended to clarify, which identify feeling tone of patient or which avoid negating or confronting patient feelings

From: "Making the grades as a test-taker," by N. Dickenson-Hazard, (1989) *Pediatric Nursing, 15,* p. 303. Adapted from: *Nurse's guide to successful test-taking* by M. B. Sides and N. B. Cailles, 1989. Philadelphia: J. B. Lippincott, Co., pp 59–70, 199–203. Copyright 1989 by A. J. Jannetti, Inc. Reprinted by permission.

As related to testing situations, the thought process from memory to analysis occurs quite quickly. Some examination items are designed to test memory and comprehension while others test application and analysis. An example of a memory question is as follows:

Non insulin dependent diabetes results from dysfunction of the:

a) liver
b) *pancreas*
c) adrenal glands
d) kidneys
e) pituitary gland

To answer this question correctly, the individual has to retrieve a memorized fact. Understanding the fact, knowing why it is important or analyzing what should be done in this situation is not needed. An example of a question which tests comprehension is as follows:

> You are taking a history on a 67 year old white female during a routine health assessment visit. She reports that in the past four weeks she has had little or no appetite and has lost weight. She complains that she is thirsty a lot of the time and has to urinate frequently. You would most likely suspect which of the following?
>
> a) Urinary tract infection
> b) Hyperthyroidism
> c) Type I diabetes mellitus
> d) Hyponatremia
> e) *Type II diabetes mellitus*

In order to answer this question correctly, an individual must retrieve facts about the physiology of diabetes mellitus in order to understand and differentiate the presenting symptoms.

In a higher level of thinking examination question, individuals must be able to recall a fact, understand that fact in the context of the question, apply this understanding to explaining why one answer is correct after analyzing the answer choices as they relate to the situation (Sides & Cailles, 1989). An example of an application analysis question is as follows:

> A 68 year old diabetic woman wants to enroll in a low-impact aerobics class. Her diabetes is being well managed with twice daily insulin injections. Your best advice is to:
>
> a) Increase daily doses of insulin
> b) *Have an extra snack before exercise class*
> c) Administer a dose of regular insulin after exercise is completed
> d) Tell her participating in the class is not advisable

To answer this question correctly, the individual must recall physiologic facts of insulin dependent diabetes, understand what is happening in this situation, consider each option and how it applies to the patient's condition and analyze why each advice option works or doesn't work for this patient. Application/analysis questions require the examinee to use logical rationale, which demonstrates the ability to analyze a relationship, based on a well defined principle or fact. Problem solving ability becomes important as the examinee must think through each question option, deciding its relevance and importance to the situation of the question.

Building your thinking skills: Effective memorization is the cornerstone to learning and building thinking skills (Olney, 1989). We have all experienced "memory power outages" at some time, due in part to trying to memorize too much, too fast, too ineffectively. Developing skills to improve memorization is important to increasing the effectiveness of your thinking and subsequent test performance.

Technique #1: Quantity is NOT quality, so concentrate on learning important content. For example, it is important to know the various pharmacologic agents appropriate for the management of chronic obstructive pulmonary disease (COPD), not the specific dosages for each medication.

Technique #2: Memory from repetition, or saying something over and over again to remember it usually fades. Developing memory skills which trigger retrieval of needed facts is more useful. Such skills are as follows:

Acronyms: These are mental crutches which facilitate recall. Some are already established such as PERRL (pupils equal, round, reactive to light), or PAT (paroxysmal atrial tachycardia). Developing your own acronyms can be particularly useful since they are your own word association arrangements into a singular word. Nonsense words or funny, unusual ones are often more useful since they attract your attention.

Acrostics: This mental tool arranges words into catchy phrases. The first letter of each word stands for something which is recalled as the phrase is said. Your own acrostics are most valuable in triggering recall of learned information since they are your individual situation associations. An example of an acrostic is as follows:

Mom **C**arried **N**ell **E**very **P**lace **S**he **W**ent stands for the areas of assessment for a cast check: **M**ovement, **C**olor, **N**umbness, **E**dema, **P**ulse, **S**ensation and **W**armth.

ABCs: This technique facilitates information retrieval by using the alphabet as a crutch. Each letter stands for a symptom, which when put together creates a picture of the clinical presentation of the disease. For example, the characteristics of the disease and symptoms of osteoarthritis using the ABC technique is as follows:

a) Aching or pain
b) Being stiff on awakening
c) Crepitus
d) Deterioration of articular cartilage
e) Enlargements at distal interphalangeal joints

f) Formation of new bone at joint surface
g) Granulation inflammatory tissue
h) Heberden's nodes

Imaging: This technique can be used in two ways. The first is to develop a nickname for a clinical problem which when said produces a mental picture. For example, "a wane, wheezy pursed lip" might be used to visualize a patient with pulmonary emphysema who is thin, emaciated, experiencing dyspnea, with a hyperinflated chest, who has an elongated expiratory breathing phase. A second form of imaging is to visualize a specific patient while you are trying to understand or solve a clinical problem when studying or answering a question. For example, imagine an elderly man who is experiencing an acute asthma attack. You are trying to analyze the situation and place him in a position which maximizes respiratory effort. In your mind you visualize him in various positions of side lying, angular and forward, imaging what will happen to the man in each position.

Rhymes, music & links: The absurd is easier to remember than the most common. Rhymes, music or links can add absurdity and humor to learning and remembering (Olney, 1989). These retrieval tools are developed by the individual for specific content. For example, making up a rhyme about diabetes may be helpful in remembering the predominant female incidence, origin of disease, primary symptoms and management as illustrated by:

There once was a woman
    whose beta cells failed
She grew quite thirsty
    and her glucose levels sailed
Her lack of insulin caused her to
    increase her intake
And her increased urinary output
    was certainly not fake
So she learned to watch her diet
    and administer injections
That kept her healthy, happy
    and free of complications.

Setting content to music is sometimes useful to remembering. Melodies which are repetitious jog the memory by the ups and downs of the notes and the rhythm of the music.

Links connect key words from the content by using them in a story. An example given by Olney (1989) for remembering the parts of an eye is: IRIS watched a PUPIL through the LENS of a RED TIN telescope while eating CORNEA on the cob.

Additional memory aids may also include the use of color or drawing for improving recall. Use different colored pens or paper to accentuate the material being learned. For example, highlight or make notes in blue for content about respiratory problems and in red for cardiovascular content. Drawing assists with visualizing content as well. This is particularly helpful for remembering the pathophysiology of the specific health problem.

The important thing to remember about remembering is to use good recall techniques.

Technique #3: Improving higher level thinking skills involves exercising the application and analysis of memorized fact. Small group review is particularly useful for enhancing these high level skills. It allows verbalization of thought processes and receipt of input about content and thought processes from others (Sides & Cailles, 1989). Individuals not only hear how they think, but how others think as well. This interaction allows individuals to identify flaws in their thought process as well as to strengthen their positive points.

Taking practice tests are also helpful in developing application/analysis thinking skills. They permit the individual to analyze thinking patterns as well as the cause and effect relationships between the question and its options. The problem solving skills needed to answer application/ analysis questions are tested, giving the individual more experience through practice (Dickenson-Hazard, 1990).

STRATEGY #3 Know The Content

Your ability to study is directly influenced by organization and concentration (Dickenson-Hazard, 1990). If effort is spent on both of these aspects of exam preparation, examination success can be increased.

Preparation for studying: Getting organized. Study habits are developed early in our educational experiences. Some of our habits enhance learning while others do not. To increase study effectiveness, organization of study materials and time is essential. Organization decreases frustration, allows for easy resumption of study and increases concentrated study time.

Technique #1: Create your own study space. Select a study area that is yours alone, free from distractions, comfortable and well lighted. The ventilation and room temperature should be comfortable since a cold room makes it difficult to concentrate and a warm room makes you sleepy (Burkle & Marshak, 1989). All your study materials should be left in your study space. The basic premise of a study space is that it facilitates a mind set that you are there to study. When you interrupt study, it is best to leave your materials just as they are. Don't close books or put away notes as you will just have to relocate them, wasting your study time, when you do resume study.

Technique #2: Define and organize the content. From the test giver, secure an outline or the content parameters which are to be examined. If the test giver's outline is sketchy, develop a more detailed one for yourself using the recommended text as a guideline. Next, identify your available study resources: class notes, old exams, handouts, textbooks, review courses, or study groups. For national standardized exams, such as initial licensing or certification, it is best to identify one or two study resources which cover the content being tested and stick to them. Attempting to review all available resources is not only mind boggling, but increases anxiety and frustration as well. Make your selections and stay with them.

Technique #3: Conduct a content assessment. Using a simple rating scale of

1 = requires no review
2 = requires minimal review
3 = requires intensive review
4 = start from the beginning

Read through the content outline and rate each content area (Dickenson-Hazard, 1990). Table 2 provides a sample exam content assessment. Be honest with your assessment. It is far better to recognize your content weaknesses when you can study and remedy them, rather than thinking during the exam how you wished you had studied more. Likewise with content strengths: if you know the material, don't waste time studying it.

Table 2

Sample Content Assessment

Exam Content: Cardiovascular Health Problems of the Elderly	
Category: Provided by Test Giver	*Rating: Provided by Examinee*
I. Age Related Cardiovascular Changes	
A. Structure	2
B. Physiology	2
II. Coronary Artery Disease	
A. Etiology	3
B. Pathophysiology	3
C. Symptomatology	2
D. Management	3
E. Nursing Interventions	2
III. Hyper and Hypotension	
A. Etiology	2
B. Pathophysiology	2
C. Symptomatology	1
D. Management	2
E. Nursing Interventions	1
IV. Stroke and Transient Ischemic Attacks	
A. Etiology	3
B. Pathophysiology	4
C. Symptomatology	3
D. Management	4
E. Nursing interventions	3
V. Congestive Heart Failure	
A. Etiology	3
B. Pathophysiology	4
C. Symptomatology	3
D. Management	4
E. Nursing Interventions	3
VI. Arrhythmias and Conduction Disorders	
A. Etiology	3
B. Pathophysiology	4
C. Symptomatology	4
D. Management	4
E. Nursing Interventions	3
VII. Peripheral Vascular Disease	
A. Etiology	2
B. Pathophysiology	3
C. Symptomatology	2
D. Management	2
E. Nursing Interventions	1
VIII. Varicosities and Chronic Venous Insufficiency	
A. Etiology	3
B. Pathophysiology	3
C. Symptomatology	3
D. Management	3
E. Nursing Interventions	2

Technique #4: Develop a study plan. Coordinate the content which needs to be studied with the time available (Sides & Cailles, 1989). Prioritize your study needs, starting with weak areas first. Allow for a general review at the end of the study plan. Lastly, establish an overall goal for yourself; something that will motivate you when it is brought to mind.

Table 3 illustrates a study plan developed on the basis of the exam content assessment in Table 2. Conducting an assessment and developing a study plan should require no more than 50 minutes. It is a wise investment of time with potential payoffs of reduced study stress and exam success.

Technique #5: Begin now and use your time wisely. The smart test taker begins the study process early (Olney, 1989). Sit down, conduct the content assessment and develop a study plan as soon as you know about the exam. DON'T PROCRASTINATE!

Getting Down To Business: The Actual Studying. There is no better way to prepare for an examination than individual study (Dickenson-Hazard, 1989). The responsibility to achieve the goal you set for this exam lies with you alone. The means you employ to achieve this goal do vary and should begin with identifying your peak study times and using techniques to maximize them.

Technique #1: Study in short bursts. Each of us have our own biologic clock which dictates when we are at our peak during the day. If you are a morning person, you are generally active and alert early in the day, slowing down and becoming drowsy by evening. If you are an evening person, you don't completely wake up until late morning and hit your peak in the afternoon and evening. Each person generally has several peaks during the day. It is best to study during those times when your alertness is at its peak (Dickenson-Hazard, 1990).

During our concentration peaks, there are mini peaks, or bursts of alertness (Olney, 1989). These alertness peaks of a concentration peak occur because levels of concentration are at their highest during the first part and last part of a study period. These bursts can vary from ten minutes to one hour depending on the extent of concentration. If studying is sustained for one hour there are only two mini peaks; one at the beginning and one at the end. There are eight mini peaks if that same hour is divided into four, 10-minute intervals. Hence it is more helpful to study in short bursts (Olney, 1989). More can be learned in less time.

Table 3

Sample Study Plan

Goal: Achieve a "B" on the Geriatric Cardiovascular Health Problem Test Time Available: 2 Weeks

Objective	*Activity*	*Date Accomplished*
Review age related changes	Review notes and re-read Chapter 22	Feb 5, 1 hour
Master arrhythmia and conduction disorder content	Read Chapter 26	
	Take notes on chapter content according to content outline	Feb 5 & 6—1 hour
	Review class notes combined with chapter notes	Feb 6—1 hour
	Review sample test questions	Feb 6—1 hour
Understand content on congestive heart failure	Read Chapter 25	
	Take notes on chapter content according to content outline	Feb 7—2 hours
	Review class notes combined with chapter notes	Feb 8—1½ hours
	Review sample test questions	Feb 9—1½ hours
Master content on stroke and TIA	Read Chapter 24	
	Take notes on chapter content according to content outline	Feb 10—2 hours
	Review class notes combined with chapter notes	Feb 11—1½ hours
	Review sample test questions	Feb 12—1½ hours
Know material on varicosities and chronic venous insufficiency	Scan Chapter 27	
	Review class notes supplementing with text notes	Feb 14—2 hours
Know material on coronary artery disease	Scan Chapter 23	
	Review class notes, supplementing with text notes	Feb 15—2 hours
Know material on peripheral vascular disease	Scan Chapter 28	
	Review highlights and important concepts	Feb 16—2 hours
Know material on hyper and hypotension	Scan Chapter 29	
	Review highlights and important concepts	Feb 17—2 hours
Demonstrate understanding of all material	Review with another person	Feb 18—2 hours
	Review all notes	Feb 19—1½ hours
	Take sample test questions	Feb 19—1½ hours
Think positively	SMILE	ON GOING
	Take frequent breaks	Reward myself after each study session
	Keep my goal in mind	

Technique #2: Cramming can be useful. Since concentration ability is highly variable, some individuals can sustain their mini-peaks for 15, 20 or even 30 minutes at a time. Pushing your concentration beyond its peak is fruitless and verges on cramming, which in general is a poor study technique. There are, however, times when cramming, a short term memory tool, is useful. Short term memory generally is at its best in the morning. A quick review or cram of content in the morning can be useful the day of the exam (Olney, 1989). Most studying, however, is best accomplished in the afternoon or evening when long term memory functions at its peak.

Technique #3: Give your brain breaks. Regular times during study to rest and absorb the content is needed by the brain. The best approach to breaks is to plan them and give yourself a conscious break (Dickenson-Hazard, 1990). This approach eliminates the ''day dreaming'' or ''wandering thought'' approach to breaks that many of us use. It is better to get up, leave the study area and do something non-study related for longer breaks. For shorter breaks of five minutes or so, leave your desk, gaze out the window or do some stretching exercises. When your brain says to give it a rest, accommodate it! You'll learn more in less stress free time.

Technique #4: Study the correct content. It is easy for all of us to become bogged down in the detail of what we are studying. However, it is best to focus on the major concepts or the ''state of the art'' content. Leave the details, the suppositions and the experience at the door of your study area. Concentrate on the major textbook facts and concepts which revolve around the subject matter being tested.

Technique #5: Fit your studying to the test type. The best way to prepare for an objective test is to study facts, particularly anything printed in italics or bold. Memory enhancing techniques are particularly useful when preparing for an objective test. If preparing for an essay test, study generalities, examples and concepts. Application techniques are helpful when studying for this type of an exam (Burkle & Marshak, 1989).

Technique #6: Use your study plan wisely. Your study plan is meant to be a guide, not a rigid schedule. You should take your time with studying. Don't rush through the content just to remain on schedule. Occasionally study plans need revision. If you take more or less time than planned, readjust the plan for the time gained or lost. The plan can guide you, but you must go at your own pace.

Technique #7: Actively study. Being an active participant in study rather than trying to absorb the printed word is also helpful. Ways to be active include: taking notes on the content as you study; constructing questions then answering them;

taking practice tests or; discussing the content with yourself. Also using your individual study quirks are encouraged. Some people stand, others walk around and some play background music. Whatever helps you to concentrate and study better, you should use.

Technique #8: Use study aids. While there is no substitute for individual studying, several resources, if available, are useful in facilitating learning. Review courses are an excellent means for organizing or summarizing your individual study. They generally provide the content parameters and the major concepts of the content which you need to know. Review courses also provide an opportunity to clarify not-well-understood content, as well as to review known material (Dickenson-Hazard, 1990). Study guides are useful for organizing study. They provide detail on the content which is important to the exam. Study groups are an excellent resource for summarizing and refining content. They provide an opportunity for thinking through your knowledge base, with the advantage of hearing another person's point of view. Each of these study aids increases understanding of content and when used correctly, increase effectiveness of knowledge application.

Technique #9: Know when to quit. It is best to stop studying when your concentration ebbs. It is unproductive and frustrating to force yourself to study. It is far better to rest or unwind, then resume at a later point in the day. Avoid studying outside your A.M. or P.M. concentration peaks and focus your study energy on your right time of day or evening.

STRATEGY #4 Become Test-wise

Most nursing examinations are composed of multiple choice questions (MCQs). This type of question requires the examinee to select the best response(s) for a specific circumstance or condition. Successful test taking is dependent not only on content knowledge but on test taking skill as well. If you are unable to impart your knowledge through the vehicle used for its conveyance, i.e. the MCQ, your test taking success is in jeopardy.

Technique #1: Recognize the purpose of a test question. Most test questions are developed to examine knowledge at two separate levels: memory (or recall) and comprehension (or application). A memory question requires the examinee to recall facts from their knowledge base while an application question requires the examinee to use and apply the knowledge (ABP, 1989). Memory questions test recall while application questions test synthesis and problem-solving skills. When taking a test you need to be aware of whether you are being asked a fact or to use that fact.

Table 4

Anatomy Of A Test Question

Background Statement:	A 70 year old woman comes for a health assessment visit with complaints of weakness, fatigue, and weight loss. A palpable abdominal mass is found on physical examination and laboratory studies reveal the patient is anemic. Barium enema and colonoscopy confirm a malignancy.
	Stem: The most likely anatomic site of the cancer is the:
	Options: (A) Rectum (B) Sigmoid colon (C) Left colon (D) Transverse colon (E) *Cecum*

Table 5

Test Question Key Words And Phrases

First	Significant	Counseling
Best	Immediate	Facilitative
Most	Helpful	Indicative
Initial	Closely	Suggestive
Important	Priority	Appropriate
Major	Advice	Accurately
Common	Approach	Likely
Least	Consideration	Characteristics
Except	Management	True Statements
Not	Expectation	Correct Statements
Greatest	Intervention	Contributing to
Earliest	Assessment	Of the following
Useful	Contraindication	Which of the following
Leading	Evaluation	Each of the following

From ''Anatomy of a test question'' by N. Dickenson-Hazard, 1989, *Pediatric Nursing 15,* p. 395. Copyright 1989 by A. J. Jannetti, Inc. Reprinted by permission.

Technique #2: Recognize the components of a test question. Multiple choice questions may include the basic components of a background statement, a stem and a list of options. The background statement presents information which facilitates the examinee in answering the question. The stem asks or states the intent of the question. The options are 4 or 5 possible responses to the question. The correct option is called the keyed response and all other options are called distractors (ABP, 1989). Knowing the components of a test question help you shift through the information presented and to focus on the questions intent (see Table 4).

Technique #3: Identify the key word(s) in a test question. Key words are generally included in the stem of a test question, whereas key concepts or conditions appear in the background statement. You should pay particular attention to the key words in the stem and their impact on the intent of the question (See Table 5).

Technique #4: Recognize the item types. Basically two styles of MCQs are used for examinations. One requires the examinee to select the one best answer; the other requires selection of multiple correct answers. Among the one best answer styles there are three types. The A type requires the selection of the best response among those offered. The B type requires the examinee to match the options with the appropriate statement. C type items require the examinee to compare or contrast two related conditions. The X type asks the examinee to respond either true or false to each option (ABP, 1989). Table 6, on the following page illustrates these item types. **Most standardized tests, such as those used for nursing licensure and certification, are composed of four or five option-A type questions.**

Technique #5: Read the directions to the questions carefully. Since an examination may have several types of questions, it is imperative to read the directions carefully. If different item types are used on an exam, they are generally grouped together by type and marked clearly with directions. Be on the lookout for changing item types and be sure you understand the directions on how you are to answer before you begin reading the question.

Technique #6: Apply the basic rules of test taking. Examination candidates can avert many problems associated with test taking if they give thought to the mechanics of sitting down, reading the question and noting their answers. Timing yourself to avoid spending too much time on a question, returning to difficult questions, and not changing your answers are all techniques that can improve performance. Table 7, on the next page provides helpful hints for the basic rules of test-taking. Review these and apply them to the testing situation.

Technique #7: Practice, practice, practice. Taking practice tests can improve performance. While they can assist in evaluation of your knowledge, their primary benefit is to assist you with test taking skills. You should use them to evaluate your thinking process, your ability to read, understand and interpret questions, and your skills in completing the mechanics of the test.

Technique #8: Be prepared for exam day. It is important to familiarize yourself with the test site, the building, the parking and travel route prior to the exam day. If you must travel, arrive early to allow time for this familiarization. It is helpful to make a list of things you need on the exam day: pencils, admission card, watch and a few pieces of hard candy as a quick energy source. On exam day allow yourself plenty of time to arrive at the site. Wear comfortable clothes and have a good breakfast that morning. The night before the exam, go to bed at a reasonable hour;

TABLE 6

Item Type Examples

A TYPE

Directions for One Best Choice Items: This item-type requires that you indicate the one best answer from the lettered alternatives offered for each item. After you have decided on the one BEST answer, completely blacken the corresponding lettered circle on the answer sheet.

1 A 68 year old man gives a history of bilateral proximal and distal leg pain. He is also experiencing weakness on prolonged standing. This is most suggestive of:
- a. Arthritis
- b. *Lumbar spinal stenosis*
- c. Peripheral neuropathy
- d. Diskitis
- e. Peripheral vascular disease

B TYPE

Directions: Each group of questions below consists of five lettered headings followed by a list of numbered words or statements. For each numbered word or statement, select the one lettered heading that is most closely associated with it and fill in the circle beneath the corresponding letter on the answer sheet. Each lettered heading may be selected once, more than once, or not at all.

#2–4

Medication types:
- a. Beta-adrenergic blockers
- b. Diuretics
- c. Digoxin
- d. Angiotensin-converting enzyme inhibitors
- e. Calcium antagonists

Most useful for treatment of:
- 2. Supraventricular tachy arrhythmias (e)
- 3. Congestive heart failure (b)
- 4. Myocardial infarction (a)

C TYPE

Directions: Each set of lettered headings below is followed by a list of numbered words or phrases. For each numbered word or phrase fill in the circle on the answer sheet under:
- a. If the item is associated with (A) only,
- b. If the item is associated with (B) only,
- c. If the item is associated with both (A) and (B),
- d. If the item is associated with neither (A) nor (B).

(A) Diabetic acidosis
(B) Insulin shock
(C) Both
(D) Neither

#5—Elevated bicarbonate level in serum (D)
#6—The duration of the condition before proper treatment is begun may influence the prognosis (C)
#7—Deep breathing (A)
#8—Coma (C)
#9—Moist skin characteristic (B)

X TYPE

Directions: Each of the questions or incomplete statements below is followed by five suggested answers or completions. For EACH lettered alternative completely blacken one lettered circle in either column T or F on the answer sheet.

Which of the following tests are useful for differentiating anemia associated with a chronic disease from iron deficiency anemia?
- a. Serum iron levels (F)
- b. Bone marrow examination (T)
- c. Reticulocyte count (F)
- d. Serum transferrin level (F)
- e. Serum ferritin level (T)

From ''Anatomy of a test question.'' by N. Dickenson-Hazard, 1989, *Pediatric Nursing 15,* p. 396. Copyright 1989 by A. J. Jannetti, Inc. Adapted by permission.

Table 7

Basic Rules For Test Taking

Basic Rule	*Helpful Hints*
Use time wisely and effectively	Allow no more than 1 minute per question—If you can't answer question, make an intelligent guess
Know the parts of a question Background statement: Informational scenario Stem: Specific question or intent statement	Select the option that best completes question or solves the problem Relate options to question and balance against each other Consider all options
Read question carefully	Understand stem first, then look for answer Underline key words in background information and stem (i.e. first, best, initial, early, most, appropriate, except, least, not).
Identify intent of item based on information given	Don't assume any information not given Don't read in or add any information not given Actively reason through question
Answer difficult questions by eliminating obviously incorrect options first	Select the best of the viable, available options using logical thought Re-read stem; select strongest option Skip difficult questions and return to them later or make an educated guess
Select responses guided by principles of communication	Choose therapeutic, respectful, communication enhancing options Avoid inappropriate, punitive responses
Know the principles of nursing practice	Select options that relate to common need or the population in general Select options that are correct without exception Select options which reflect nursing judgement
Know and use test-taking principles	Avoid changing answers without good reason Attempt every question Don't rely on flaws in test construction Be systematic and use problem-solving technique in answering questions

From "Making the grade as a test-taker" by N. Dickenson-Hazard, 1989. *Pediatric Nursing 15,* p. 304. Adapted from *How to take tests.* (pp 15-57) by J. Millman and W. Paul, 1969, New York: McGraw-Hill Co. and from *Nurses's guide to successful test taking.* (pp 43–53) by M.B. Sides and N.B. Cailles, 1989, Philadelphia: J. B. Lippincott Co. Copyright 1989 A.J. Jannetti, Inc. Reprinted and adapted by permission.

avoid last minute cramming; and avoid excessive drinking or eating (Sides & Cailles, 1989). The idea is to arrive on time at the test site, prepared and as rested as possible.

STRATEGY #5 Psych Yourself Up: Taking tests is stressful

While a little stress can be productive, too much can incapacitate you in your studying and test taking (Divine & Kylen, 1979). Your attitude and approach to test taking and studying can influence the results you achieve. Psyching yourself up can have a positive effect and make examinations a non-anxiety laden experience (Dickenson-Hazard, 1990). The following techniques are based on the principles of successful test taking as presented by Sides & Cailles (1989). Incorporation of these techniques can improve response and performance in examination situations.

Technique #1: Adopt an "I can" attitude. Believing you can succeed is the key to success. Self belief inspires and gives you the power to achieve your goals. Without a success attitude, the road to your goal is much harder. We all stand an equal chance of success in this world. It is those who believe they can who achieve it. This "I can" attitude must permeate all your efforts in test taking, from studying, to improving your skills, to actually writing the test.

Technique #2: Take control. By identifying your goal, deciding how to accomplish it and developing a plan for achieving it, you take control. Do not leave your success to chance; control it through action and attitude.

Technique #3: Think positively. Examinations are generally based on a standard which is the same for all individuals. Everyone can potentially pass. Performance is influenced not only by knowledge and skill but by attitude as well. Those individuals who regard an exam as an opportunity or challenge will be more successful.

Technique #4: Project a positive self-fulfilling prophecy. While preparing for an examination, project thoughts of the positive outcomes you will experience when you succeed. Self-talk is self-fulfilling. Expect success, not failure, of yourself.

Technique #5: Feel good about yourself. Without feeling a sense of positive self worth, passing an examination is difficult. Recognize your professional contributions and give yourself credit for your accomplishments. Think "I will pass," not "I suppose I can."

Technique #6: Know yourself. Focus exam preparation and test taking on your strengths. Try to alter your weaknesses instead of becoming hung up on them. If you tend to overanalyze, study and read test questions at face value. If you're a speed demon when taking a test, slow down and read more carefully.

Technique #7: Failure is a possibility. We all have failed at something at some point in our lives. Rather than dwelling on the failure, making excuses and believing you'll fail again, recognize your mistakes and remedy them. Failure is a time to begin again; use it as a motivator to do better. It is not the end of the world unless you allow it to be. It is best to deal with the failure and move on, otherwise it interferes with your success.

Technique #8: Persevere, persevere, persevere! Endurance must underlie all your efforts. Call forth those reserve energies when you've had all you think you can take. Rely upon yourself and your support systems to help you maintain a sense of direction and keep your goal in the forefront.

Technique #9: Motivation is muscle. Most individuals are motivated by fear or desire. The fear in an exam situation may be one of failure, the unknown or discovery of imperfection. Put your fear into perspective; realize you are not the only one with fear and that all have an equal opportunity for success. Develop strategies to reduce fear and use fear to your advantage by improving the imperfections. Desire is a powerful motivator and you should keep the rewards of your desire foremost in your mind. Whatever motivates you, use it to make you successful. Reward yourself during your exam preparation and once the exam has been completed. You alone hold the key to success; use what you have wisely.

This chapter has provided concepts, strategies and techniques for improving study and test taking skills. Your first task in improvement is to know yourself: how you study and how you take a test. You should use your strengths and remedy the weaknesses. Next you need to develop your thinking skills. Work on techniques to improve memory and reasoning. Now you need to organize your study and concentrate on using your strengths and these new and improved skills to be successful. Create a study space, develop a plan of action, then implement that plan during your periods of peak concentration. Before taking the exam be sure you understand the components of a test question, can identify key words and phrases and have practiced. Apply the test taking rules during the exam process. Finally, believe in yourself, your knowledge and your talent. Believing you can accomplish your goal facilitates the fact that you will.

BIBLIOGRAPHY

American Board of Pediatrics. (1989). *Developing questions and critiques.* Unpublished material.

Burke, M. M., & Walsh, M. B. (1992). *Gerontologic nursing,* St. Louis: Mosby Year Book.

Burkle, C.A., & Marshak, D. (1989). *Study program: Level 1.* Reston, Va: National Association of Secondary School Principals.

Conaway, D. C., Miller, M. D., & West, G. R. (1988). *Geriatrics.* St. Louis: Mosby Year Book.

Dickenson-Hazard, N. (1989). Making the grade as a test taker. *Pediatric Nursing, 15,* 302–304.

Dickenson-Hazard, N. (1989). Anatomy of a test question. *Pediatric Nursing, 15,* 395–399.

Dickenson-Hazard, N. (1990). The psychology of successful test taking. *Pediatric Nursing, 16,* 66–67.

Dickenson-Hazard, N. (1990). Study smart. *Pediatric Nursing, 16,* 314–316.

Dickenson-Hazard, N. (1990). Study effectiveness: Are you 10 a.m. or p.m. scholar? *Pediatric Nursing, 16,* 419–420.

Dickenson-Hazard, N. (1990). Develop your thinking skills for improved test taking. *Pediatric Nursing, 16,* 480–481.

Divine, J. H., & Kylen, D. W. (1979). *How to beat test anxiety.* New York: Barrons Educational Series, Inc.

Millman, J., & Paul, W. (1969). *How to take tests.* New York: McGraw-Hill Book Co.

Millonig, V. L. (Ed.). (1991). *The adult nurse practitioner certification review guide* (rev. ed). Potomac, MD: Health Leadership Associates.

Olney, C. W. (1989). *Where there's a will, there's an A.* New Jersey: Chesterbrook Educational Publishers.

Sides, M., & Cailles, N. B. (1989). *Nurse's guide to successful test taking.* Philadelphia: J. B. Lippincott Co.

Demographics, Theories & Nursing Process

Catharine A. Kopac

Demographics of Older Adults

- Population statistics (A Profile of Older Americans, 1992)
  1. Persons 65 years or older numbered 31.8 million
     a. 12.6 % of U.S.; one in every eight Americans
     b. Increase of 24% (6.1 million) since 1980
  2. Sex ratio 148 women for every 100 men
     a. Increases with age
     b. Ratio of 123/100 for 65–69 group
     c. Ratio of 259/100 for 85 and older
  3. Percentage of older Americans has increased since 1900
     a. 4.1% in 1900
     b. 12.6% in 1991
  4. Older population itself is getting older
     a. In 1991 the 65–74 age group (18.3 million) was eight times larger than in 1900
     b. The 75–84 group (10.3 million) was 13 times larger
     c. The 85+ group (3.2 million) was 25 times larger
  5. In 1990, persons reaching age 65 had an average life expectancy of an additional 17.3 years
  6. A child born in 1990 could expect to live 75.4 years, about 8 years longer than a child born in 1900.
  7. By 2030, there will be about 66 million older persons (2 and 1/2 times their number in 1990)
  8. By 2000, persons 65+ are expected to represent 13.0% of the population; by 2030, 21.8%.
  9. Factors affecting decreased mortality: improved nutrition, improved sanitation, social improvements, disease prevention, health promotion/wellness movement
- Marital Status and Living Arrangements
  1. Older men are twice as likely to be married as older women (77% of men; 41% of women)

2. Half of all older women are widows (48%); five times as many widows (8.5 million) as widowers (1.8 million)
3. Of the 65+ group 5% are divorced; these numbers have increased three times as fast as the older population as a whole since 1980 (2.1 times for women, 3.8 times for men)
4. Majority (67%) of noninstitutionalized persons live in a family setting
5. Of noninstitutionalized persons, 31% (9.4 million) live alone (7.2 million women, 1.9 million men)
6. In 1987, 5% (2.0 million) of the 65+ population lived in nursing homes; with age the percentage increases dramatically: 1% for persons 65–74 years, 5% for persons 75–84 years, 25% for persons 85+

- Racial & Ethnic Composition and Geographic Distribution
  1. Eighty-nine percent of persons 65+ are white; 8% black; 4% Hispanic; 3% other races
  2. Fifty-two percent of persons 65+ live in nine states: California, Florida, New York, Pennsylvania, Texas, Illinois, Ohio, Michigan, New Jersey
  3. Persons 65+ constitute 14.0% or more of the total population in ten states: Florida (18.3%), Pennsylvania (15.5%), Iowa (15.4%), Rhode Island & West Virginia (15.1% each), Arkansas (14.9%), South Dakota (14.7%), North Dakota (14.5%), Nebraska (14.1%), and Missouri (14.1%)
  4. Of the elderly, 74% live in metropolitan areas
     a. Thirty percent live in central cities
     b. Forty-four percent live in suburbs
- Income and Poverty
  1. Median income (1991), persons 65+, $14,357 for men and $8,189 for women
  2. Median income (1991), households headed by persons 65+, $24,865
     a. $25,741 for Whites
     b. $15,977 for Blacks

   c. $19,633 for Hispanics
   d. Twenty-three percent had incomes less than $15,000
   e. Thirty-nine percent had incomes more than $30,000

3. In 1991, 48% of persons living alone, or with nonrelatives, had an income of $10,000 or less; 10% had incomes under $5,000. Median income was $10,420
   a. $10,934 for Whites
   b. $ 6,794 for Blacks
   c. $ 7,019 for Hispanics
4. Major sources of income (1990)
   a. Social Security (37%)
   b. Asset income (25%)
   c. Earnings (18%)
   d. Public & private pensions (18%)
   e. All other sources (3%)
5. Of older households, 12% have one or more members covered by Medicaid
6. Of older renter households, 29% live in publicly owned or subsidized housing
7. Median net worth of older households (1988) was $73,500
   a. Seventeen percent had net worth below $10,000
   b. Fourteen percent had net worth above $250,000
8. Twenty percent of the older population was poor or near-poor in 1990
   a. There were 3.8 million below poverty level
   b. There were 2.3 million (7%) classified as "near poor"
   c. Ten percent of elderly Whites poor
   d. Thirty-four percent of elderly Blacks poor
   e. Twenty-two percent of elderly Hispanics poor

   f. Poverty rate of older women—16%

   g. Poverty rate of older men—8%

- Education and Employment

  1. Have been steadily increasing; between 1970 and 1991 the percentage who had completed high school rose from 28% to 58%. About 12% had four or more years of college.

  2. Percentage who had completed high school (1990) varied by race and ethnic origin

     a. Of Whites—61%

     b. Of Blacks—28%

     c. Of Hispanics—26%

  3. Three and a half million older Americans (12%) were in labor force (working or actively seeking work) in 1991; 2.0 million men (16%) and 1.5 million women (9%)

     a. Constitute 2.8% of U.S. labor force

     b. Three percent unemployed

     c. Fifty-four percent of workers over 65 employed part-time

        (1) Women—49%

        (2) Men—60%

- Health and Health Care

  1. Number of days in which usual activities are restricted due to illness or injury increases with age—the average is 31 such days

     a. Days for males—28

     b. Days for females—34

     c. Days for Whites—30

     d. Days for Blacks—47

  2. Six million (23%) older people living in the community had health-related difficulty with one or more personal care activities (bathing, dressing, eating, etc.)

  3. Over seven million (27%) had difficulty with one or more home management activities (shopping, managing money, doing housework, etc.)

4. Most older people have at least one chronic condition and many have multiple conditions; the most frequently occuring conditions (1990):
   a. Arthritis (47%)
   b. Hypertension (37%)
   c. Hearing impairments (32%)
   d. Heart disease (29%)
   e. Orthopedic impairments (17%)
   f. Sinusitis and cataracts (15%)
   g. Diabetes (9%)
5. Older people accounted for 34% of all hospital stays and 45% of all days of care (1990)
   a. Average length of stay—8.7 days
   b. Average number of physician contacts—9
6. In 1987 the 65+ group represented approximately 12% of the population but accounted for 36% of total personal health care expenditures; expenditures totaled $162 billion and averaged $5,360 per year per older person. Approximately 25% came from direct "out-of-pocket" payments by older persons.
7. Hospital expenses are the largest portion of health expenditures (42%); followed by physicians (21%) and nursing home care (20%).

Theories of Aging

- Biological—Attempts to explain three in-vivo biocomponents: Cells that undergo miosis throughout life (e.g., white blood cells (WBCs), epithelial cells); cells incapable of division and renewal (e.g., neurons); and noncellular material with little turnover and that is under integrated physiologic control (e.g., collagen). A unifying theory does not exist that explains the underlying mechanics and causes of aging.
  1. Genetic theories
     a. Gene—one or more harmful genes in the organism become active in later life, causing failure of the organism to survive.

   b. Error—decreased bond over time in protein synthesis; weakening of organic synthesis produces defective cells, leading to successive generations of faulty cells.

   c. Somatic mutation—when cells are exposed to x-ray radiation or chemicals, a cell-by-cell alteration of DNA occurs, thereby increasing the incidence of chromosomal abnormalities.

   d. Programmed (biologic clock)—internal, genetic control determines aging process; a set time to live, winds down over time.

2. Nongenetic theories

   a. Immunologic—changes in lymphoid tissue leads to an imbalance in T cells and subsequent cellular immune function decrease; results in autoantibody production and immune deficiencies.

   b. Free radical—unstable free radicals from environmental pollutants alter biological system, causing changes in chromosomes, pigment, and collagen.

   c. Cross-link—collagen molecules and chemicals alter tissue functioning, leading to stiffness & rigidity of tissues.

3. Physiologic theories

   a. Stress adaptation—accumulated damage results from stress response activation.

   b. Wear-and-tear—after repeated injury/use, body structures and functions deteriorate from stress.

- Social—behavioristic; examines how one most successfully experiences late life

  1. Disengagement—"aging is an inevitable, mutual, withdrawal or disengagement, resulting in decreased interaction between the aging person and others in the social system he belongs to" (Cummings & Henry, 1961, p 2)

     a. Progressive social disengagement occurs with age

     b. Mutual, acceptable to individual and society

     c. Studies done since this theory was proposed have found:

        (1) Theory does not hold true for the majority

(2) Degree of disengagement varies with personality and life activity pattern

(3) Social involvement is a lifelong pattern that remains constant

(4) Health, energy income and roles affect disengagement and activity pattern

2. Activity—theory purports that the maintenance of regular activity, roles (formal and informal), and social supports is positively correlated to life satisfaction and positive self concept.

   a. Theory does not take into account diversity of outlook and life-style

   b. Studies done since this theory was proposed have found that the quality and meaningfulness of activity are more important than the number of social activities

3. Continuity—focuses on the relationship between life satisfaction and activity as an expression of enduring personality traits

   a. Assumes stability of patterns over time

   b. Recognizes that the ''self'' remains the same despite life changes

   c. Focuses on personality and individual behavior over time

- Developmental

1. Psychosocial—(Erik Erickson, 1963)

   a. Adult development is based on successful resolution of basic psychosocial conflicts

   b. The crisis facing the mature adult is that of generativity versus stagnation, or self-absorption

   c. Final crisis faced is integrity versus despair

2. Developmental Tasks—(Havinghurst, 1972) Adult development encompasses a number of developmental tasks:

   a. Tasks of later maturity (60—death)

      (1) Adjusting to decreasing physical strength and health

      (2) Adjusting to retirement and reduced income

      (3) Adjusting to death of spouse or partner

(4) Establishing an explicit affiliation with one's age group

(5) Adopting and adapting social roles in a flexible way

(6) Establishing satisfactory physical living arrangements

3. Adaptation Theory—views development as age-appropriate adaptation to social expectations and norms; healthy adaptation is determined within the context of three dimensions of time: historical time, life time (chronological age), and social time, all of which are interwoven (Neugarten, 1968).

4. Life Transitions—the life transitions that occur in adulthood provide a useful framework for explaining adult development; transformation is the central concept of adult development; believes people have an innate drive to grow and change (Gould, 1978); general themes for 50–60 year olds:

   a. Mellowing and decreased negativeness

   b. Realization of mortality and concern for health

   c. Less responsibility and concern for children

Nursing: History, Theory, Process, and Practice

- History: Landmarks in Gerontological Nursing

  1. 1904—First article published on care of the aged (American Journal of Nursing)
  2. 1961—American Nurses Association (ANA) recommendation for formation of specialty group for geriatric nurses
  3. 1962—First national meeting of ANA's Conference Group on Geriatric Nursing Practice (Detroit)
  4. 1966—Formation of Geriatric Nursing Division (ANA)
  5. 1969—Standards of Geriatric Nursing developed
  6. 1970—Standards of Geriatric Nursing published
  7. 1975—First nurses certified in geriatric nursing
  8. 1975—Journal of Gerontological Nursing first published
  9. 1976—Geriatric Nursing Division changes title to Gerontological Nursing Division

10. 1976—Standards of Geriatric Nursing Care redefined as Standards of Gerontologic Nursing Practice

11. 1981—Statement on Scope of Gerontological Nursing Practice issued by ANA

12. 1987—Revision of the ANA Scope & Standards of Gerontological Nursing Practice—Broadens the standards of 1976 from the nursing process and nurse-client responsibilities to organization of nursing service, research, ethics, and professional development. (See Standards of Gerontological Nursing Practice in Professional Issues, Role Functions, Health Policy Chapter)

- Theory—As nursing continues to evolve nurses theorize about the nature of nursing practice, principles on which practice is based, and the goals and functions of nursing in society.

  1. Theory provides:
     a. Goals for assessment, diagnosis and planning
     b. Common ground for communication
     c. Professional autonomy & accountability
  2. Nursing theoretical models have emerged; the goals of these models are to:
     d. Develop curriculum plans for education
     e. Guide development of nursing care delivery systems
     f. Guide research to provide an empirical base for practice
     g. Establish criteria for measuring the quality of care, education, and research
  3. Nurse theorists have had a major influence on the nursing profession since Florence Nightingale's time; contemporary theory began to emerge in the late 1950s and 1960s. Selected nurse theorists include:
     a. Dorthea Orem—Self-care deficit theory. Nursing care becomes necessary when client is unable to fulfill biological, psychological, developmental, or social needs. Goal is to care for client and help client attain self-care.
     b. Martha Rogers—"Unitary man" evolving along a life process. Client continually changes and coexists with environment.

Goal is to maintain and promote health, prevent illness, care for and rehabilitate through ''humanistic science of nursing.''

c. Sister Callista Roy—Adaptation model based on four adaptive modes: physiological, psychological, sociological, and dependence-independence. Goal is to identify types of demands placed on client, assess client's adaptation to demands and help client adapt.

- Nursing Process—systematic broad theoretical framework that draws from humanities and biological and social sciences; logical and deliberate, yet fluid and dramatic; provides a structure for approaching clients and addressing their responses to actual or potential health problems in a systematic and deliberate manner; process is dynamic, cyclical, interdependent, flexible and often overlapping; five steps to the process that are sequential but not necessarily linear are:

1. Assessment—the act of appraising or reviewing; involves collecting information from and about a client and identifying relevant cues

   a. Information types: Subjective, objective, current, historical

   b. Methods: Nursing history, observation, inspection, palpation, percussion, auscultation, consultation

   c. Screening: Anemia, Cancer (breast, cervical/uterine, colon, lung, oral), Cardiac Disease (arteriosclerosis, hypertension), Endocrine imbalance (diabetes mellitus), Hearing impairments, Liver damage (alcoholism), Pulmonary disease (emphysema), Visual impairments (Glaucoma and cataracts).

2. Diagnosis—the analysis and synthesis of data to formulate impressions about client's responses to actual or potential health problems; the impressions are NURSING DIAGNOSES; when possible, nursing diagnoses should be selected from the most recent nursing diagnosis taxonomy approved by the North American Nursing Diagnosis Association (NANDA), shown on following page.

3. Planning—the planning phase begins once the nursing diagnoses have been formulated

   a. Client goals and objectives are formulated

   b. Priorities are assigned

   c. Nursing actions are selected

d. Alternative intervention strategies are planned

e. Plan of care is recorded in client record

Approved Nursing Diagnoses:

North American Nursing Diagnosis Association, June 1992

Activity intolerance Activity intolerance, potential Adjustment, impaired Airway clearance, ineffective Anxiety Aspiration, potential for Body image disturbance Body temperature, altered, potential Bowel incontinence Breastfeeding, effective Breastfeeding, ineffective Breastfeeding, interrupted Breathing pattern, ineffective Cardiac output, decreased Caregiver role strain Caregiver role strain, high risk for Communication, impaired verbal Constipation Constipation, colonic Constipation, perceived Coping, defensive Coping, family: potential for growth Coping, ineffective family: compromised Coping, ineffective family: disabling Coping, ineffective individual Decisional conflict (specify) Denial, ineffective Diarrhea Disuse syndrome, potential for Diversional activity deficit Dysreflexia Family process, altered Fatigue Fear Feeding pattern, infant: ineffective Fluid volume deficit (1) Fluid volume deficit (2) Fluid volume deficit, potential Fluid volume excess Gas exchange, impaired Grieving, anticipatory	Grieving, dysfunctional Growth and development, altered Health maintenance, altered Health-seeking behaviors (specify) Home maintenance management, impaired Hopelessness Hyperthermia Hypothermia Incontinence, functional Incontinence, reflux Incontinence, stress Incontinence, total Incontinence, urge Infection, potential for Injury, potential for Knowledge deficit (specify) Mobility, impaired physical Neurovascular dysfunction, peripheral, high risk for Noncompliance (specify) Nutrition, altered: less than body requirements Nutrition, altered: more than body requirements Nutrition, altered: potential for more than body requirements Oral mucous membrane, altered Pain Pain, chronic Parental role conflict Parenting, altered Parenting, altered, potential Personality identity disturbance Poisoning, potential for Post-trauma response Powerlessness Protection, altered Rape-trauma syndrome Rape-trauma syndrome: compound reaction Rape-trauma syndrome: silent reaction Relocation stress syndrome	Role performance, altered Self-care deficit, bathing/hygiene Self-care deficit, dressing/grooming Self-care deficit, feeding Self-care deficit, toileting Self-esteem disturbance Self-esteem, chronic low Self-esteem, situational low Self-mutilation, high risk for Sensory/perceptual alterations (specify) (visual, auditory, kinesthetic, gustatory, tactile, olfactory) Sexual dysfunction Sexuality patterns, altered Skin integrity, impaired Skin integrity, impaired, potential Sleep pattern disturbance Social interaction, impaired Social isolation Spiritual distress (distress of the human spirit) Suffocation, potential for Swallowing, impaired Therapeutic regimen, individual: ineffective management of Thermoregulation, ineffective Thought processes, altered Tissue integrity, impaired Tissue perfusion, altered (specify) (cardiopulmonary, cerebral, gastrointestinal, peripheral, renal) Trauma, potential for Unilateral neglect Urinary elimination, altered patterns Urinary retention Ventilation, spontaneous, inability to sustain Ventilatory weaning response, dysfunctional Violence, potential for: self-directed or directed at others

Note. From *North American Nursing Diagnosis Association.* Copyright 1992 by North American Nursing Diagnosis Association. Reprinted by permission.

4. Implementation—the doing or intervening phase
   a. Initiate and complete nursing actions
   b. Supervise delegated care
   c. Organize supplies, equipment, teaching materials, personnel
   d. Document nursing actions in client record
5. Evaluation—focuses on client's behavioral changes and compares them with outcomes stated in objectives
   a. Monitor client response to care
   b. Revise plan of care
   c. Document response, achievement of outcomes, revisions in plan of care

- Practice—Nurses in all speciality areas except pediatrics and obstetrics are likely to find that more than half of their clients are over age 65. A nurse who cares for the aged may be a generalist or specialist.
  1. Generalist—functions in a variety of settings (hospital, home, or community); draws on the expertise of the specialist
  2. Specialist—works primarily with older people in varied situations; has a master's degree in gerontological nursing; can perform all the functions of a generalist, but has developed substantial clinical expertise with individuals, families, and groups, and in formulating health and social policy, and planning, implementing, and evaluating health programs. Graduate programs in gerontological nursing prepare nurses to function in one of three roles:
     a. Gerontological nurse practitioner—prepared for physical examination and assessment, health monitoring, and management
     b. Community health nurse—focus on direct client care, biopsychosocial support, discharge planning, counseling, and referral
     c. Clinical specialist—prepared to teach and to coordinate and consult in speciality units and service agencies

Questions

1. The older population can be described as being

   a. Predominately female
   b. Becoming a smaller percentage of the total population
   c. Comprised of a decreased number of "old-old"
   d. Predominantly male

2. Most older adults

   a. Live alone
   b. Reside in a nursing home
   c. Reside in a group home
   d. Live in a family setting

3. Which statement best describes widowhood in the United States?

   a. It is a fact of life for most older men
   b. It is a fact of life for most older women
   c. Widowers outnumber widows in old age
   d. Few women over age 75 are widowed

4. The major source of income for most older persons is

   a. Savings
   b. Earnings
   c. Social security
   d. Pensions

5. Which statement is most accurate about income in the elderly?

   a. Older Blacks have more income than their White counterparts
   b. Older women have more income than their male counterparts
   c. Twenty percent of the elderly have incomes less than $15,000
   d. Thirty-nine percent of the elderly have incomes greater than $30,000

6. Which statement is the most accurate?

   a. Older people account for 50% of all hospital stays
   b. The largest portion of health care expenditures for the aged is nursing home care
   c. Approximately 50% of older people living in the community have health-related difficulty with one or more personal care activities

d. The over 65 age group accounts for 36% of total health care expenditures

7. Mr. Smith lives in a senior high rise apartment building. He is infrequently seen at the Geriatric Clinic for problems related to an enlarged prostate. One of the social workers at the clinic has commented that Mr. Smith lives in "one of those nice places where the old people live; most of them prefer it that way." This type of thinking is most consistent with which theory?

   a. Continuity
   b. Developmental
   c. Disengagement
   d. Activity

8. During reminiscing, Mrs. Gato talks about the many quilts that she has made and the number of women that she had taught to quilt. She reflects that she has done much for future generations. This thinking is consistent with the theory of:

   a. Neugarten
   b. Gould
   c. Havinghurst
   d. Erickson

9. The theory that views biological aging as being under internal genetic control is:

   a. Free radical theory
   b. Immunologic theory
   c. Programmed theory
   d. Stress adaptation theory

10. Mr. Johnson, a 75 year old man, is admitted to the hospital with symptoms of vomiting and diarrhea. He is 5 feet and 4 inches tall and weighs 130 pounds. During admission the nurse focuses on the assessment component of the nursing process; this includes all of the following except:

   a. The nursing history
   b. Inspection
   c. Revising the plan of care
   d. Auscultation

11. Mr. Johnson has a nursing diagnosis of "fluid volume deficit." In formulating this diagnosis the nurse used all of the following except:

a. Objective data (height and weight)
b. Subjective data ("I feel very weak and tired.")
c. Teaching materials (Mr. Johnson was taught about fluid replacement.)
d. Current history (The client had vomiting & diarrhea for three days before he was admitted to the hospital.)

12. During the planning phase of Mr. Johnson's care, the nurse remembers that Mrs. Johnson has expressed her fears about being unable to care for her husband. Which of the following is not an appropriate action at this time?

    a. Revising the plan of care to include Mrs. Johnson
    b. Having Mrs. Johnson's fears high on the priority list
    c. Establishing a pattern of communication so that Mrs. Johnson remains informed about her husband's condition
    d. Recording the plan of care for Mr. Johnson

13. Prior to discharge, the nurse evaluated Mr. Johnson's care; the evaluation phase includes which of the following?

    a. Supervising delegated care
    b. Taking the nursing history
    c. Selecting nursing actions
    d. Documenting the achievement of outcomes

Answers:

1. a
2. d
3. b
4. c
5. d
6. d
7. c
8. d
9. c
10. c
11. c
12. a
13. d

Bibliography

A Profile of Older Americans (1992). Washington, D.C.: Program Resources Department, American Association of Retired Persons in cooperation with the Administration on Aging.

Carnevali, D. L., & Patrick, M. (1986). *Nursing management for the elderly* (3rd ed.). Philadelphia: J. B. Lippincott.

Christ, M. A., & Hohlock, F. J. (1988). *Gerontological nursing, a study and learning tool.* Springhouse PA: Springhouse Publishing.

Chenitz, W. C., Stone, J. T., & Salisbury, S. (1991). *Clinical gerontological nursing: A guide to advanced practice.* Philadelphia: W. B. Saunders.

Cummings, E. & Henrey, W. (1961). *Growing old.* New York: Basic Books.

Ebersole, P., & Hess, P. (1990). *Toward healthy aging, human needs and nursing response* (4th ed.). St. Louis: C.V. Mosby.

Eliopoulos, C. (1991). *Gerontological nursing review, a self-instructional text* (2nd ed.). Baltimore: National Health Publishing.

Erickson, E. (1963). (2nd. ed.) *Childhood and society.* New York: W. W. Norton.

Gould, R. (1978). *Transformations.* New York: Simon & Schuster

Havinghurst, R. (1972). *Developmental tasks and education.* New York: David McKay.

Hogstel, M. O. (1992). *Clinical management of gerontological nursing.* St. Louis: Mosby-Year Book.

Kozier, B., Erb, G., & Olivieri, R. (1991). *Fundamentals of nursing, concepts, process, & practice.* Redwood City, CA: Addison-Wesley.

Neugarten, B. (1968). Adult personality: Toward a psychology of the lifecycle. In Neugarten, B. (Ed.) *Middle age and aging.* Chicago: University of Chicago Press.

Potter, P., & Perry, A. (1989). *Fundamentals of nursing, concepts, process, and practice.* St. Louis: C.V. Mosby.

Yura, H., & Walsh, M. B. (1988). *The nursing process, assessing, planning, implementing, evaluating* (5th ed.). Norwalk, CT: Appleton & Lange.

Health Assessment of the Elderly/Health Promotion

Karen Cassidy King

Health assessment is a deliberate, ordered process of examination. Physical, objective evidence of disease is determined to be absent, or quantified if present. Assessment is accomplished by interview, inspection, palpation, percussion and auscultation.

Health assessment of the elderly client is multidimensional because of the complex problems of the elderly. Problems are prioritized and interventions employed only if benefits outweigh risks. Sensitivity is needed to small changes over time. Health assessment is most effective if performed in a private, well lighted room with minimal background noise.

Take advantage of every encounter with the client, no matter how brief. Valuable information can be obtained from observation and informal interview about the client's changing status, the effectiveness of the interventions and the development of new problems.

Observe posture, gait and balance. Observe the ability to rise from a chair, ambulation, and the use of any assistance devices. Be mindful that guidelines for referral vary with the practice setting.

History

Subjective information is gathered through a comprehensive history. Information is used to determine areas to focus on during the physical examination.

Taking a health history from an older adult involves assessment and special awareness of the normal sensory changes of aging. The health history may be difficult to obtain due to hearing and memory deficits.

The interview frequently includes family and caregiver. Old medical records may be useful. Encourage the client to bring all medications, prescription and over the counter, to the examination in a brown bag (sack test).

- Content of the Health History
  1. Health Status or Present Health Problems
     a. Personal perception of health status, feeling of well being now and in past
     b. Present health problems—clear, comprehensive narrative
        (1) Initial onset of the problem

(2) Setting in which it developed

(3) Alleviating factors

(4) Aggravating factors

(5) Symptoms

(a) Location

(b) Quality

(c) Severity

(d) Duration

(e) Frequency

(f) Effect on activity

(6) Client's understanding of symptoms

(7) Treatment

(8) Meaning and impact problem has on client's life

2. Past Health History (include date and treatment for each)

a. Communicable disease, especially tuberculosis (TB), influenza, measles, streptococcal infections, sexually transmitted diseases (STD).

b. Operations and hospitalizations

c. Accidents and injuries (including falls)

d. Allergies and drug sensitivities

e. Emotional/mental problems

3. Health Habits

a. Tobacco use

b. Alcohol use

c. Coffee/tea/caffeine

d. Drug use—over the counter, prescription, home remedies, addictive.

e. Exercise patterns

f. Sleep patterns

g. Elimination habits

h. Use of safety measures, such as seat belts

4. Health Promotion Practices/Preventive Care

a. Health examination frequency

(1) Complete physical examination every two years

(2) Female: Self Breast Examination (SBE) every month Mammogram yearly, Papanicolaou smear yearly

(3) Male: Self Testicular Examination (STE) every month, Prostate examination yearly

(4) Sigmoidoscopy every four years

(5) Stool guaiac yearly

(6) Tonometry (intraocular pressure) yearly

b. Immunizations

(1) Pneumovax (one dose only)

(2) Influenza (annual in late fall if over 65)

(3) Tetanus/diphtheria toxoid (once every 10 years)

(4) *Hemophilus influenzae*

5. Family History

a. Age and health, or age and cause of death, of parents, siblings, and children

b. Psychosocial history may be more important than family history in elderly

c. Recent physical problems in family members

d. Occurrence of diabetes, TB, heart disease, high blood pressure, stroke, kidney disease, cancer, arthritis, anemia, headaches, epilepsy, mental illness, alcoholism, drug addiction, and any symptoms like those of the client

e. Assessment of the family may be appropriate, depending on family members and caregivers. Tools for family assessment are available.

6. Personal and Social History
    a. Hobbies, recreation, occupational history—type and frequency of each, exposure to occupational hazards
    b. Educational background—literacy level
    c. Religious practices—spirituality, church membership, clergy of choice
    d. Cultural influences—primary language
    e. Socioeconomic status—income sources, ability to meet basic needs
    f. Relationships with family and community
    g. Outlook on present and future, concerns, self esteem

- Review of Systems

A systematic collection of subjective data about the parts and systems of the body. The review of systems may be conducted as a separate section of the assessment or incorporated during the physical examination.

Disease often presents atypically in the elderly. To accurately correlate information from subjective and objective data collection and make clinical decisions, the nurse must know the physiological changes expected to occur in aging and atypical presentations.

Keep in mind that infection presents uniquely in the elderly client. The client may not have a fever or leukocytosis, but may present with lethargy, confusion or anorexia.

Physical Examination

Use a systematic approach, either a "head to toe" method or the major body system method. The basic assessment techniques used in examining the elderly client are no different from those used in examining adults of any age.

- General Survey

1. Apparent state of health, signs of distress, skin color, weight by appearance, posture, motor activity, gait, dress, grooming and personal hygiene, odors of breath or body, facial expressions, speech

2. Vital signs
   a. Temperature
      (1) Unreliable sign of infection in elderly
      (2) If dyspneic, use rectal/axillary measurement
      (3) If hypothermic, (below 96 degrees F) evaluate cause immediately
   b. Respiratory Rate
      (1) Assess rate, depth, rhythm, quality
      (2) Periods of apnea followed by deep breaths may occur normally during sleep
      (3) Following periods of exercise, respiratory rate may increase and take longer to return to normal range
      (4) May be a reliable sign of infection and congestive heart failure (CHF), especially if tachypneic
   c. Pulse Rate
      (1) Apical pulse counted for one full minute is most accurate
      (2) Incidence of dysrhythmias (premature ventricular contractions and atrial fibrillations) increase with age
   d. Blood Pressure (BP)
      (1) Take routinely in the supine and upright positions
      (2) Changes reflect several physiologic age related changes: gradual increase in systolic and diastolic values and widening of pulse pressure due to increased arterial rigidity and decreased blood vessel resiliency
      (3) Assess postural blood pressure changes: measure and document BP in each arm lying, sitting, and standing. Use arm with higher pressure consistently for routine baseline checks. Tendency toward orthostatic hypotension when standing
   e. Weight
      (1) Gradual weight gain may occur over the years.

BP 120/90

(2) Weight gain also indicative of certain diseases e.g., CHF and depression

(3) Weight loss of over 10% of the typical weight in a six month time period, evaluate further.

- Integumentary System

1. Inspect scalp, head, neck, trunk, limbs
2. Note color, skin tears, lacerations, scars, lesions, ulcerations, edema, and tone
3. Palpate for temperature, moisture, thickness, texture, and turgor
4. Subcutaneous tissue decreases in older adults. Skin turgor may not be a reliable sign of hydration
5. Fat pad protection decreases with resulting increased likelihood of pressure sores over bony prominence
6. Status ulceration of legs secondary to chronic venous insufficiency common
7. Common Normal Age Related Changes
   a. Seborrheic or senile keratoses (raised dark, warty, areas on trunk, face, neck, hands)
   b. Senile lentigine (liver spots or age spots: flat brown macules on hands, arms, neck, face)
   c. Cherry angiomas (small round, red spots) and senile purpura (vivid purple patches)
8. Common disorders: keratosis, pruritis, ulceration, dehydration, corns, calluses, ingrown toenails, bruising, skin cancers, actinic keratosis

- Hair

1. Inspect: Color, quantity, distribution, and texture
2. Hypothyroidism and hyperthyroidism cause changes in hair distribution and texture: Loss of pigment, fine, brittle
3. Hair thins and becomes finer with age.

- Nails
  1. Inspect fingernails: Color, shape, thickness, presence of lesions, capillary refill
  2. Hypertrophy of nails common: Results in nail thickness
  3. Fungal infection (onychomycosis) commonly produces thickened, friable nails, yellow color.
  4. Abnormal nail bed colors: Red (infection), cyanotic (respiratory distress/heart disease)
- Head
  1. Inspect size, contour, symmetry. Size and shape do not change with age. Soft tissue swelling indicates recent head trauma.
  2. Observe facial expressions. Note masklike facies or blank stare, indicative of Parkinson's Disease.
  3. Palpate skull. Note tenderness, masses, lesions.
- Eyes
  1. Assessment of the eyes includes: Visual acuity, visual fields, extraocular eye movement, external and internal structures.
     a. Visual acuity—test each eye separately and both eyes together using Snellen Chart at 20 feet.
     b. Visual fields—examiner and client cover opposite eyes with opaque card. Visualization of objects should be simultaneous for client and examiner when object is above, below and from each side. Changes occur with transient ischemic attack (TIA), cardiovascular accident (CVA), or glaucoma. Scotoma: Blind area in visual field often accompanies glaucoma.
     c. External structures (inspect eyebrows, eyelids, eye lashes, lacrimal apparatus, conjunctiva, sclera, pupils and iris.)
        (1) Eyelids—common eyelid problems—ptosis: Partially or completely cover pupil, entropion (inversion) and ectropion (eversion).
        (2) Lacrimal apparatus-note discharge, redness, edema, excessive tearing, tenderness. Common: Decreased tear production.
        (3) Conjunctiva-light pink/pale color normal in older adults.

(4) Sclera-usually creamy white, due to presence of fat; sclera and conjunctiva may appear yellow. Pinguecula-yellowish thickenings of the bulbar conjunctiva that are triangular, occur on inner and outer margins of cornea.

(5) Pupils—Observe accommodation response by having client shift gaze from far to near. Eyes should converge, pupils constrict, and lenses thicken. Use pen light to assess pupillary response to light. Note size, equality, shape, reaction to light. Pupils should constrict equally with direct light (direct response) and opposite pupil should constrict when light is shined on other (consensual response).

(a) Senile miosis: Pupils smaller that usual

(b) Cataracts: Ophthalmoscopic examination may reveal gross opacity due to clouding of crystalline lens.

d. Internal Structures: (Funduscopic (Ophthalmoscopic) Examination.)

(1) Inspect retina, retinal blood vessels, optic disc, macula and fovea centralis.

(2) Red reflex: Clouding and opacity are abnormal. Pale, narrowed arterioles common. Disc margins should be distinct, physiologic cup yellow-white.

(3) Background eye changes characteristic of common diseases in elderly: Diabetes, hypertension, arteriosclerosis.

2. Common Normal Age Related Changes

a. Progressive relaxation of eyelids

b. Arcus senilis: thin grayish-white ring at the corneal margin

c. Lens becomes less transparent

d. Dry appearance due to decreased lacrimal duct production

e. Cornea clouds with aging

f. Loss of peripheral vision

g. Opthalmoscopic examinations show mildly narrowed vessels and granular pigment in macula

- Ears

1. Inspect auricle. Palpate auricle, auricular lymph nodes, and mastoid process. Note color, temperature, discharge, tenderness, and lesions.
2. Otoscope Examination
   a. Inspect external canals, tympanic membrane (T.M.), and light reflex; Normal T.M. should appear gray and translucent.
      (1) T.M. may lose mobility and increase in opacity. Atrophy of T.M. causes exaggerated landmarks.
      (2) Assessment of Hearing Function
         (a) Whisper Test: Evaluate higher range acuity
         (b) Rinne Test: Compare air to bone conduction
         (c) Weber Test: Note conduction deficit and/or sensory neural deficit.
3. Incidence of hearing loss, especially high frequency loss increases with age.
4. Common Normal Age Related Changes
   a. Ability to hear high frequency sounds decreases
   b. Auricle loses elasticity, lobe may elongate and develop linear oblique wrinkles
   c. T.M. may lose mobility, increase in opacity, lose luster
   d. Cerumen may be drier and harder
   e. Increased hair growth in auditory canal
   f. Senile atrophy of T.M. may make landmarks appear exaggerated
5. Common disorders: Presbycusis, impacted cerumen, otoscelerosis, tinnitus, conductive hearing loss

- Nose and Sinus

1. Inspect
   a. External—septum, vestibule, bridge
   b. Internal—with penlight: mucosa for color, discharge, swelling,

bleeding; turbinates for discoloration, enlargement, inflammation and lesions

2. Palpate
   a. External—note tenderness, swelling in frontal and maxillary sinuses

3. Common Normal Age Related Changes
   a. Decreased sense of smell common

- Mouth and Pharynx
  1. Inspect
     a. Observe hydration status, ability to chew food and presence of disease, ie. oral cancer, vitamin deficiencies.
     b. Inspect oral cavity, remove dentures before inspection
        (1) Lips: Dry, parched lips—dehydration, cheilosis—poor fitting dentures, cheilosis with reddened lips—B complex deficiency, persistent coated tongue or bleeding tongue—suspect leukoplakia.
        (2) Tongue: Color, size, texture and coating.
            (a) Macroglossia: Enlarged tongue-hypothyroid
            (2) Deviation to left or right-suggest TIA/CVA
        (3) Condition/presence/absence of tonsils
        (4) Side effects from psychotropic drugs: Involuntary movements, e.g., lip smacking, tongue protrusion and slow rhythmic movements of tongue, lips and jaws. Decreased production of saliva and taste sensations are normal.
        (5) Reduced taste sensation in advanced old age due to papillae atrophy on lateral edges of tongue
  2. Palpate
     a. Note tenderness or crepitus of temperomandibular joint (TMJ)
     b. Note lesions, color, tenderness or swelling of posterior and lateral surfaces of tongue

3. Common Normal Age Related Changes
   a. Loss of taste buds, especially for sweet and sour
   b. Decreased salivary gland activity, drying the oral mucosa

- Neck
  1. Inspect scars, masses, symmetry. Thyroid gland should not be observable.
  2. Palpate thyroid, trachea, and lymph nodes.
     a. Thyroid gland
        (1) Decrease in size and activity normal.
        (2) Heart failure with atrial fibrillation and proximal muscle weakness may be due to hyperthyroidism.
        (3) Hypothyroidism may be present with nonspecific symptoms, e.g., fatigue, bradycardia, dry skin, coarse voice.
        (4) Usual symptoms of thyroid disease may be absent or atypical.
        (5) Hyperthyroid patients over sixty present with a triad of weight loss, anorexia, and constipation (a GI presentation). The classic signs of Graves Disease (goiter and exophthalmos) are uncommon.
     b. Trachea—should be midline, without tenderness
     c. Lymph nodes—note tenderness, mobility, and size. Normal findings include less than 1 cm, nontender, soft and discrete and good mobility.
        (1) Lymph nodes of head and neck: Pre-auricular, post auricular, submental, submandibular, supramandibular, post cervical, occipital, superficial cervical, deep cervical chain.
     d. Cervical spine—note crepitus, tenderness, lesions.
- Chest and Lungs
  1. Inspect—shape and symmetry of anterior and posterior chest, note anteroposterior (AP) to lateral diameter. Examination is best performed with the client in the sitting position.

a. Observe for bulging, retraction, barrel shape. Bulging of intercostal spaces on exhalation and barrel chest indicate chronic obstructive pulmonary disease (COPD).

b. Inspect breasts. Note mass, nodule, dimpling, nipple retraction, symmetry.

2. Palpate temperature, tenderness, masses, lumps

   a. Local tenderness over costochondral junction suggests costochondritis, a frequent cause of chest pain in the elderly.

   b. Palpation includes chest excursion, tactile fremitus and breast palpation.

      (1) Chest excursion

         (a) Anterior—place thumbs along costal margins, push toward xiphoid

         (b) Posterior—place thumbs on lateral chest with thumbs at level of 10th rib.

         (c) Thumbs should move symmetrically on both sides as client takes deep inhalation

      (2) Tactile fremitus

         (a) Vibratory tremors felt through chest wall, most evident near tracheal bifurcation

         (b) Client says one-two-three, or ''99'', examiner uses palmar surfaces starting at apices and moving down. Compare side to side laterally, posteriorly and anteriorly.

      (3) Breast palpation—use palmar surface of fingers

         (a) Lymph Nodes—with client sitting, use light and deep palpation.

         (b) Breast—with client supine, palpate separately using rotary motion in either concentric circles or inward from periphery (spokes of wheel pattern). Squeeze nipple for discharge.

            (i) Bimanual palpation for women with large breasts

(ii) Note location, size, mobility, consistency, tenderness of any masses

c. Common findings in the elderly women include breasts feeling stringy, granular, and nodular from glandular tissue changes. Men may have increase in fatty breast tissue.

3. Percussion

a. Compare side to side percussing at 5 cm intervals. Note duration, tone and pitch. Normal lung fields: resonant percussion; dullness over bony prominences

4. Auscultation

a. With the diaphragm of stethoscope, auscultate from bases to apices, anterior and posterior and in a symmetrical fashion.

b. Normal findings

(1) Vesicular sounds over most lung fields

(2) Bronchovesicular sounds over main bronchi, between scapulae and below clavicles

(3) Bronchial sounds over trachea

c. Adventitious sounds

(1) Rhonchi—continuous sound; usually clears with coughing

(2) Friction rub—grating sound, coughing has no effect

(3) Rales or crackles—best heard on inspiration

(a) With rales, ask client to cough. Rales secondary to CHF will not clear with coughing, rales caused by immobility may not clear. Pulmonary fibrosis or interstitial lung disease often present with "velcro-type" rales.

(b) Adventitious lung sounds (rales, rhonchi) with dullness on percussion indicate consolidation. Egophony confirms consolidation. Ask client to say EEE while auscultating, AAA sounds are positive.

5. Common Normal Age Related Changes
   a. Kyphosis may be present from osteoporosis and collapse of vertebra
   b. Chest wall less compliant
   c. Inspiration less deep, decreased inspiratory reserve volume
   d. Expiration requires active use of accessory muscles
6. Common disorders: COPD, pulmonary edema, pneumonia, chronic respiratory acidosis, pulmonary emboli, breathlessness upon exertion. Swallowing dysfunction and poor dentition predispose to aspiration pneumonia.

- Cardiovascular
  1. Inspect and Palpate
     a. Point of maximal impulse (PMI), in elderly may be displaced downward to the left, usually palpated around 5th or 6th left intercostal space at the midclavicular line.
     b. Location of heart sounds and PMI may be different if client has kyphosis or scoliosis. Assess the client from the supine and right side.
  2. Auscultate
     a. With diaphragm of stethoscope listen in the following areas: Aortic, pulmonic, tricuspid, mitral areas, Erb's point. Listen for S_1 and S_2 over each area, in three of four positions: Sitting, supine, left lateral, sitting leaning forward.
        (1) S_1: "Lub" sound most audible over mitral area with bell in left lateral position. Normal S_1 splitting heard in tricuspid area.
        (2) S_2: "Dub" sound most audible through diagram in aortic area with client sitting and leaning over. Normal S_2 splitting heard on inspiration in pulmonic area.
        (3) S_3: (Ventricular gallop) not normal in older adults. Most audible through bell in mitral area after beginning of diastole with client supine. Sound is short, dull, low and soft. Not a reliable sign of CHF in the elderly.

(4) S_4: (Atrial gallop) most audible in late systole over apex.

b. Cardiac murmurs

(1) Murmur not necessarily abnormal in elderly. Common secondary to valvular heart disease: Aortic stenosis, aortic sclerosis, mitral regurgitation and idiopathic hypertrophic subaortic stenosis.

(2) Listen one full minute over apex of heart. Murmurs may occur in any valve. Note location, position most audible, timing in the cardiac cycle, and loudness.

(a) Subjective grading scale

Grade I: Soft, not heard every beat

Grade II: Soft, heard every beat

Grade III: Loud

Grade IV: Loud, with thrill

Grade V: Very loud, with thrill

Grade VI: Audible with stethoscope off the chest

3. Common Normal Age Related Changes

a. Slower heart rate (rate can range from 44 to 108 beats per minute)

b. Valves become thick and rigid

c. Difficult contraction and dilation of cardiac muscle due to decreased elasticity and increased rigidity

d. EKG changes: possible decreased voltage of all waves, slight prolongation of all intervals, left axis deviation

e. Posterior tibial and dorsalis pedis pulses are difficult to palpate

f. Functional systolic murmurs increase with age, heard best at base or aortic area

g. Peripheral vessels may be tortuous and distended

4. Common cardiac disorders: Hypertension, valvular disease, coronary artery disease with insufficiency or eventual myocardial infarction

(MI), CHF, arteriosclerosis, atherosclerosis, CVA, thrombophlebitis, arrhythmias.

- Peripheral Vascular System

1. Inspect

   a. Inspect neck for jugular vein pulsation or distention in sitting position.

   b. Extremities: Note visible pulsation, venous bulging, edema

2. Palpate

   a. Arteries: Carotid, temporal, brachial, radial, femoral, popliteal, dorsalis pedis, and posterior tibial. Palpate one at a time, note rate, rhythm, strength, symmetry, temperature, tenderness, edema. Use care in carotid palpation due to increased sensitivity of baroreceptors and atherosclerotic changes of vessels.

   b. With aging, arteries may be tortuous, feel stiff, and appear kinked. There may be decreased venous return and competency.

   c. Pallor may indicate arterial insufficiency. Erythema may be secondary to contact dermatitis, cellulitis, lymphangitis or superficial or deep vein phlebitis. Cyanosis or mottling may indicate arterial occlusion. Brown discoloration may indicate longstanding venous insufficiency.

   d. Temperature: Heat indicates thrombosis, but temperature may be decreased in elderly.

   e. Edema: Indicates CHF, lymphatic obstruction, renal failure, hypoalbuminemia and inflammation. In the elderly, lower leg edema is usually attributed to chronic venous disease. Best assessed over body prominences and most pronounced in dependent areas of body.

   f. Trophic changes: Decreased hair in distant extremities. Seen in arterial disease, neuropathies, diabetes.

   g. Varicosities: Twisted, swollen veins, typically in legs.

3. Auscultate

   a. Blood Pressure (see vital signs)

   b. Carotid and femoral arteries for bruits using bell of stethoscope. Adventitious sounds are high pitched. Differentiate between carotid bruit and transmitted heart murmur by inching up the artery with stethoscope starting at the base of the neck. Bruits: louder as auscultate slowly up neck, murmurs loudest at base of neck, bruits are higher pitched.

- Gastrointestinal

  1. Inspection and auscultation BEFORE percussion and palpation in supine position. Percussion and palpation increases bowel motility and sounds.
  2. Inspect shape, symmetry, scars, masses, distention, and striae.
  3. Auscultate bowel sounds in all four quadrants using diaphragm. Normal sound—high-pitched and gurgling. Listen for aortic bruits with bell of stethescope.
  4. Percuss for presence of air or fluid, size of liver, and bladder distention.
     a. Tympanic sound—lower pitched over gastric bubble, high pitched over gas-filled bowel, dull sound indicates fluid. Distention with a tympanic sound indicates fecal impaction.
     b. Dullness over liver 6 to 12 cm in midclavicular line and 4 to 8 cm in midsternal line. Dullness over spleen sixth to ninth rib in left midaxillary line.
     c. Shortened liver span on percussion in elderly.
  5. Palpate: Light and deep
     a. Light palpation: Fingertip exam in all four quadrants. Note tenderness or spasms.
     b. Deep palpation: Bimanual method with two hands or using distal half of palmar surface. Note pain or distention.
     c. Liver border more easily palpated in elderly.
  6. Common Normal Age Related Changes
     a. Weaker intestinal musculature
     b. Esophageal mobility increases
     c. Decreased peristalsis

d. Liver smaller in size and reduced in storage capacity

e. Altered rates of insulin release

7. Common disorders: Periodontal disease, poor mastication with ill fitting dentures or failure to replace lost teeth, dysphagia, hiatal hernia, malnutrition, anemia, constipation, fecal impaction, intestinal obstruction, diverticulosis, cancer of GI tract.

- Genitourinary

1. Male

a. Inspect pubic hair, glans of uncircumcised penis, penile shaft, scrotum and inguinal canals for bulging, masses, lesions, inflammation, edema, and discoloration.

b. Palpate

(1) Penis: Note masses or induration

(2) Scrotum: Note tenderness, mobility, texture, symmetry, and firmness of testes.

(3) Inguinal ring: Assess for hernia with client standing. Note masses when client bears down.

2. Female

a. Inspect: External and internal

(1) External: Perineum for rash, lesions, or nodules. Inspect labia majora, labia minora, clitoris, and urethral and vaginal orifices for color, shape, size and discharge.

(2) Internal: Cervix, Os, walls and vagina using speculum.

b. Palpate

(1) Bimanual examination—palpate vagina, uterus, ovaries. Note smoothness, mobility, tenderness.

(2) Recto-vaginal exam—palpate all rectal walls. Note nodules or masses and sphincter tone.

3. Common Normal Age Related Changes

a. Pubic hair thins and grays

   b. Decreased bladder capacity; frequency of urination, nocturia, stress incontinence, dribbling
   c. Atrophic changes in vaginal mucosa
   d. Decrease in size and elasticity of vagina
   e. Decreased vaginal secretions
   f. Slight testicular atrophy
   g. Prostate gland enlargement. May have urinary frequency
   h. Elongation of scrotal sac

4. Sexuality: Correct underlying medical problems, diabetes, CVA, cardiac disease, musculoskeletal disease. Change offending medications if possible, esp. hypertensive drugs.

5. Common disorders: Urinary tract infection (UTI), urgency and frequency, urinary incontinence, atrophic vaginitis (women), benign prostatic hypertrophy (BPH), (men).

- Rectum
  1. External (inspect hair distribution, opening, color, drainage, color, and mucosa)
  2. Internal
     a. Client lying on left side. Palpate and note masses, nodules, lesions, hemorrhoids. Note sphincter tone and condition of rectal walls. In males, palpate prostate gland at anterior surface for size, consistency, shape, surface and symmetry.
  3. Examination should never be "deferred." Occult bleeding, rectal cancer and hemorrhoids can be missed, as well as BPH and prostate cancer in men.
- Musculoskeletal
  1. Inspect gait, posture, station.
     a. Assess balance and strength. Romberg test, heel to toe
     b. Inspect joints of hands, wrists, elbow, shoulders, neck, hips, knees, and ankles. Note enlargement, swelling, tenderness,

crepitus, temperature changes or deformity. Pain with movement and stiffness with range of motion is indicative of degenerative joint diseases.

c. Common foot deformities: Hallux valgus, prolapsed metatarsals, hammer toes, accentuated dorsal spine curve (kyphosis), loss of muscle bulk and strength, partial ROM of spine, neck, extremities, decrease in height.

d. Tremors

(1) Resting tremors and pin-rolling tremors indicate Parkinson's Disease

(2) Intention tremors indicate cerebellar disorders

e. Note color, temperature, varicosities of legs, trophic changes of digits.

2. Palpate

a. Note swelling, tenderness, deformity, symmetry, crepitus, weakness.

b. Assess muscle strength testing muscle groups head to toe. Passive ROM resistance indicates hypertonicity.

3. Assess rapid, rhythmic, alternating movements for coordination. Speed reduced in elderly. Generalized decrease in sensation, coordination and voluntary movements are slowed.

4. Common Normal Age Related Changes

a. Normal reduction of muscle mass

b. Loss of bone beginning at fourth decade of life

c. Decreased muscle strength

d. Slower reaction time

e. Poorer coordination

f. Increased muscle fatigue

5. Common disorders: Osteoarthritis (Heberden's nodes), rheumatoid arthritis, gout, osteoporosis (kyphosis of spine), hip fracture, hallus valgus (bunions), hammer toes.

- Neurological (Assessment includes: Cerebral functioning, cranial nerves, cerebellar functioning, motor system functioning, sensory system functioning, and reflexes.)

1. Cerebral functioning
    a. Mental Status
        (1) Cognitive: Level of consciousness, memory, orientation, concentration, judgment, reasoning
            (a) Level of consciousness (center of the clients level of attention)
                (i) Consciousness: Fully alert, aware, oriented
                (ii) Delirium: Acute confusion, common in dementia
                (iii) Lethargy: Arousable with stimuli
                (iv) Stupor: Partial or near complete unconsciousness; response to strong stimuli only
                (v) Semicoma: No verbal response, withdraws body part in response to pain
                (vi) Coma: State of unconsciousness; No response to painful stimuli.
            (b) Memory (Clients who complain that they have memory problems usually do not have dementia.)
                (i) Immediate (does information register)
                (ii) Recent (can information be retained)
                (iii) Remote (can information be recalled)
            (c) Orientation: Person, time, place, circumstances
            (d) Concentration, judgment, reasoning
    b. Emotional: Mood and affect, appearance, behavior
        (1) Mood: Normal, calm, depressed, elated, anxious, agitated
        (2) Affect: Flat, inappropriate (flat affect: failing to show emotions, symptoms of disease of basal ganglia, e.g., Parkinson's disease)
    c. Thought processes: Appropriate perceptions and thoughts

(1) General knowledge and vocabulary, knowledge of current news or family events. Vocabulary and general knowledge increase with age.

(2) Psychiatric conditions are composed of any combination of disordered thinking, feeling, or behaving. Any of these can be on a functional or organic level.

d. Cortical functions

(1) Sensory recognition

(2) Skilled motor ability

(3) Skilled language and speech functions

(a) Speech disorders usually occur due to circulatory disorders, e.g., acute CHF secondary to emboli or bleeding. Can be detected via casual conversation.

2. Cranial Nerves: Examine sequentially I to XII. Few changes occur with normal aging. Most are assessed in appropriate body system assessment).

a. I. Olfactory: Identification of variety of smells

b. II. Optic: Visual acuity, visual fields, fundoscopic exam without pathology

c. II, III. Optic, Oculomotor: Pupillary reactions

d. III, IV, VI. Oculomotor, Trochlear, Abducens: Extraocular movements

e. V. Trigeminal: Teeth clench, corneal reflexes, jaw movements

f. VII. Facial: Facial movements

g. VIII. Acoustic: Hearing

h. IX, X. Glossopharyngeal, Vagus: Swallowing, rise of palate, voice, gag reflex

i. XI. Spinal Accessory: Phonation; head, neck and shoulder movements

j. XII. Hypoglossal: Tongue movements

3. Cerebellar Functioning

a. Gross motor and balance testing

(1) Gross motor

(a) Romberg test

(b) Heel to toe test

(c) Balance on one foot, then another

b. Fine motor/upper extremities

(1) Rapid alternating of index finger to nose, eyes open, then closed

(2) Rapid alternating touching of index finger to nose, then to examiner's finger.

c. Fine motor/lower extremities

(1) Run each heel down opposite shin in smooth motion

4. Motor System Functioning (see Musculoskeletal Section)

5. Sensory System Functioning

a. Primary sensory: Pain perception, temperature, light touch, vibration, position

b. Discriminary sensation: Stereognosis (objects), graphesthesia (numbers in palms), and two point discrimination

6. Reflexes

a. Rate rapidity and strength of contraction and compare bilaterally the following tendons:

(1) Triceps (above olecranon process)

(2) Biceps (in fossa of bent elbow)

(3) Brachioradialis (proximal to styloid process of elbow)

(4) Patella (below patella)

(5) Achilles (above heel)

b. Rating scale:

(1) 0: Absent

(2) 1+: Minimal, sluggish

(3) 2+: Brisk (normal)

(4) 3+: Brisker

(5) 4+: Hyperreactive, perhaps clonus

c. Babinsky reflex

7. Common Normal Age Related Changes
   a. Response time may be slower with age
   b. Sense of smell and taste may be diminished
   c. Sensations and reflexes in feet and ankles may be diminished
   d. Decreased response to pain stimuli
   e. Generalized decreased and slow reflexes
8. Common disorders: Delirium, Dimentia, Parkinson's Disease, CVA

Functional Assessment

- Definition—the measure of physical and mental capabilities commonly used in physical, psychosocial and economic self management in daily life.

1. Purpose—to determine the ability to perform the activities of daily living.

2. Two major categories—physical and social functioning
   a. Physical Functioning
      (1) Generalized physical health or absence of illness
         (a) Reliable and valid instruments
            (i) Index of Illness (Shanas, 1962)
            (ii) Older Americans Research and Service (OARS)
      (2) Activities of daily living (ADL)—activities needed for self-care
         (a) Reliable and valid instruments
            (i) Katz Index of ADL
            (ii) Barthel Index

(iii) Kenny Self-Care Evaluation

(iv) OARS ADL

(3) Instrumental activities of daily living—activities needed for individual living, e.g., cooking, shopping, laundry.

(a) Reliable and valid instruments

(i) Instrumental Activities of Daily Living Scale

(ii) Pilot Geriatric Arthritis Project Functional Status Measure

(iii) Performance Test of Activities of Daily Living (PADL)

b. Social Functioning

(1) Social interactions and resources

(a) Reliable and valid instruments

(i) Kerckhoff's Mutual Support Index

(ii) OARS Social Resources Scale

(iii) Bennet Social Isolation Scales

(2) Subjective well being and coping

(a) Reliable and valid instruments

(i) Philadelphia Geriatric Center Morale Scale

(ii) Coping with Stress Sentence Completion

(iii) Geriatric Scale of Recent Life Events

(3) Person-environment fit

(a) Reliable and valid instruments

(i) Satisfaction With Nursing Home Scale

(ii) Sheltered Care Environment Scale

(4) Multidimensional Assessment Instruments

(a) Provide information about functioning across many domains. Give an overall picture of the status of the individual.

(b) Barriers—lengthy, staff training necessary to administer and interpret

(c) Reliable and Valid Instruments

(i) Older Americans Resources and Services Group (OARS)

(ii) Comprehensive Assessment and Referral Evaluation (CARE)

(iii) Patient Appraisal and Care Evaluation (PACE)

4. Choosing an Instrument

a. Consider population being assessed, purpose of measurement, role of the user, knowledge of content of instrument, and history of use of instrument.

b. Use in clinical settings

(1) Screening or case finding—focus on population at risk

(2) Assessment—focus on diagnosis or description of condition

(3) Monitoring—rescreening or retesting at specific intervals

c. Observational measures most appropriate for clinical use with elderly clients. Self-report measures (e.g., OARS ADL Scale) more appropriate as screening tool or for identifying at risk populations.

Standard Laboratory Values That Change With Age

Test		Range
Hematology		
Hemoglobin	Decreases to lower limits of normal	M-12.4-14.9 g/100 ml F-11.7-13.8 g/100ml
Hematocrit	Decreases to lower limits of normal	M-42%-54%, F-38%-46%
Sedimentation rate	Mild increase	0-20 units
Chemistry		
Albumin	Decreases	3.3-4.9 g/100ml
Creatinine	Increases	0.6-1.8 mg/100ml
BUN	Increases	M-8-35 mg/100ml F-6-30 mg/100ml
Potassium	Increases	Upper standard range
Glucose	Mild increase	150 mg/100 ml upper limit
Calcium	Changes occur	Stays in ranges
Uric Acid	Mild increase	7.7 mg/100 ml upper limit
Enzymes		
Alkaline phosphatase	Increases	M-80 units average F-79 units average
Urine chemistry		
Creatinine clearance	Calculate for age related changes	
Specific gravity	Decreases	1.028-1.024
Blood gasses		
PCO_2	Increases	
PO_2	Decreases	
Hormones		
Thyroid stimulation hormone	Increases	

Laboratory Values That Remain Constant With Age

Platelet Count
Magnesium
Bilirubin
Lactic dehydrogenase (LDH)
Chloride
Bicarb
Sodium
Aspartate aminotransferase (AST)
(formerly SGOT)

Note. From *Clinical Manual of Gerontological Nursing* (p.26) by M. O. Hogstel, 1992, St. Louis: Mosby Year Book. Copyright 1992 by Mosby Year Book. Adapted by permission.

Questions

1. When taking the health history of Mrs. King, age 62, the nurse finds that she smokes a pack of cigarettes a day. Mrs. King has smoked since her adolescence. Upon physical examination, the nurse would expect to find which of the following?:

   a. Barrel chest
   b. Local tenderness
   c. Resonant percussion
   d. Vesicular sounds over most lung fields

2. Assessment of respiratory expansion provides information about:

   a. Breath sounds
   b. Chest movement
   c. Vibrations
   d. Voice sounds

3. Assessment of the mobility of the tongue tests the motor function of the following:

   a. Cranial nerve VI
   b. Cranial nerve IX
   c. Cranial nerve X
   d. Cranial nerve XII

4. Asking a client to distinguish familiar objects by touch is called:

   a. Extinction
   b. Graphesthesia
   c. Stereognosis
   d. Two-point discrimination

5. The expected response to a deep tendon reflex is graded as:

   a. 1+
   b. 2+
   c. 3+
   d. 4+

6. General mental status can be assessed by asking the client to do all of the following except:

   a. Give name, date and location
   b. Interpret a proverb
   c. Perform the Romberg Test
   d. Demonstrate recall of past, recent and immediate events

7. The pupils should constrict when changing focus from a distant object to a near object. This is called:

   a. Accommodation
   b. Consensual response
   c. Convergence
   d. Oculomotor response

8. The normal tympanic membrane should appear:

   a. Amber and translucent
   b. Gray and opaque
   c. Gray and translucent
   d. White and opaque

9. The gag reflex tested during the oropharyngeal exam is testing:

   a. Hypoglossal
   b. Trigeminal
   c. Vagal only
   d. Vagal and glossopharyngeal

10. The Rinne Test is done to note:

    a. A conduction deficit and/or sensory neural deficit
    b. The comparison between air and bone conduction
    c. If the client has problems with balance

11. Fine muscle twitching that often occurs with lower motor neuron dysfunction is called:

    a. Tics
    b. Clonus
    c. Nystagmus
    d. Tremors

12. To assess cerebellar functioning, the examiner primarily evaluates

    a. Proprioception
    b. Motor coordination
    c. Muscle strength
    d. Deep tendon reflexes

13. The best position to hear an S_3 is for the client to be:

    a. Supine
    b. Sitting
    c. Leaning forward
    d. Standing

14. The correct sequence of assessment techniques in the abdominal examination is:

    a. Auscultation, inspection, palpation, percussion
    b. Inspection, palpation, percussion, auscultation
    c. Inspection, auscultation, percussion, palpation
    d. Inspection, percussion, palpation, auscultation

15. Tactile fremitus or vibratory tremors felt during palpation are most evident in the following locations:

    a. Lower lungs
    b. Directly above abdomen
    c. Near tracheal bifurcation
    d. In the middle of the back

16. The nurse knows that pulmonary infections are more common in patients with chronic bronchitis and emphysema. If an elderly client has an infection, the nurse can expect all of these symptoms except:

    a. Fever
    b. Lethargy
    c. Anorexia
    d. Confusion

17. Mr. F comes to the clinic complaining of blurred vision, distortion, and glare. The nurse should suspect

    a. Diabetic retinopathy
    b. Cataract

c. Glaucoma
d. Macular degeneration

18. The most common findings in the assessment of hyperthyroidism in the elderly are:

    a. Diffuse enlargement, exophthalmos, pretibial myxedema
    b. Dull facial expression, periorbital swelling
    c. Forgetfulness, tachycardia, tremor, dry skin
    d. Weight loss, anorexia, and weakness

19. Brown discoloration in the lower extremities may indicate:

    a. Arterial insufficiency
    b. Longstanding venous insufficiency
    c. Arterial occlusion
    d. Deep vein thrombosis

20. A 67 year old patient complains of dizziness. He felt well until about a week ago. He says he is dizzy when he stands up, but is better when he sits down. One time, he nearly lost consciousness. He says this has never happened in the past. He has no history of nausea or vomiting or blood loss. PE: BP 140/85 supine, 110/50 standing, pulse: 80 supine, 80 standing. The rest of the PE and laboratory are normal. He takes hydrochlorothiazide and guanethidine for his hypertension. The client most likely has:

    a. Alcoholism
    b. Dementia
    c. Orthostatic hypotension
    d. TIAs

21. A carotid bruit can be differentiated from a transmitted heart murmur by

    a. Tactile fremitus
    b. Auscultation at neck
    c. Diaphragmatic excursion
    d. Auscultation at Erb's point

22. Mr. P. is a 78 year old man who has forgotten to take his digoxin and hydrochlorothiazide for the past week. He comes to the clinic with an annoying cough and complains of difficulty getting on his shoes. The nurse listens to his lungs and hears some discrete noncontinuous sounds late in inspiration. These sounds are

a. Rales
b. Rhonchi
c. Wheezes
d. Friction rubs

23. Mr. J.is a 73 year old man with an indirect inguinal hernia. To examine the hernia, the nurse should ask Mr. B to:

    a. Sit
    b. Stand
    c. Lie down
    d. Lie on affected side

24. Mr. D. is an 85 year old man with suspected pneumonia in the right lower lobe. The nurse would expect which of the following notes on percussion:

    a. Dullness
    b. Flatness
    c. Hyperresonance
    d. Tympany

25. In the elderly, it is important to assess the following health promotion practice annually:

    a. Complete physical examination
    b. Sigmoidoscopy
    c. Breast self examination
    d. Stool guaiac

26. The following is a reliable sign of infection in the elderly:

    a. Fever
    b. Tachypnea
    c. Hypertension
    d. Leukocytosis

27. Hyperthyroidism in the elderly should be expected with all of the following symptoms except:

    a. Weight loss
    b. Anorexia
    c. Constipation
    d. Fatigue

28. The major categories in a functional assessment are:
    a. Physical and social
    b. Physical and environmental
    c. Mental and physical
    d. Physical and economic

29. Common normal aging changes related to the cardiac system include all of the following except:
    a. Slower heart rate
    b. Decreased voltage of all EKG waves
    c. Distended peripheral vessels
    d. Ventricular gallop (S_3)

30. All of the following are laboratory values that change with age except:
    a. Hemoglobin decreases to lower limits of normal
    b. Hematocrit decreases to lower limits of normal
    c. Sedimentation rate mildly decreases
    d. Glucose mildly increases

Answers

1. a	11. d	21. b
2. b	12. b	22. a
3. d	13. a	23. b
4. c	14. c	24. a
5. b	15. c	25. d
6. c	16. a	26. b
7. a	17. b	27. d
8. c	18. d	28. a
9. d	19. b	29. d
10. b	20. c	30. c

Bibliography

Ahronheim, J. C. (1990). *Case studies in geriatrics.* Baltimore: Williams & Wilkins.

Bates, B. (1991). *A pocket guide to physical examination and history taking.* Philadelphia: J. B. Lippincott.

Chenitz, W. C., Stone, J. T. & Salisbury, S. A. (1991). *Clinical gerontological nursing: A guide to advanced practice.* Philadelphia: W. B. Saunders.

Eliopoulos, C. (1990). *Health assessment of the older adult.* Redwood City, CA: Addison Wesley.

Goldenberg, K., & Faryna, A. (1990). *Geriatric medicine for the house officer.* Baltimore: Williams & Wilkins.

Hogstel, M. O. (1992). *Clinical manual of gerontological nursing.* St. Louis: Mosby Year Book.

Humphrey, C. J. (1986). *Home care nursing handbook.* Norwalk, CT: Appleton-Century-Crofts.

Newman, D. K. (1991). *Geriatric care plans.* Springhouse, PA: Springhouse Corporation.

Weber, J. (1988). *Nurses' handbook of health assessment.* Philadelphia: J. B. Lippincott.

Yurick, A. G. & Spier, B. E. (1989). *The aged persona and the nursing process.* Norwalk, CT: Appleton & Lange.

Dermatologic Disorders

Molly English

Xerosis (dry skin)

- Definition
  1. Dry, scaly, rough, pruritic skin widespread especially on anterior shins
- Etiology
  1. Most common cause of pruritis in the elderly
  2. Unclear as to exact cause
  3. Possible increase in water loss through stratum corneum or decrease in water content of aging skin
  4. Exacerbated by sun exposure, swimming pools, dry cold winter air, hot dry air of central heating
- Incidence
  1. Especially severe in elderly
  2. Can be precipitated by admission to a hospital (harsh soaps, air conditioning, heating)
  3. Very high after age 70 years
- Signs and Symptoms: Dry, rough, scaly skin with enhanced "itching" (pruritis) sensation
- Differential Diagnosis: Rule out other causes of xerosis such as metabolic/endocrine problems, chronic renal disease, or drug ingestion.
- Physical Findings
  1. Skin is dry, rough, scaly especially over anterior shins
- Diagnostic Evaluation/Findings
  1. Complete health history including allergies, medications, and any systemic disease. Include questions such as: When did itching begin?, Severity of itching?, Body areas involved?, What makes itching better or worse?
  2. Obtain CBC, urinalysis, and chemistry to rule out systemic disease
  3. Perform a thorough assessment of all skin surfaces, skinfolds, mucous membranes and hair

- Management/Treatment
  1. Minimize frequency of hot baths
  2. Encourage use of oatmeal baths and topical emollients
  3. Avoid harsh soaps, rubbing alcohol, and other drying agents
  4. Referral/consultation to physician for skin that does not respond to conservative treatment
- Nursing Considerations
  1. Instruct client to avoid overexposure to sun
  2. Encourage use of sun screens
  3. Emphasize need to avoid intense cold or wind
  4. Limit use of swimming pools
  5. Encourage daily application of body lotion when skin still moist especially in winter
  6. Advise clients to keep air in home as humid as possible

Contact Dermatitis

- Definition: Any reactionary, pruritic disorder that occurs when the skin comes in contact with a particular substance.
- Etiology
  1. Inflammation of epidermis due to direct toxin or delayed hypersensitivity reaction.
  2. Can be due to an allergic reaction resulting from contact with poison ivy or contact with perfumes, clothing, lotions, or topical antibiotic ointments.
- Incidence
  1. Especially prevalent in elderly.
  2. Often subdued due to muted inflammatory response and decreased sensory perception of skin in elderly patient.
- Signs and Symptoms: Skin with erythema, pruritis, scaling, patches, fissures and plaques, form linear or sharp bordered pattern limited to site of exposure.

- Differential Diagnosis
  1. Rule out other causes of dermatitis such as systemic disorder, insect bites, or drug eruption
- Physical Findings (can range from mild to extreme)
  1. Mild: erythema, dryness, and pruritis of skin area
  2. Severe: blistering, erosions, crusts, scales, ulcers of affected area with increased irritation
- Diagnostic Evaluation/Findings
  1. A complete history is imperative in order to identify the causative agent. The history should focus on exposure to common allergic agents. Elicit information regarding exposure to agents in household, at place of work, and outside environment.
  2. Diagnosis can be based on history of exposure and distribution pattern of pruritic lesions.
  3. A thorough physical exam, medical history, and interpretation of any biopsy specimens is beneficial in determining a diagnosis.
- Management/Treatment
  1. Cool compresses
  2. Lotions
  3. Oral antihistamines
  4. Topical or oral steroids if necessary
  5. Referral/consultation with a dermatologist if not responsive to initial treatment
- Nursing Considerations
  1. Educate patient to recognize and avoid causative agent
  2. Encourage patient to use protective gloves if exposure is unavoidable
  3. Emphasize that dermatitis can last up to three weeks
  4. Provide clear written instructions for use of any medication prescribed
  5. Follow-up evaluation one week after treatment initiated

Seborrheic Dermatitis

- Definition: A chronic, recurrent inflammatory response causing a scaly eruption in areas where sebaceous glands are abundant.
- Etiology:
  1. The exact cause of seborrheic dermatitis is unknown, the exacerbations associated with emotional stress and neurologic disease suggest a role of the central nervous system.
- Incidence
  1. Predominantly seen in adults as a chronic condition with increased incidence after 50 years.
  2. Genetic factors may play a role in severity and incidence of the disorder, as well as stress.
  3. Seborrheic dermatitis is often worse during the fall and winter months.
  4. More severe and more difficult to treat in patients with Parkinson's disease.
- Signs and Symptoms: Scaling, flaking, and pruritis distributed over eyebrows, scalp, external auditory canals, groin, chest, and nasolabial fold
- Differential Diagnosis
  1. Tinea cruris
  2. Tinea capitis
  3. Candidiasis
  4. Psoriasis
- Physical Findings
  1. Lesions may be mild (erythema, dryness) to severe (thick, yellow, oily, crusting, scaling).
  2. Patches often begin on the scalp and can migrate to eyebrows, eyelids, external ear and chest area.
  3. Eczema and inflammation of the epidermis may be present as well as thick, yellow, greasy scales.
- Diagnostic Evaluation/Findings: Diagnosis is based on the presence and recognition of characteristic plaques (erythema, oily, scales)

- Management/Treatment
  1. Medicated antiseborrheic shampoos (tar)
  2. Anti-infective agents
  3. Topical corticosteroid lotions or solutions
  4. Keratolytic agents
- Nursing Considerations
  1. Emphasize control rather than cure for seborrheic dermatitis
  2. Encourage frequent use of medicated shampoos (tar)
  3. Instruct in use of medications and preparations and plan of care
  4. Educate patient to avoid excessive heat, perspiration, and external irritants
  5. Encourage patient to wear nonirritating fabrics such as cotton

Herpes Zoster (Shingles)

- Definition
  1. An acute viral infection resulting from reactivaton of the dormant varicella (chicken pox virus)
  2. The reactivation begins at the nerve root ganglia with neuralgia stemming from the involved dermatome
  3. The initial infection is followed by an outbreak of cutaneous vesicular skin lesions
- Etiology
  1. Reactivation of the varicella virus causes an eruption of herpes zoster resulting in an acute infection
  2. During the lifetime of the individual, the virus lies dormant in the sensory root ganglia and resurfacing of the virus can be initiated at any time
  3. Reactivation can be sparked by acute systemic illness, psychological upset, deficient immunological state, or chronic fatigue and debilitation

- Incidence

1. The elderly are more susceptible to developing herpes zoster due to a diminished immunological state. At age 80 years, the annual rate of incidence surpasses 10 per 1000 in population. By age 85 years, individual has 50% chance of developing herpes zoster
2. Individuals over age 50 comprise two thirds of cases of herpes zoster.

- Signs and Symptoms

1. Common initial complaints include myalgia and fever followed by itching, burning, and pain along the affected dermatome.
2. Eruption of lesions often follow in four to five days. Lesions are usually restricted to the skin surface of a single dermatome, but one or two dermatomes near by can be involved.

- Differential Diagnosis

1. Contact dermatitis
2. Herpes simplex virus infection
3. Cellulitis
4. Presence of pain without lesions, rule out renal colic, herniated disc, sciatica, temporal arteritis, pleurisy

- Physical Findings

1. Most common in the trunk region
2. Various sizes of erythematous lesions arise and evolve into purulent, fluid-filled vesicles stemming from the reddened base
3. The eruption continues to appear for about seven days and lasts up to three to four weeks
4. One can always see a straight line of demarcation initiating at the midline and a clear pattern of lesions at the dermatome. The outbreak never crosses over the midline.
5. Postherpetic neuralgia (chronic pain at site for many years)
6. Increases in incidence in the elderly client

- Diagnostic Evaluation/Findings
    1. Diagnosis is based on the presentation of painful, itching clusters of vesicles grouped on a reddened base in a dermatomal pattern.
    2. The classic appearance of unilateral disease, history of previous varicella infection, presence of pain and prodromal symptoms will aid in making a diagnosis.
    3. A tzanck smear can reveal multinucleated giant cells.
    4. Viral cultures or direct viral antigen smears can also be performed to assist in confirmation of herpes zoster.
- Management/Treatment—aimed at symptomatic relief and preventional control of secondary infections
    1. Analgesic agents (acetaminophen) for pain
    2. Antiviral agents (acyclovir)
    3. Topical care (burow's solution; idoxuridine)
    4. Systemic steroids (prednisone) for inflammation
    5. Oral narcotics (codeine) for severe pain
    6. Psychotrophics as needed for anxiety and depression
- Nursing Considerations
    1. Educate patient regarding course of disease process
    2. Instruct patient in use of oral medications and topical solutions
    3. Explain possibility of development of postherpetic neuralgia and methods of pain control
    4. Emphasize careful hygiene measures and risk of infecting those who have not had chicken pox.
    5. Referral/consultation with physician for patients who do not respond to treatment, develop bacterial infection, or who have other concurrent illnesses.
    6. Follow-up evaluation of treatment within one week.

Skin Cancers and Keratoses

- Definition

    1. Skin cancer is an abnormal condition resulting from uncontrolledgrowth of cells in one skin layer. Aging skin is especially susceptible to development of skin cancer.

    2. Types of skin cancer are distinguished by the kinds of cells the tumors resemble. The three most prevalent classes of skin cancer include basal cell carcinoma, squamous cell carcinoma, and malignant melanoma.

- Etiology

    1. Basal cell carcinoma is the most common skin cancer seen in the elderly population, especially caucasians

        a. The germinative layer of the epidermis is the beginning site for basal cell carcinoma.

        b. Basal cell is generally slow growing and is often detected and treated in the primary stage.

        c. Metastasis is rarely observed, however can be locally invasive

        d. This type of cancer is prevalent in people with chronic sun exposure, fair skin, and immunosuppression.

    2. Squamous cell is the second most common form of skin cancer

        a. Lesions are slow growing and often appear as scaly, raised, irregular nodules.

        b. Squamous cell has the potential for metastasis especially if treatment is delayed.

        c. This form of cancer can arise from actinic keratoses, which are premalignant lesions found in sun exposed areas of the body.

        d. Squamous cell can also originate from areas of chronic irritation or trauma.

    3. Malignant melanoma is the third and least common type of skin cancer, but is very serious and highly metastatic

        a. It stems from melanocytes found in nevi or other pigmented lesions.

b. Associated with sunlight or irritation of mole

c. Any bleeding or change in a mole can signal melanoma and should be investigated.

d. The face and hands are primary areas for melanoma in the elderly.

e. Fair skinned caucasians of European descent most at risk

- Incidence

1. Eighty percent of non melanoma skin cancers are basal cell carcinoma. It is five times more prevalent than squamous cell and there is a higher incidence among men.
2. Squamous cell carcinoma ranks second to basal cell and usually occurs at a later age. This form of skin cancer appears to be more prevalent in women.
3. The third and least common type of skin cancer is malignant melanoma. It is the most dreaded of skin cancers because it often metastasizes to other parts of the body. Melanoma is responsible for about seventy-five percent of all deaths from skin cancer, but early detection can decrease the death rate.

- Signs and Symptoms

1. Skin cancers often begin as elevations on the skin that are red and itchy. They can appear as abrasions that will not heal.

- Differential Diagnosis

1. Rule out benign lesions such as seborrheic keratoses and premalignant patches known as actinic keratoses.

- Physical Findings

1. Basal cell carcinoma

a. Lesions frequently originate as pearly gray papules with a waxy, raised border.

b. The nose, eyelid, and cheek are most often affected as well as the neck, back of hands, and trunk.

c. Penetration of the skin is primarily local

d. The nodule may have a central induration and telangiectasias

2. Squamous cell carcinoma
    a. Papule or nodule appears reddened, scaly, and wart-like with a wide, depressed border.
    b. Lesions often stem from areas of actinic keratoses on the neck, ears, arms, and hands.
3. Malignant melanoma
    a. Nodular lesion can be tan, black, brown, gray, white, red, or blue, and often < 1 cm in diameter
    b. Area is flat or somewhat raised with irregular shape and stems from a pigmented mole.
4. Actinic keratoses (Senile or solar keratoses)
    a. Premalignant, irregular lesion with red, brown, pink, or tan coloring. Approximately 20% develop into squamous cell carcinoma but rarely metastasize.
    b. Area is often raised and scaly and found on sun exposed parts of the body.
5. Seborrheic keratoses (Benign)
    a. Waxy, wart-like, raised growths often found in groups on the face, trunk, shoulder and groin regions. Usually found in unexposed areas.
    b. Can be brown, black, yellow, or tan in color and vary in size.

- Diagnostic Evaluation/Findings
    1. Careful inspection and evaluation should be made of any lesions demonstrating change in size, shape, or color as well as presence of ulceration or bleeding.
    2. A family history, history of sun exposure, and any medications or allergies are part of the medical history.
    3. Onset of the skin lesion, accompanying symptoms, past medical history, and any past treatment should be included in the work up.
    4. Complaints of pain, paresthesia, or pruritis can help distinguish skin lesions.
    5. Any skin lesion suspected to be cancerous should be referred to a dermatologist for biopsy and conclusive diagnosis.

- Management/Treatment

  1. Basal cell carcinomas and squamous cell carcinomas are often treated with surgery (scalpel excision), medications (anti-neoplastic), or procedures such as radiotherapy, cryotherapy, or electroexcision.
  2. Malignant melanomas are frequently managed with deep excision of primary lesion, antineoplastic agents, anti-infective agents, radiotherapy, or hyperthermic isolation perfusion.

- Nursing Considerations

  1. A complete examination of the elderly client's skin may reveal a host of dermatologic lesions.
  2. Correct identification of premalignant and malignant tumors is mandatory for complete and appropriate care of the older adult patient.
  3. The ability to diagnose these lesions and provide proper medical intervention is an essential element in care of the elderly.
  4. Education of the elderly client is also a key factor in preventing skin lesions from becoming a threat to the health of the individual.
  5. Emphasize the need for regular self examination as well as routine physical examinations with a health care provider.
  6. Instruct the client in general skin care such as types of soaps and moisturizers best suited for aging skin.
  7. Inform clients of the need to protect their skin from sun exposure with the use of sunscreens and protective clothing when outside.
  8. Encourage avoidance of excessive exposure to the sun and limit exposure to ionizing radiation and ultraviolet light especially midday between 10 a.m. and 3 p.m.
  9. Instruct client to avoid the sun if using photosensitizing drugs.
  10. Remind individuals to be alert to reflection from sand, snow, and water because of increased radiation.
  11. It is important for the health care provider to be informed and prepared to answer any questions or concerns regarding care of aging skin and skin cancers.
  12. Because malignancies of the skin are common in the elderly, all suspicious skin lesions should be referred to a dermatologist for evaluation in order to enhance early detection and prompt treatment.

Adult Candidiasis

- Definition: A superficial fungal infection of the skin
- Etiology: *Candida albicans*
- Incidence: Prevalent fungal infecton commonly seen in the compromised elderly patient. More common in women and persons who are obese, diabetic, or taking systemic antibiotics
- Signs and Symptoms: Itching, burning pain often seen especially in the vulval area and in uncontrolled diabetics
- Differential Diagnosis: Rule out other fungal infections and seborrheic dermatitis.
- Physical Findings
  1. Shiny red macerated placques outlined by pustules and papules with satellite lesions
  2. Found in warm, moist, intertriginous skin areas
- Diagnostic Evaluation/Findings
  1. The level of glucose in the urine and blood should be measured to determine possible presence of diabetes mellitus.
  2. The lesions can be prepared with potassium hydroxide to isolate the fungus candida under microscopic examination
  3. Cultures of vaginal secretions should also be obtained if the diagnosis is not clear.
- Management/Treatment
  1. A suspected diabetic or known uncontrolled diabetic should be referred to and evaluated by a physician.
  2. Intertriginous candida can be treated with Nystatin, Miconazole, or Clotrimazole cream twice daily.
  3. Monitor weekly until infection clears
  4. Referral/consultation should be made to a physician if the candida does not resolve in approximately two weeks.
- Nursing Considerations
  1. Instruct in methods of keeping the skin clean and dry

2. Encourage frequent change of clean clothing to prevent reinfection.
3. Discuss use of loose, cotton undergarments and stockings to control moisture.
4. Educate the client to apply medicated creams to prevent further maceration.
5. Emphasize need to avoid use of cornstarch which can enhance the growth of candida organisms.
6. Assist in controlling underlying diabetes if indicated.

Folliculitis

- Definition: A superficial or deep bacterial infection involving irritation and possibly destruction of the hair follicle.
- Etiology: *Staphylococcus aureus*
- Incidence: Can result from such systemic factors as obesity, diabetes mellitus, immunosuppressed state, malnutrition
- Signs and Symptoms: Edema, redness, and pain localized at the site of the lesion
- Differential Diagnosis
    1. Pseudomonal folliculitis
    2. Pseudofolliculitis
    3. Insect bite
    4. Infection due to foreign object
- Physical Findings
    1. Scalp and extremities most often affected
    2. Pustule surrounding hair shaft
    3. Redness at site of nodule
    4. Edema and exudate present at lesion
    5. Crusted exudate following rupture of pustule
- Diagnostic Evaluation/Findings
    1. Gram stain test of exudate can confirm diagnosis.

2. Culture and sensitivity of the lesion is usually not necessary.

- Management/Treatment
  1. Warm compresses
  2. Anti-infective agents
  3. Oral or systemic antibiotics
  4. Topical antibiotics
  5. Incision and drainage of lesions
  6. Follow-up evaluation
  7. Referral/consultation with a dermatologist if no improvement

- Nursing Considerations
  1. Patient Education
     a. Daily bath with bacteriostatic soap
     b. Individual use of towels, clothes, and linen
     c. Daily washing of linens and clothes
     d. Instruct in proper use of antibiotic therapy and warm compresses
     e. Emphasize meticulous handwashing and hygiene
     f. Inform patient that drainage can last for several days
     g. Teach signs and symptoms of systemic infection such as fever and red streaks
     h. Educate patient not to pick at lesions

Questions

1. A yellow, oily, scaling eruption of the skin on the scalp, face, and chest area most likely describes:
   a. Contact dermatitis
   b. Basal cell carcinoma
   c. Seborrheic keratoses
   d. Seborrheic dermatitis

2. Folliculitis is an infection of the:
   a. Lymph gland
   b. Sebaceous gland
   c. Hair follicle
   d. Skin tag

3. What body area is xerosis most likely to be found?
   a. Face
   b. Neck
   c. Anterior shins
   d. Hands

4. Contact dermatitis is often subdued in the elderly because:
   a. Skin has decreased elasticity
   b. Skin is often dry
   c. Increased sensitivity to irritants
   d. Decreased sensory perception
   e. Both c and d

5. Mr. Smith is a 70 year old white male who comes to the clinic with a slightly raised, scaly pink, irregular lesion on his scalp. Mr. Smith is a farmer and works outdoors all day. You suspect an actinic keratoses. What recommendation would you give him?
   a. Ignore the sore and it will go away
   b. Instruct him to use a nonprescription cream to dry up the lesion
   c. Tell him to come back in a month if it doesnt go away
   d. Explain to Mr. Smith that the lesion looks suspicious and refer him to a dermatologist as soon as possible

6. Which of the following skin lesions is least common, but most serious?

a. Squamous cell carcinoma
b. Malignant melanoma
c. Seborrheic keratoses
d. Basal cell carcinoma

7. Mrs. Brown is a 65 year old widow who is worried about several waxy, yellowish-brown, wart-like growths on her back. What advice would you give to Mrs. Brown?

a. Tell her to see a doctor because the growths are cancer
b. Instruct her to ignore the lesions and they will disappear
c. Inform her that she should have the growths removed
d. Reassure Mrs. Brown that the growths are called seborrheic keratoses and are not harmful to her

8. Which of the following dermatologic conditions results from reactivation of the varicella virus that has been dormant?

a. Candidiasis
b. Basal cell carcinoma
c. Herpes zoster
d. Actinic keratoses

9. Dry, rough, scaly skin with the presence of an enhanced "itching" sensation can best be described as:

a. Shingles
b. Sqamous cell carcinoma
c. Seborrheic keratoses
d. Xerosis

10. The tzanck prep is a laboratory study often used to diagnose which of the following disorders?

a. Contact dermatitis
b. Herpes zoster
c. Candidiasis
d. Malignant melanoma

11. Mr. Wood is a 69 year old white male who comes to the office with a scaly, pruritic, red rash over both forearms and hands. Mr. Wood states that he has

been pulling weeds and fixing his garden. After further investigation you determine that Mr. Wood has poison ivy. What would be the best initial treatment for Mr. Wood?

a. Instruct him to do nothing
b. Advise him to apply cold compresses to the affected areas four to six times a day for 20 minutes and apply over the counter hydrocortizone cream (1%) after each compress
c. Tell him to see a dermatologist immediately because he has a rare skin disorder.
d. Emphasize that he should give up gardening

12. Mrs. Boone is a 75 year old white female who comes to the outpatient clinic complaining of a red, painful rash over the left side of her back. She says that she often has a burning sensation and has noticed some drainage from the spots. What initial diagnosis would you make for Mrs. Boone?

a. Candidiasis
b. Shingles
c. Seborrheic dermatitis
d. Sqamous cell carcinoma

13. What initial treatment would be indicated for Mrs. Boone?

a. Calamine lotion
b. Cold compresses
c. Systemic steroids
d. Analgesic agent and antiviral medication
e. None of the above

14. A smooth, round nodule with a pearly grey border and central induration best describes which type of the following skin lesions?

a. Seborrheic keratoses
b. Malignant melanoma
c. Basal cell carcinoma
d. Herpes zoster

15. Which of the following is true regarding the treatment of Candidiasis?

a. Use of cold, moist compresses and cornstarch to the affected area
b. Systemic steroids and hot packs to the involved skin
c. Calamine lotion
d. Topical antifungal cream

16. Mr. Jones is a 68 year old widower who has just recently started dating again. He comes to the office complaining of a red, scaly, weepy rash over both sides of his neck and under his chin. What would be the initial assessment?

    a. Tell Mr. Jones to ignore the rash
    b. Explain to Mr. Jones that the rash is due to "nerves"
    c. Obtain a biopsy of the lesions
    d. Obtain a complete medical history including medications and recent use of new soaps, lotions, colognes, etc.

17. During the course of the interview, Mr. Jones tells you that he has been using a new cologne because he wants to "smell good" for his date. What would be an initial diagnosis for Mr. Jones?

    a. Seborrheic dermatitis
    b. Shingles
    c. Contact dermatitis
    d. Psoriasis

18. Candidiasis is caused by which of the following organisms?

    a. *Pseudomonas aeruginosa*
    b. *Staphylococcus aureus*
    c. *Escherchia coli*
    d. *Candida albicans*

19. A chronic, recurrent inflammatory response causing a scaling eruption in areas where sebaceous glands are prevalent best describes:

    a. Malignant melanoma
    b. Shingles
    c. Contact dermatitis
    d. Seborrheic dermatitis

20. Mrs. Harper is a 72 year old white female who comes to the clinic complaining of dry, scaly, itchy skin over her lower legs. Mrs. Harper states that she takes "a warm bath" every night to clean off the dead skin. Which of the following is a likely diagnosis for Mrs. Harper?

    a. Poison ivy
    b. Contact dermatitis
    c. Xerosis
    d. Candidiasis

21. What recommendations would you give Mrs. Harper?

    a. Continue warm baths every day
    b. Apply calamine lotion to stop the itching
    c. Limit warm baths to two to three times a week and apply a topical emollient to lower legs once a day and after bathing
    d. None of the above

22. Which of the following best describe why the elderly are more susceptible to developing herpes zoster?

    a. Age related changes
    b. Diminished immunological state
    c. Sensitive skin
    d. Reason is unknown

23. The etiology of contact dermatitis can best be attributed to:

    a. Increased water loss through stratum corneum
    b. Yeast like fungus
    c. Inflammation of epidermis due to toxin or delayed hypersensitivity reaction
    d. Reactivation of varicella virus

24. Treatment modalities for contact dermatitis include all of the following except:

    a. Lotions
    b. Oral antihistamines
    c. Topical steroids
    d. Warm compresses

25. Hilda is an 82 year old white female who comes to the clinic complaining of fever and muscle aches. During the examination, you notice a line of vesicular lesions on the right side of her back. After further evaluation, you determine that Hilda has herpes zoster or shingles. She wants to know if it is common for other people her age to get shingles. Your best response to her would be:

    a. "Yes, older adults have sensitive skin."
    b. "No, this is a rare disorder."
    c. "I don't know."
    d. "Yes, the elderly are more susceptible to shingles due to a diminished immune state."

26. Which of the following best describes adult candidiasis?

a. Dry, scaly pruritic skin over anterior shins
b. Pearly gray papule with a waxy raised border
c. Thick, yellow greasy scales
d. Shiny red macerated plaques outlined by pustules and papules with satellite lesions

27. A raised, irregular lesion, that is often black, brown, or blue and stems from a pigmented mole best describes:

a. Seborrheic keratoses
b. Folliculitis
c. Malignant melanoma
d. Basil cell carcinoma

28. All of the following can be used in the management and treatment of seborrheic dermatitis except:

a. Keratolytic agents
b. Antiviral agents
c. Antiinfective agents
d. Topical corticosteroid lotions or solutions

Answers:

1. d
2. c
3. c
4. d
5. d
6. b
7. d
8. c
9. d
10. b
11. b
12. b
13. d
14. c
15. d
16. d
17. c
18. d
19. d
20. c
21. c
22. b
23. c
24. d
25. d
26. d
27. c
28. b

Bibliography

Burke, M. M. & Walsh, M. B. (1992). *Gerontologic nursing: Care of the frail elderly.* St. Louis: Mosby Year Book.

Chenitz, W. C., Stone, J. T., & Salisbury, S. (1991). *Clinical gerontological nursing: A guide to advanced practice.* Philadelphia: W. B. Saunders.

Delafuente, J. C., & Stewart, R. B.(Eds.) (1988). *Therapeutics in the elderly.* Baltimore: Williams and Wilkins.

Gambert, S. R. (Ed.). (1987). *Handbook of geriatrics.* New York: Plenum.

Goldstein, B. G., & Goldstein, A. O. (1992). *Practical dermatology. St. Louis: Mosby Year Book.*

Hogstel, M. O. (Ed.). (1992). *Clinical manual of gerontological nursing.* St. Louis: Mosby Year Book.

Hoole, A. J., Greenberg, R. A., & Pickard Jr., C. G. (Eds.). (1988). *Patient care guidelines for nurse practitioners.* Boston: Little, Brown and Company.

Patterson, J. A. K. (1989). *Aging and clinical practice: Skin disorders.* New York: Igaku-Shoin.

Smoller, J., & Smoller, B. R. (1992). Skin malignancies in the elderly: Diagnosable, treatable, and potentially curable. *Journal of Gerontological Nursing. 18,* (5), 19–24.

Thompson, J. M., Mcfarland, G. K., Hirsch, J. E., Tucker, S. M., & Bowers, A. C. (1989). *Mosby's manual of clinical nursing.* St. Louis: C. V. Mosby.

Respiratory Disorders

Catharine Kopac

Chronic Obstructive Pulmonary Disease (COPD)

- Definition: A progressive respiratory disease syndrome composed of one or more of the following conditions
    1. Emphysema (resulting in "air trapping" and permanent destruction of alveolar tissue);
    2. Chronic bronchitis (an inflammatory process of the bronchi accompanied by increased mucous production); and
    3. Bronchoconstriction.

    Majority of clients have mixed pathology, although one characteristic usually predominates.

- Etiology: Cause is generally unknown; chronic irritation of the lung is the primary physiologic finding; epidemiologic studies show association between COPD and cigarette smoking. Exposure to chemical or environmental irritants and chronic respiratory infections may also be causative agents. Heredity and aging may also play a part in susceptibility.

- Incidence: Affects approximately ten percent of population. Respiratory failure, due to COPD, is fifth leading cause of death. Men are affected more than women although discrepancy between sexes is narrowing because of increased cigarette smoking in women.

- Signs and Symptoms
    1. Shortness of breath and cough
    2. Use of accessory muscles of respiration
    3. Prolonged expiration
    4. Increased sputum production
    5. Restlessness or twitching
    6. Hyperemia of hands
    7. Cyanotic or clubbed fingers
    8. Fatigue (due to the increased work necessary to breathe)
    9. Difficulty in sleeping
    10. Intermittent productive cough
    11. Increase of the anteroposterior diameter of the chest

12. Distant breath sounds
13. Wheezing

- Differential Diagnosis: Includes acute bronchitis, allergic asthma, and congestive heart failure.
- Physical Findings

1. Type A COPD (Emphysema)
    a. Inspection
        (1) Thin, muscle wasted appearance
        (2) Absent central cyanosis, "pink puffer"
        (3) Hypertrophy of accessory muscles of respiration
        (4) "Barrel chest"; slight to moderate increase in AP diameter in older adults in general
        (5) Decreased effective cough
    b. Percussion
        (1) Hyperresonance
        (2) Decreased diaphragmatic excursion
    c. Auscultation
        (1) Distant diminished breath sounds
2. Type B COPD (Chronic Bronchitis)
    a. Inspection
        (1) Body appearance is typically overweight
        (2) Central cyanosis, "blue bloater"
        (3) Minimal use of accessory muscles
    b. Percussion
        (1) Resonant percussion note is usually produced
    c. Auscultation
        (1) Adventitious breath sounds, primarily wheezes

- Diagnostic Evaluation/Findings
  1. Chest x-ray in
     a. Emphysema—findings are hyperinflation, flat diaphragm, small/normal heart, widened intercostal margins.
     b. Chronic bronchitis—findings are cardiac enlargement, normal or flattened diaphragm, evidence of chronic inflammation, and congested lung fields.
  2. Spirometry in
     a. Emphysema—findings include increased total lung capacity (TLC), increased residual volume (RV), decreased vital capacity (VC), and decreased forced expiratory volume (FEV_1).
     b. Chronic bronchitis—findings include normal or only slightly increased TLC, increased RV, decreased VC, and decreased FEV_1.
     c. If FEV_1 is less than 70 percent of the forced vital capacity, then significant obstruction is present.
  3. Arterial blood gases in
     a. Emphysema—near normal, mild hypoxemia.
     b. Chronic bronchitis—moderate to severe hypoxemia and hypercapnia.
  4. Electrocardiogram in
     a. Emphysema—normal.
     b. Chronic bronchitis—may include right axis deviation, or right ventricular hypertrophy.
  5. Sputum culture—helpful in chronic bronchitis to identify bacterial agent.
  6. Hemoglobin (Hgb) and Hematocrit (Hct) in
     a. Emphysema—normal until late in disease.
     b. Chronic bronchitis—Hgb and Hct are usually increased.

- Management/Treatment: Management addresses five basic areas
  1. Improve ventilation
     a. Drugs (intravenous, oral, or topical)—xanthines and other bronchodilators; steroids, anticholinergics
     b. SHOULD AVOID RESPIRATORY DEPRESSANTS
     c. Oxygen as indicated by arterial blood gases (low flow—less than 5 liters/minute per nasal cannula)
  2. Improve airway clearance
     a. Maintain high fluid intake. (Patients with cardiac disease still need thin secretions—diuretic may be necessary to avoid overload.)
     b. Postural drainage and percussion during acute phases for all patients and daily for people with chronic bronchitis.
     c. Smoking cessation
     d. Aerosol therapy (Nebulizer mist)
     e. Pursed-lip breathing
  3. Prevent or treat infection
     a. Avoid exposure to infection
     b. Treat infection early with appropriate antibiotics
  4. Improve strength and exercise tolerance
     a. Gradually increase patient's activity.
     b. Teach energy conservation techniques
     c. Ensure adequate nutrition; encourage weight loss prn
  5. Reduce depression and anxiety
     a. Encourage activity rather than solitary behaviors
     b. Provide counseling.
     c. Avoid sedatives and tranquilizers.

- Nursing Considerations: The nursing goal is to relieve signs and symptoms, prevent complications and assist with adjustment to life-style changes. The nursing implications parallel the treatment
  1. Improve ventilation
     a. Administer bronchodilators, antibiotics, and steroids. Be aware of drug side effects and teach medication's side effects and what drugs to avoid, especially respiratory depressants.
     b. Administer oxygen. Teach purpose of oxygen therapy, how to use and clean equipment, and signs and symptoms of carbon dioxide narcosis, if oxygen therapy is continued at home.
  2. Improve airway clearance
     a. Encourage 2 to 3 liters of fluid daily to mobilize secretions (clients with cardiac problems need to be monitored for fluid overload—the actual fluid intake may need to be specified and diuretic therapy monitored); humidifiers, vaporizers, and nebulizers may also be used.
     b. Perform postural drainage, chest percussion, and vibration to mobilize secretions and improve ventilation. (Be aware that positions used in maneuvers to drain lung segments can be uncomfortable and/or harmful to the elderly client).
     c. Smoking cessation and avoidance of other respiratory irritants
  3. Prevent or treat infection
     a. Instruct on need to avoid other people with known respiratory infections and seek treatment early when infection does occur.
     b. The following signs and symptoms indicate that a health care provider should be contacted
        (1) Any change in regular symptoms, e.g.,
           (a) Increase in shortness of breath, wheezing, coughing
           (b) Chest discomfort occurs or increases
           (c) Increased difficulty in sleeping, due to respiratory problems

(d) Changes in color, amount, or character of sputum, or more difficulty in bringing up sputum

(2) If new symptoms occur, e.g.,

(a) Chills and/or fever

(b) Sudden weight gain

(c) Swelling of feet

(d) Increased intolerence to exercise

c. Instruct client on the need for regular immunizations.

(1) Pneumonia

(2) Influenza

d. Provide instruction on how to improve strength and exercise tolerance

(1) Gradually increase activity

(2) Teach energy conservation techniques

(3) Ensure adequate nutrition and encourage weight loss prn

(4) Teach use of bronchodilator before activities

(5) Teach use of pursed-lip breathing

e. Focus on reducing depression and anxiety

(1) Encourage social activity

(2) Provide counseling

(3) Avoid sedatives and tranquilizers

Asthma

- Definition: Acute reversible (episodic) obstructive airway disease that involves inflammation and edema of respiratory mucosa, excessive sputum production, and bronchospasm. Recognition of asthma depends upon demonstration of increased airway responsiveness to a variety of stimuli and reversibility of airway obstruction either spontaneously or with therapy.
- Etiology: Certain extrinsic factors may initiate or provoke predisposed individual into an attack; mechanism is not clear: Viral respiratory infec-

tion, irritants (eg., tobacco smoke, perfume, air pollutants), allergens, aspirin and other prostaglandin inhibitors, exercise, cold air, and emotional factors.

- Incidence: Small percentage of asthmatics have onset of disease after age 60 and 70.

- Signs and Symptoms
  1. Wheezing and dyspnea (usual presenting symptoms); however, older client may present with
  2. Paroxysmal nocturnal dyspnea and/or
  3. Episodic cough

  Depending on the etiology other symptoms may occur

  4. Fever
  5. Upper respiratory infection, rhinorrhea
  6. Allergic rash
- Differential Diagnosis: Includes acute bronchitis, foreign body aspiration, pneumonia, pulmonary emboli, congestive heart failure, anaphylactic reaction to some allergen (e.g., drug, food, inhalant), upper airway compression-tumor, extrinsic compression, or foreign body.
- Physical Findings
  1. Inspection
     a. Use of accessory muscles of respiration
     b. Intercostal, sub/suprasternal retractions
     c. Nasal flaring
     d. Cyanosis
     e. Tachypnea
     f. Diaphoresis
  2. Auscultation
     a. Prolonged expiration
     b. Expiratory wheezing
     c. Occasionally, some inspiratory wheezing
     d. Distant breath sounds

3. Percussion

   Hyperresonant percussion note may be produced

- Diagnostic Evaluation/Findings: The diagnosis of asthma depends upon documentation of reversible airway obstruction.

  1. Spirometry—valuable aid in establishing diagnosis, severity of illness, response to treatment, and the need for hospitalization. Peak Expiratory Flow Rate can determine the severity of an attack; for an adult general outcome criteria are as follows

     a. 200 Liters/min. or greater—mild obstruction

     b. 100–200 Liters/min—moderate obstruction; observe in response to treatment

     c. 60 100 Liters/min—severe obstruction; hospitalization is necessary

  2. Chest x-ray (P.A. and lateral)—may show a hyperinflation of lung tissue or signs of pulmonary infection

  3. White blood cell count with differential

     a. Total eosinophil count helpful in diagnosis, as well as monitoring treatment and/or course of the illness. Rise in eosinophil rate frequently occurs prior to onset of symptoms.

     b. Elevated WBC count may indicate an acute infection.

  4. Arterial blood gases (ABGs)—

     a. Early in attack ABGs show hypoxemia and hypocapnia; as hypoxia increases, hyperventilation in an attempt to raise the pO_2; this blows off excess CO_2 and lowers the pCO_2 to well below the normal 35 to 45 mm Hg.

     b. During the course of the attack, as fatigue sets in, ability to hyperventilate is diminished and the pCO_2 gradually rises.

     c. When pCO_2 is at high edge of normal, there is danger of respiratory failure.

  5. Sputum—The most common cause of acute illness in the asthmatic client is infection.

     a. Gram stain—polymorphonuclear leukocytes and/or bacteria may indicate acute infection.

b. Wright's—increased eosinophils when allergic reaction is the precipitant.

c. Sputum culture—may reveal pathogenic bacteria

- Management/Treatment: Strategies are directed toward preventing attacks when possible and managing the attacks when they occur. The management addresses three specific areas

1. Prevent attacks when possible

a. Encourage healthy lifestyle

b. Maintain a high fluid intake

c. Administer bronchodilators

d. Avoid over the counter medications, especially, aspirin and sedatives

e. Avoid exposure to infection

f. Seek treatment for infection early

g. Avoid respiratory irritants and allergens

2. Manage the attack when it occurs; prompt treatment to avoid "status asthmaticus"

a. Improve ventilation with xanthines and other bronchodilators (intravenous, topical), and steroids (during attack).

b. Oxygen as indicated by ABGs

c. Treat infection, if present

d. Improve airway clearance by high fluid intake, postural drainage, percussion, and eliminating smoking.

3. Improve strength and exercise tolerance

a. Ensure adequate nutrition; weight loss prn

b. Establish plan for resting when fatigued or short of breath

c. Bronchodilator inhaler before activities prn

d. Avoid use of respiratory depressants—sedatives, tranquilizers, narcotics.

- Nursing Considerations: Nursing goal is to relieve symptoms, prevent complications and assist the client to understand how to manage the disease and prevent attacks

1. Prevent attacks when possible
    a. Client education re: Avoidance of stimuli responsible for attack, adequate nutrition and exercise, pursed lip breathing, high fluid intake, appropriate use of drugs, drugs to avoid, and necessity of reporting symptoms of bronchospasm and infection early
2. Manage the attack when it occurs
    a. Administer xanthines and other bronchodilators (intravenous,topical), and/or steroids (intravenous during attack)
    b. Oxygen therapy prn as indicated by ABGs
    c. Keep secretions thin by high fluid intake
    d. Postural drainage and percussion
    e. Eliminate smoking
3. Improve strength and exercise tolerance
    a. Ensure adequate nutrition, encourage weight loss prn
    b. Stress importance of rest periods when tired or short of breath (SOB)
    c. Teach use of bronchodilator prior to activities that cause wheezing or SOB
    d. Avoid use or respiratory antidepressants, e.g., sedatives, tranquilizers, narcotics

Pneumonia

- Definition: A bacterial or viral lung infection for which the elderly, particularly those with COPD are at high risk. Bacterial pneumonias are the type most commonly found in the elderly. *Streptococcus pneumoniae* is the cause of bacterial pneumonia in 50% to 90% of community acquired pneumonia. Pneumonia can also be caused by gram-negative aerobic bacteria, viruses, fungi, or *mycobacteria tuberculosis* (infrequently). Most commonly identified pathogen is the pneumococcus.
- Etiology: Pneumococcus is a normal inhabitant of nose and throat. Pneumonia results when there is an imbalance in the interactions between the

number and virulence of the bacteria and host defenses. Elderly are particularly vulnerable to pneumonia and certain conditions increase the risk: COPD, congestive heart failure, influenza, alcoholism, and pulmonary neoplasm. Upper respiratory infections increase the risk of pneumonia; about 60 to 75% of those who acquire pneumococcal pneumonia have had a preceding upper respiratory infection. Aspiration of infected material into lower respiratory tract can begin infectious process. Viral respiratory infections damage normal lung defenses and make them vulnerable to bacterial invasion.

- Incidence
    1. Lower respiratory tract infections are found in 25 to 60 percent of elderly at autopsy
    2. Annual rate of hospitalization for pneumonia (per 10,000 persons)—30 to 60 cases during three year period for persons over 65 years compared to 5 to 15 cases for all other age categories (Glezen, Decker, Perotta, 1987)
    3. Long term care facilities have an incidence of 100 cases per 1000 patient years (Bentley, 1981)
- Signs and Symptoms
    1. Elderly can exhibit a classic pneumonia syndrome which includes
        a. Sudden onset
        b. Shaking chills
        c. Fever
        d. Pleuritic chest pain
        e. Cough productive with purulent sputum; may be blood tinged
    2. However, it is not unusual for the elderly to exhibit rather subtle clinical findings:
        a. Low grade fevers (or perhaps no fever)
        b. No pleuritic pain
        c. Non-productive and/or weak cough
        d. Change in sensorium
- Differential Diagnosis: Includes tuberculosis, bronchial asthma, foreign

body obstruction, atelectasis, pulmonary embolism with infarction, and congestive heart failure

- Physical Findings
  1. Inspection
     a. Cyanosis
     b. Intercostal, sub/suprasternal retractions
     c. Nasal flaring
     d. Tachypnea
     e. Tachycardia
  2. Auscultation
     a. Bacterial pneumonia presents with
        (1) Diffuse crackles and wheezes
        (2) Bronchial breath sounds
        (3) Pleural friction rub
        (4) Whispered pectoriloquy
     b. Viral, non-bacterial pneumonia presents with fine crackles
  3. Palpation
     a. Increase in tactile fremitus over areas of consolidation
  4. Percussion
     a. Dull note over areas of consolidation
- Diagnostic Evaluation/Findings
  1. Sputum must be collected before starting antibiotics; needed for Gram stain, culture and sensitivity.
  2. Chest x-ray—a PA and lateral chest x-ray are mandatory; bacterial pneumonia is associated with consolidation, effusions, and/or abscess formation. True interstitial infiltrate supports viral etiology.
  3. WBC count with differential
     a. Normal WBC may be present in Mycoplasma/Pneumococcal
     b. May be elevated in bacterial pneumonia

   c. Polymorphonuclear leukocytosis is found in bacterial pneumonia

4. Blood gases may be indicated

- Management/Treatment: Strategies directed at early diagnosis and prompt treatment since it is a leading causes of death in older persons

1. Identify and treat causative organism with appropriate antibiotics
2. Provide adequate ventilation/oxygenation
   a. Bronchodilators (systemic and inhaled)
   b. Give oxygen as indicated by ABGs
   c. Reduce metabolic demands (bed rest, long rest periods, light diet, reduce fever)
3. Improve airway clearance
   a. Hydration (oral, intravenous, mist)
   b. Postural drainage
   c. Percussion
   d. Suction
   e. COUGH SUPPRESSANTS ARE CONTRAINDICATED
4. Relieve pain with mild analgesics that will not depress respirations

- Nursing Considerations: Nursing goals: (1) relieve signs and symptoms, (2) prevent complications, and (3) assist in recovery from the illness. Nursing care parallels the treatment.

1. Identify and treat causative organism
   a. Blood and sputum specimens for culture must be collected prior to commencement of treatment
   b. Aseptic technique: respiratory isolation as needed
   c. Antibiotics according to prescribed schedule to maintain appropriate blood levels
2. Provide adequate ventilation
   a. Administer oxygen as ordered

b. Elevate head of bed; support arms as necessary to improve diaphragmatic action, open airways and allow use of shoulder girdle for inspiration

c. Reduce metabolic demands with bedrest, long rest periods, light diet, and fever reduction

d. Mild analgesia as ordered to facilitate respirations and coughing

e. Relaxation techniques to reduce discomfort

3. Improve airway clearance

   a. Encourage fluids as indicated, up to 2 to 3 liters/day

   b. Monitor quantity and character of secretions

   c. Assess respiratory status at least every four hours

   d. Perform postural drainage and percussion

   e. Turn, cough, and deep breathe at least every two hours

4. Relieve pain and discomfort

   a. Antipyretics and other measures prn; monitor response

   b. Mild analgesics as ordered; monitor response

   c. Monitor levels of discomfort, splinting

   d. Monitor respiratory rate, depth, and character

5. Instruct client on need for vaccine

   a. Pneumonia

   b. Influenza

Tuberculosis

- Definition: An infection which occurs in richly oxygenated tissues, especially the lungs. Can also occur in the kidneys and meninges. Usually results from reactivation of microorganism after a previous exposure; reinfection with *tubercule bacilli* is a problem among elderly persons whose infection is so remote and completely healed that the immune memory of the T cells has been lost.
- Etiology: *Mycobacterium tuberculosis,* a gram-positive, acid-fast bacillus.

Primary infection acquired via airborne droplet nuclei released by an infected person; casual exposure generally does not result in transmission of bacilli. Secondary cases develop with repeated, close contact (e.g., family, fellow workers, fellow residents in long term care facilities). Most infectious prior to diagnosis; by the time treatment has been continued for a week the client is usually noninfectious. Bacilli can spread quickly through lymphatic channels to regional lymph nodes via the thoracic duct to the circulating blood. Spread often occurs before body has sufficiently mounted cellular response.

- Incidence: Has been on the decline; however, increased incidence since 1985. Two thirds of the active cases are among Hispanics, Native Americans, Blacks, and Asians. Homeless, immunosuppressed (HIV infection, diabetes, or chronic renal failure), malnourished, and people on chemotherapy or steroid treatment are at increased risk. About 5% of all infected persons experience some recurrence of active disease.
- Signs and Symptoms
    1. More than 90% of clients are asymptomatic at time of primary infection and have been identified by a positive tuberculin skin test. Among those who are symptomatic the symptoms will vary and may include
        a. Fever
        b. Cough (may be nonproductive)
        c. Pleuritic chest pain
        d. Occasional dyspnea.
    2. In postprimary tuberculosis, client is usually debilitated and presents with more clinical symptoms including
        a. Anorexia
        b. Weight loss
        c. Night sweats
        d. Fever (usually low grade) with chills
        e. Persistent productive cough with thick sputum
        f. Hemoptysis
        g. Extrapulmonary disease may produce symptoms which affect

the genitourinary tract, musculoskeletal system and the lymph nodes.

3. Postprimary tuberculosis (reactivation) can occur within a few months, years or even decades after the initial infection.

- Differential Diagnosis: Includes acute bacterial pneumonia, viral pneumonia, and pleurisy.
- Diagnostic Evaluation/Findings

1. Skin testing—A positive skin test does not mean active disease, but only that an initial primary infection has occurred and the immune system has responded to it.
    a. False positives occur when
        (1) Client has had another mycobacterial disease
        (2) Client has received (BCG) vaccine
    b. False negatives occur when
        (1) Insufficient time has elapsed between exposure and skin test
        (2) Immune system is depressed
        (3) Client is taking steroids
        (4) Client is malnourished
        (5) Client has had a recent immunization or viral disease
        (6) Initial exposure and immune response were many years ago; sensitivity to the skin test diminishes with time
    c. False negative and positive readings may also result from improper reading of skin test.
2. Chest x-ray—Required for all who demonstrate positive tuberculin skin testing, and should be done with all symptomatic clients.
    a. Reticulonodular infiltration in apicoposterior segments of one or both upper lobes, with or without cavitation, (common in reactivation)
    b. Bilateral distribution of nodular infiltration in upper zones of lungs

c. Extensive consolidation of a lobe of the lung may occur (tuberculosis pneumonia)

d. Infiltration in the mid- and lower lung fields rather than apical zones (progressive primary infection)

3. Sputum smear—

a. Microscopic examination of gram-stained sputum smears for acid-fast bacilli is usually the initial evidence of tubercle bacilli

b. Other organisms also acid-fast, so must be followed up by sputum cultures

c. Failure to identify the mycobacterium in sputum does not rule out tuberculosis

4. Sputum culture—

a. Three sputum specimens usually cultured for six weeks to give positive diagnosis (Drug therapy is begun in the interim)

b. Sputum cultures are also used for follow-up to determine absence of tuberculosis

5. Bronchoscopy—If hemoptysis occurs for no apparent reason, should be included in the pulmonary workup.

6. CBC with differential, urinalysis and liver function tests (particularly alkaline phosphatase) may provide evidence of active disease

7. Tissue biopsy—Used for diagnosis of extrapulmonary disease

- Management/Treatment: Strategies are directed toward prompt diagnosis and treatment to prevent further destruction of lung tissue and alleviate symptoms

1. Treat the infection

a. Usually, drug therapy with a combination of three or more drugs is begun on initial diagnosis which includes clinical signs and symptoms, and a positive chest x-ray and sputum smear. Drug therapy usually continues for six months after the client's sputum is negative, which makes a total treatment period of about nine months. Isoniazid (INH) and Rifampin are the two most common drugs that are used in combination.

b. Once drug therapy is begun, client is considered noninfectious within a week

c. Regular monthly monitoring for side effects and evaluation of the progress of the disease is necessary.

(1) Check for nausea and vomiting

(2) If decrease in visual acuity—do funduscopic examination

d. Clients who have converted from a negative to a positive skin test within the last two years should be considered for prophylactic treatment with INH.

e. All diagnosed cases of tuberculosis should be reported to the Center for Disease Control.

2. Promote immune response and optimal general health

3. Manage symptoms by identifying and treating any particular medical problems that are present.

- Nursing Considerations: The nursing goal is to relieve signs and symptoms and assist the client in compliance with drug therapy. The nursing care parallels the treatment.

1. Treat the infection

a. Administer drugs as ordered

b. Teach about the use of the medication (why used, when to take and possible side effects) (Hepatotoxicity is a particular hazard of INH)

c. Teach about the chronic nature of disease; emphasize the importance of adhering to drug treatment and follow-up schedules

d. Minimize the potential for spread of infection

(1) Isolation during first week of hospitalization only

(2) Family members and close contacts should be tested

(3) Client and family should be taught proper disposal of sputum and tissues

2. Promote immune response and optimal general health

a. Instruct on importance of nutritious, high-carbohydrate, varied diet
b. Assistance in planning daily schedule that includes adequate rest and exercise

3. Manage symptoms
   a. Encourage fluids to decrease viscosity of respiratory secretions
   b. Monitor temperature at least every four hours; administer antipyretics, provide cool liquids, and give tepid baths

Lung Cancer

- Definition: Is a disease of older individuals who have a long smoking history. After cigarette smoking, asbestos is the next most common exposure that leads to lung cancer. Cancers of lung may be primary or secondary; i.e., they may originate in lung or may metastasize to lung from other areas of the body.
- Etiology: About 95% of lung cancers originate in airways and are classified as bronchogenic cancers. Other lung cancers include squamous cell or epidermoid carcinoma, small cell carcinoma, and bronchiolar or alveolar carcinoma (the adenomas). In general, cancers form over a very long period of irritation from factors such as smoking or inhalation of asbestos.
- Incidence: Number one cancer killer of both men and women; there is a continuous increase in mortality for both men and women with advancing age. By 1984 lung cancer deaths in women had exceeded those from breast cancer.
- Signs and Symptoms
  1. Most clients seek treatment because of lower respiratory symptoms
     a. Change in a chronic cough
     b. Hemoptysis
     c. Onset (or progression) of dyspnea
     d. Chest pain.
  2. Small cell carcinoma and rapidly advancing epidermoid, squamous, and adenocarcinoma may first be recognized by onset of symptoms of distant metastases (brain, bone, liver)

a. Brain
    (1) Headache
    (2) Focal weakness
    (3) Seizures
b. Bone: Persistent pain in the spine and ribs
c. Liver: Dull aching in right upper quadrant
d. Nonspecific fatigue and anorexia may also be present

- Differential Diagnosis: Includes pneumonia and bronchitis.
- Physical Findings: Clients may present with any of previously mentioned symptoms; physical findings will be dependent upon stage of disease
- Diagnostic Evaluation/Findings: Clients in whom possibility of lung cancer is suspected undergo evaluation to determine three things: First, whether the lung cancer is primary; second, if the lung cancer is primary, whether it is localized, and third, if it is localized, can the client tolerate a resection
    1. Chest x-ray
    2. Computed tomography
    3. Sputum cytology
    4. Urine and stool specimens (test for occult blood × 3 to minimize possibility that an occult extrathoracic lesion is responsible for a chest x-ray nodule)
    5. Spirometry and ABGs
    6. Lymph node biopsy
    7. Bronchoscopy with needle aspirate biopsy
    8. WBC with differential-Elevated WBCs
    9. Serum chemistries
- Management/Treatment: Depends upon desires of client and family, how advanced cancer is when discovered, and whether client can tolerate surgery. Lung cancer discovered before onset of symptoms in some clients may result in survival of two to five years or more; slower growing lung

cancers are more common in elderly. Surgical section is hardly ever justified after age 70 if an estimate of postoperative pulmonary function predicts that remaining FEV_1 will be less than 1.0 liter or if any degree of CO_2 retention is present. Management addresses three basic areas

1. Curing of the cancer
    a. Thoracotomy
    b. Resection
    c. Radiotherapy/chemotherapy—when used without surgery is primarily a palliative measure
2. Pain control
3. Improve ventilation
    a. Bronchodilators
    b. Fluid therapy
    c. Oxygen therapy

- Nursing Considerations: The nursing goal is to assist client in adjusting to diagnosis of lung cancer and provide a supportive atmosphere with minimum discomfort.

1. Curing of cancer
    a. Pre-operative and post-operative care following a thoracotomy/resection
    b. Instruction on side effects of chemotherapy/radiation; assistance in managing side effects
    c. Highly nutritious diet
2. Pain control
    a. Analgesia as ordered
    b. Monitor levels of discomfort, use splinting
    c. Monitor vital signs and other parameters to determine comfort level of client
    d. Teach relaxation techniques to reduce discomfort
3. Improve ventilation
    a. Administer oxygen as ordered

b. Elevate head of bed; support arms prn

c. Reduce metabolic demands: Bed rest, long rest periods, light diet, reduce fever

d. Administer analgesia as ordered to relieve pain and facilitate respirations and coughing

e. Encourage fluids (2 to 3 L/day) to decrease viscosity of secretions

f. Assess respiratory status at least every 4 hours

g. Turn, cough, and deep breathe at least every 2 hours

4. Prevent or treat infection

   a. Avoid exposure to known respiratory infections and seek prompt treatment

   b. Teach signs and symptoms of infection

5. Provide an atmosphere of support for life-threatening disease

   a. Listen

   b. Encourage client to express their feelings

   c. Assure client that (s)he has right to feelings

   d. Assist client to identify past coping strategies

   e. Assist client to identify support persons

   f. Refer client to American Cancer Society, hospice, and coping support groups

Questions

1. Which of the following physical findings are seen with patients who have (type A COPD) emphysema?
   a. Central cyanosis, "blue bloater"
   b. Body appearance is typically overweight
   c. Minimal use of accessory muscles
   d. Absent central cyanosis, "pink puffer"

2. Which of the following characteristics is inaccurate about COPD?
   a. Is a progressive respiratory disease syndrome
   b. Affects 10 per cent of the U.S. population
   c. Is the leading cause of death in people over 65 years
   d. Affects men more than women

3. Spirometry in COPD would show which of the following?
   a. Decreased total lung capacity (TLC)
   b. Increased residual volume (RV)
   c. Increased vital capacity (VC)
   d. Increased forced expiratory volume (FEV_1)

4. Management of COPD addresses all but:
   a. Improve ventilation
   b. Cure the disease
   c. Prevent or treat infection
   d. Improve airway clearance
   e. Improve strength and exercise tolerance

5. Nursing care for a patient with COPD includes all of the following except:
   a. Administration of oxygen
   b. Performing postural drainage
   c. Administration of respiratory depressants
   d. Encouraging increased fluid intake

6. Which of the following would not be a drug of choice for the treatment of COPD?
   a. Theophylline
   b. Guaifenesin

c. Codeine
d. Terbutaline sulfate

7. Which of the following is true concerning the use of oxygen therapy for the patient with COPD?

    a. Oxygen therapy is of little value
    b. Oxygen, if used, must be given at a flow rate of 5–10 liters/minute per nasal cannula
    c. Oxygen, if used, must be given at a flow rate less than 5 liters/minute per nasal cannula
    d. Oxygen therapy cannot be continued at home

8. Patient education for the client with COPD includes all of the following except:

    a. Use of oxygen
    b. Increased fluid intake
    c. Avoid respiratory irritants
    d. Resume smoking

9. Distant breath sounds and enlarged AP chest diameter are findings in patients with:

    a. Asthma
    b. Chronic bronchitis (Type B COPD)
    c. Bacterial pneumonia
    d. Emphysema bronchitis (Type A COPD)

10. To improve strength and exercise the patient with COPD should do all of the following except:

    a. Use energy conservation techniques
    b. Use pursed-lip breathing
    c. Gradually increase activity
    d. Use a bronchodilator after activities

11. Characteristics of asthma include all of the following except:

    a. An obstructive airway disease
    b. Reversible
    c. Typical onset after age 60 years
    d. Excessive sputum production

12. A predisposed individual can be provoked into an asthmatic attack by certain extrinsic factors which include all of the following except:

    a. Smoke
    b. Viral respiratory infection
    c. Perfume
    d. Oxygen

13. Hospitalization would be indicated for the asthmatic patient with a Peak Expiratory Flow Rate of:

    a. 250 Liters/Min.
    b. 200 Liters/Min
    c. 100–200 Liters/Min
    d. 60–100 Liters/min

14. A WBC with differential can be helpful in monitoring the asthmatic patient. Which measure is a useful marker?

    a. Basophils
    b. Eosinophils
    c. Monocytes
    d. PMN leukocytes

15. Which of the following is not a treatment strategy when managing asthmatic attacks?

    a. Give oxygen prn as indicated by ABGs
    b. Keep secretions thin by high fluid intake
    c. Wait before giving medications; bronchospasms pass spontaneously
    d. Treat infection

16. Patient education for the asthmatic includes all of the following except:

    a. Avoid respiratory irritants
    b. Use of sedatives
    c. Avoid exposure to infection
    d. Use of bronchodilator prior to exercise

17. The elderly are particularly vulnerable to pneumonia but certain conditions increase the risk; these include all of the following except:

    a. COPD
    b. Hiatal hernia

c. Congestive heart failure
d. Alcoholism

18. Signs and symptoms of pneumonia in the elderly can present with rather subtle findings including

    a. Pleuritic pain
    b. Hacking cough, productive cough
    c. Low grade fever and change in sensorium
    d. High fever

19. Physical examination for the patient with pneumonia can reveal all of the following except:

    a. Bronchial breath sounds
    b. Wheezing
    c. Areas of lung consolidation
    d. Hyperresonance

20. Nursing care for the client with pneumonia includes all of the following except

    a. Administer oxygen prn
    b. Administer mild analgesia to relieve pain
    c. Keep head of bed flat to facilitate drainage
    d. Reduce fever

21. Which of the following signs or symptoms would be present in a client presenting with a primary infection of tuberculosis?

    a. Weight loss
    b. Night sweats
    c. Hemoptysis
    d. Positive skin test

22. Postprimary tuberculosis presents with all of the following except:

    a. Anorexia
    b. Weight loss
    c. Negative skin test
    d. Persistent productive cough

23. False negatives occur in skin testing for tuberculosis; this can happen in all of the following except:

a. When the patient is taking steroids
b. When the patient is malnourished
c. When the patient is HIV positive
d. When the patient has received BCG vaccine

24. In the treatment of tuberculosis it is essential to work with the patient and the family. Which of the following should not be considered?

a. Intensive aerobic exercise program
b. Testing of family members and close contacts
c. Aseptic technique for disposal of sputum and tissues
d. Fluids to liquefy respiratory secretions

25. Which of the following statements is not true regarding sputum specimens that are obtained for tuberculosis patients?

a. It takes six weeks for the culture to grow
b. Sputum cultures are used for follow-up
c. A gram-stain sputum smear can provide initial evidence of tuberculosis
d. Failure to identify the mycobacterium in the sputum rules out tuberculosis

26. Which of the following characteristics of lung cancer is not correct?

a. It causes more deaths than breast cancer
b. It may be primary or secondary
c. It is not related to smoking
d. It is the number one cancer killer of both men and women

27. An early symptom associated with lung cancer is

a. Bone pain
b. Change in chronic cough
c. Headache
d. Focal weakness

Answers:

1. d
2. c
3. b
4. b
5. c
6. c
7. c
8. d
9. d
10. d
11. c
12. d
13. d
14. b
15. c
16. b
17. b
18. c
19. d
20. c
21. d
22. c
23. d
24. a
25. d
26. c
27. b

Bibliography

Bentley, D. W. (1981). Pneumococcal vaccine in the institutional elderly: Review of past and recent studies. *Review of infectious disease.* 3 (Suppl) 61–70.

Chenitz, W. C., Stone, J. T., Salisbury, S. (1991). *Clinical gerontological nursing: A guide to advanced practice.* Philadelphia: W. B. Saunders.

Christ, M. A., Hohlock, F. J. (1993). *Gerontological nursing, a study and learning tool. (2nd ed.)* Springhouse, PA: Springhouse Publishing.

Eliopoulos, C. (1991). *Gerontological nursing review, a self-instructional text.* (2nd ed.). Baltimore: National Health Publishing

Ebersole, P., Hess, P. (1990). *Toward health aging, human needs and nursing response.* (4th ed.). St. Louis: Mosby Year Book.

Glezen, W. P., Decker, M., Perotta, L. (1987). Survey of underlying conditions of persons hospitalized with acute respiratory disease during influenza epidemics in Houston, 1978–1981. *American review of respiratory disease.* 136, 550–555.

Hazzard, W. R., Andres, R., Bierman, E. L., Blass, J. P. (Eds). (1990). *Principles of geriatric medicine and gerontology* (2nd ed.). New York: McGraw-Hill.

Hilton, D. L. (1992). *Medical-surgical nursing: Lippincott's review series.* Philadelphia: J. B. Lippincott.

Hogstel, M. O. (1992). *Clinical management of gerontological nursing.* St. Louis: Mosby Year Book.

Newman, D. K., Smith, D. A. (1991). *Geriatric care plans.* Springhouse, PA: Springhouse Publishing.

Swartz, M. (1989). *Textbook of physical diagnosis.* Philadelphia: W. B. Saunders.

Cardiovascular Disorders

Helene M. Clark

Hypertension

- Definition/Classification

Hypertension: A persistent elevation of systolic blood pressure (SBP) and/or diastolic blood pressure (DBP) at or above the normal parameters of 140 (SBP) and 90 (DBP) on at least three consecutive readings. (National Heart, Lung, and Blood Institute, 1993).

The new classification of blood pressure in the fifth report of the Joint National Committee on Detection, Evaluation, and Treatment of High Blood Pressure published by the National Heart, Lung, and Blood Institute (N.H.L.B.) in January, 1993 de-emphasizes the terms "mild" and "moderate" hypertension used in previous classifications because these terms failed to convey the real risks of morbidity, disability and mortality of these levels and tended to delay treatment. There are two categories added to the new classification, "normal" and "high normal" and new emphasis on the importance of elevated systolic levels. The report also advises clinicians to specify target organ damage and risk factors as well as elevated blood pressure levels for better management.

1. Classification of blood pressure for adults age 18 years and older (N.H.L.B.)., 1993, p.4)

Category	Systolic (mm Hg)	Diastolic (mm Hg)
Normal	under 130	under 85
High Normal	130-139	85-89
Hypertension		
Stage 1 (Mild)	140-159	90-99
Stage 2 (Moderate)	160-179	100-109
Stage 3 (Severe)	180-209	110-119
Stage 4 (Very Severe)	210 & above	120 & above

"When systolic and diastolic pressures fall into different categories, the higher category should be selected to classify the individual's blood pressure status. For instance, 160/92mm Hg should be classified as Stage 2, and 180/120mm Hg should be classified as Stage 4" (N.H.L.B., 1993, p. 4).

2. Isolated systolic hypertension (ISH) which is the most prominent form of hypertension in the elderly is defined as SBP of 140 mm Hg or greater with a DBP of less than 90 mm Hg. ISH may also be

classified in stages using the levels of SBP for Stages 2, 3, 4 and DBP under 90 mm Hg (N.H.L.B., 1993).

In developed societies systolic and diastolic pressures tend to rise till age 60 then systolic may keep rising and diastolic tends to level off or decline. Because of the prevalence of elevated arterial pressures in the elderly in the USA, some people have labelled hypertension a harmless aging change. Recent studies (Frohlich, 1990) refute this with evidence of relationships between high arterial pressures and increased morbidity and mortality rates.

- Etiology: Exact causes in the elderly and similarities to causes at younger ages not known.
  1. Primary hypertension (85–90% of all hypertension) no identified cause, may arise from normal blood pressure mechanisms but still unproven—heterogenous process with contributing age-related factors (Carethers & Blanchette, 1989) as follows:
     a. Increased weight
     b. Increased sodium intake
     c. Increased peripheral vascular resistance
     d. Decreased vessel wall compliance and atherosclerosis
     e. Left ventricular hypertrophy
     f. Decreased renal mass and function
  2. Secondary hypertension etiology (Frohlich,1990)
     a. Renovascular e.g., renal aneurysm, renal arterial disease
     b. Renal parenchymal e.g., chronic pyelonephritis and glomerulonephritis, polycystic disease, diabetic glomerulosclerosis
     c. Hormonal e.g., hyper/hypothyroidism, Cushing's Disease, pheochromcytoma
     d. Coarctation of the aorta
     e. Drugs, chemicals, and foods e.g., excessive alcohol, salt, over the counter drugs (OTCs) such as cold preparations
     f. Secondary to specific therapy e.g., steroids, antidepressants, immunosuppressants.
- Incidence: Affects 35 to 45% of the elderly over 65, more women than

men in contrast to prevalence at younger ages, Blacks more than Whites and causes serious complications of stroke, myocardial infarction, congestive heart failure, sudden death and renal insufficiency (Applegate, 1990; Flack, Woolley, Esunge & Grimm, 1992).

- Signs and Symptoms
  1. Primary hypertension
     a. Asymptomatic most common, if uncomplicated and no target organ damage—may be picked on routine exam or screening
     b. Suboccipital headaches in a.m
     c. Epistaxis
     d. Tinnitus
     e. Fatigue
     f. Nervousness and irritability
     g. May have "cardiac awareness" (rapid heart rate, palpitations, or ectopic beats) occurs in young patients with borderline hypertension, also in older ones with more severe disease
     h. With target organ damage symptoms are also related to that organ e.g. heart, kidneys, brain
  2. Secondary hypertension—depends on target organ damage and primary disease site such as kidneys, adrenals

- Differential Diagnosis
  1. Primary hypertension
  2. Secondary hypertension

     In the elderly patient the elevated pressure should be documented on at least three different occasions with two measurements taken on each occasion (Frohlich, 1990)—both arms should be used and two positions: supine and sitting or sitting and standing. (occlusive unilateral arterial disease and orthostatic hypotension may give false readings).

- Physical Findings
  1. May have none in early stages of mild or moderate hypertension other than elevated blood pressure—most findings not present until hypertension has caused some target organ damage.

2. Retinopathy—ranging from mild, Grades I & II arteriolar constriction and arterial/venous (A/V) nicking (distinguish from sclerotic age changes—A/V nicking, copper- or silver wire arterioles often found in older people) to more severe signs, Grades III & IV, retinal flame hemorrhages and papilledema.

   Severe retinopathy is associated with poor long term prognosis and indicates need for immediate aggressive treatment (Hurst, Schant, Rockley, Sonnenblik & Wenger, 1990).

3. Bruits carotid, aortic, renal, abdominal
4. S_3 sound (ventricular gallop) may develop usually in association with S_4 (atrial gallop).
5. Harsh systolic murmer at apex
6. Rales and wheezes
7. Peripheral edema
8. Decrease in proximal muscle strength

- Diagnostic Evaluation/Findings
  1. Initial workup—thorough baseline history to assess for cardiac risk factors and identify potential target organ damage. The health history should include family and patient history of high blood pressure, cardiovascular and cerebrovascular disease, diabetes mellitus, and renal disease; assessment of dietary habits, alcohol intake and exercise; psychosocial and environmental factors which may influence blood pressure control; and effectiveness of previous antihypertensive therapy.
  2. CBC, serum electrolytes for general assessment
  3. Specific tests/Findings:
     a. Urinalysis to detect hematuria, proteinuria.
     b. BUN, creatinine and potassium levels, if elevated may indicate renal failure; decreased potassium level could indicate primary aldosteronism.
     c. Cholesterol and triglycerides if elevated, show increased risk of coronary artery disease.
     d. Elevated glucose levels may indicate diabetes mellitus.

e. Electrocardiagram (ECG)—check for left ventricular hypertrophy (LVH) or myocardial ischemia—ECG evidence of LVH more common and serious risk factor in older adults than in younger ones (Allman, 1989).

f. Chest X-ray may show cardiomegaly or aortic stenosis. They are difficult to interpret in elderly due to age related skeletal and pulmonary changes (Allman, 1989).

g. Renin levels may be measured to determine renovascular occlusive disease.

h. Intravenous Pyelogram (IVP) may identify stenosed renal arteries.

- Management/Treatment

Goals of management are the same for older persons as for younger ones but more difficult to achieve due to age changes and to frequent comorbidity—the goals of management are: achieving and maintaining a normal blood pressure for the person's age; relieving symptoms, and preventing or slowing the progression of vascular damage (complications).

There are two major types of therapy: life style modification and pharmacological.

1. Life style modification is initiated first and is based on changing life style risk factors.

   a. Weight loss

   b. Salt and alcohol restriction, and decrease fats in diet

   c. Moderate physical activity increase

   d. Stress reduction and relaxation

2. Pharmacological therapy—no consensus on ideal clinical approach for elderly patients—but general consensus, should be treated—most drugs are effective with some special precautions and monitoring (Flack, et al., 1992).

   a. Thiazide diuretics—are effective with elderly persons, can be used alone or in combination with other antihypertensives—thiazides enhance effectiveness of other antihypertensives—may confer reduction in risk of cardiovascular disease. Older people should be monitored closely however because diuretics can cause postural hypotension due to decreased volume, and vascular system doesn't respond as quickly as in younger individuals

b. Other antihypertensives: beta blockers, angiotension converting enzyme (ACE) inhibitors, calcium channel blockers, or others may be selected for older persons with equal effectiveness, but precautions are needed in use of beta blockers and calcium channel blockers which can produce negative effects on ventricular function leading to heart failure. There is also some indication of decreased effectiveness of beta blockers as anti-ischemic agents in elderly (Gerstenblith, 1990).

c. Selection of particular drug therapy is based less on age and more on: existing medical conditions, possible drug interactions, probable side effects, and cost (Flack, 1992).

d. Optimal B.P. level still not definitely established but a goal of low 140s and a diastolic of 90 or below appears reasonable for elderly without prior myocardial infarction (M.I.)

e. Individualized comprehensive management is best approach, not structured step method previously used.

- Nursing Considerations

1. Nursing goals parallel and support medical management but are focused on assisting the elderly individual to adapt in a positive way to his/her condition, physiologically and psychosocially. Long term goals are: keeping blood pressure under control through a specific treatment plan, preventing complications, and returning to optimum independence consistent with the person's life circumstances. Nursing management for the individual hypertensive patient starts with identifying actual or potential problems (Havens & Weaver, 1992)

   a. If assessment reveals signs and symptoms related to hypertension then treatment should first be directed to their relief. For instance, headache and fatigue may require medication and rest periods as well as careful monitoring.

   b. Keeping blood pressure under control

      (1) Monitor blood pressure at specified intervals.

         (a) Teach patient and family to check B.P. at home, keep a record, report results.

(2) Administer medications

(a) Dosage initially lower for elderly then gradually increase.

(b) Monitor response—generally slower for elderly.

(c) Observe for side effects, similar to those in younger people but elderly more susceptible, more often on other medications.

(d) Teach patient/family rationale for medications, need for compliance, possible side effects, provide written information and schedule if necessary.

(3) Explain and discuss life style changes such as dietary changes, weight loss, decreased salt and alcohol, increased excercise, rest and relaxation, cessation of smoking.

(4) Involve patient/family in plans to incorporate changes gradually, permanently, and realistically. Discuss available community resources such as senior center programs on exercise, stress management, nutrition, and smoking.

(5) Instruct patient/family on follow-up physician or clinic visits.

(6) Determine if cost is a problem in securing medication, transportation etc. and explore resources with patient/family.

c. Preventing complications

(1) Teach signs and symptoms of potential problems to patients/families/significant others:

(a) Decreased tissue perfusion (delayed capillary refill)

(b) Shortness of breath

(c) Increased blood pressure readings

(d) Decreased urine output

(e) Weak or absent pulses

(f) Restlessness and confusion

(g) Severe headache, dizziness or ringing in the ears

d. Return to optimum independence

(1) Reinforce patient's sense of competence in self care, provide opportunities for problem solving—give positive feedback on planning and efforts at independence.

(2) Encourage family and others to allow patient maximum autonomy where possible in care, life style, scheduling own appointments, food shopping, meal planning, taking blood pressure.

(3) Important to note however, that older people with chronic illnesses rely heavily on family for advice and support and interdependence may be a more appropriate goal than complete independence.

Coronary Artery Disease: Angina Pectoris, Myocardial Infarction

- Definition: Coronary artery disease (CAD) or ischemic heart disease—a state in which one or more of the coronary arteries has narrowing of the lumen resulting in loss of oxygen supply to the myocardium and causing ischemia, angina, and myocardial infarction.

  1. Angina Pectoris is a sensation of discomfort under the sternum described as burning, squeezing, or heavy pressure brought on by exertion and relieved by rest.

  2. Myocardial Infarction (M.I.) is necrosis of myocardial tissue caused by an obstruction of the blood flow in a coronary artery. In older adults an M.I. may be brought on by other medical problems such as infection, hypotension, bleeding or hypothermia.

- Etiology: Atherosclerosis—a lesion of the inner wall of the coronary artery containing proliferated smooth muscle tissue, increased amounts of connective tissue matrix and accumulation of intracellular and extracellular lipids is the underlying pathology of CAD. It causes progressive narrowing of the coronary artery and decrease in blood flow to the heart muscle. It is an age-related disorder which begins early and progresses over the years until clinical symptoms appear in middle or old age after the blood vessel has 50% or more occlusion. Risk factors predisposing certain individuals to CAD are listed with the first three being major risk factors

1. Hypertension—major
2. Hyperlipidemia especially low density lipoproteins (LDL) and elevated triglyceride levels—major
3. Smoking—major
4. Increasing age
5. Male gender until middle age-risk, begins to equalize for women after menopause
6. Family history
7. Obesity
8. Hyperglycemia/diabetes
9. Sedentary, high stress life style (Type A personality)

- Incidence: Although the number of deaths due to ischemic heart disease has been on the decline for several years, coronary artery disease is still the leading cause of death in the United States with 500,000 deaths annually and responsible for about 1.5 million myocardial infarctions.

  It is the leading cause of death over age 65 with more than 80% of CAD cases in this age group.

- Signs and Symptoms

  1. Angina Pectoris

     a. Characteristic burning, squeezing pain or pressure in the substernal area of the chest or may be referred to the back, lower jaw, down the inner aspect of the left arm to the fingers, or the epigastric area.

     b. Pain is brought on by exertion and relieved by rest or nitroglycerine after a few minutes.

     c. The elderly person may not have the standard pain of angina because of limited activities, diminished pain sensation or failure to recognize the pain.

     d. Pain may still occur if there is stress to the cardiovascular system such as infection.

e. Dyspnea may be as common a presenting symptom in the elderly as pain.

f. Angina associated symptoms may be diaphoresis, fatigue, shortness of breath, heart palpitations, and anxiety. These are usually transient and disappear when the pain is relieved.

2. Myocardial Infarction (M.I.)

   a. Presenting signs and symptoms in the older person may be atypical and vague resulting in failure to diagnose an M.I. Gastric distress, anorexia, complaints of not feeling well, fatigue and some dyspnea may be more evident than chest pain. Occasionally, a low grade fever may be first sign. A history of risk factors such as hypertension, hyperlipidemia and smoking may be significant

   b. Usual signs and symptoms are:

      (1) Chest pain that is severe, prolonged, different from anginal pain, and not relieved by nitroglycerine or rest. This classical symptom may be absent or greatly diminished in older patients

      (2) Nausea/vomiting

      (3) Anxiety

      (4) Diaphoresis, clammy skin, pallor

      (5) Dyspnea, orthopnea

      (6) Fatigue, dizziness, syncope

      (7) Impending feeling of doom

- Differential Diagnosis (Rossi & Leary, 1992) for both angina (chest pain) and myocardial infarction

  1. Cardiovascular problems: aortic dissection, pulmonary embolus, pericarditis, mitral valve prolapse
  2. Gastric problems: esophageal reflux and spasm, peptic ulceration, biliary colic, cholecystitis, pancreatitis
  3. Musculoskeletal problems: costochondritis, cervical osteoarthritis, chest muscle or rib injuries, strains
  4. Pulmonary problems: pleurisy, pneumothorax, pneumonia

- Physical Findings

  May be unremarkable or may include some of the following:

  1. Pallor, diaphoresis, breathlessness, cyanosis
  2. Presence of S_3 and S_4, friction rub, murmurs, rales, irregular pulse
  3. Presence of atherosclerosis in other blood vessels e.g., retinopathy, carotid bruit
  4. Anxious appearance.

- Diagnostic Evaluation/Findings

  The careful assessment of type and character of pain is an important factor in determining appropriate diagnostic tests.

  1. Angina
     a. Serum enzymes and isoenzymes/normal levels
     b. Electrocardiogram/normal or may have reversible ST or T wave changes during episode of angina.
     c. Stress tests (treadmill and/or thallium) may show evidence of ischemia.
     d. Echocardiogram/may reveal wall motion abnormalities with ischemia.
     e. Cardiac catheterization/normal arteries or varying degrees of occlusion and normal, absent, or diminished wall motion.
  2. Myocardial Infarction
     a. Serum enzymes and isoenzymes—the most important source of information to rule out M.I.—Three major enzymes released from injured myocardial tissue are: creatinine phosphokinase (CPK), lactic dehydrogenase (LDH), and serum glutamic oxalo-acetic transaminase (SGOT). The isoenzyme CPK-MB is specific to myocardial tissue. Elevations of this enzyme may not always be present in elderly patients. Findings in M.I. (Rossi & Leary, 1992):
        (1) CPK has onset 4–6hr., peaks in 16–30 hr., and returns to normal in 3–4 days. CPK-MB % of rise more specific to myocardial tissue damage.

(2) LDH has onset within 24–48 hours, peaks in 3–6 days, and returns to normal in 7–10 days.

(3) SGOT has onset in 12–18 hr., peaks in 24–48 hr., and returns to normal in 4–7 days.

b. Electrocardiogram (ECG)/varies with ischemia but will develop specific pattern with infarction—ST and T wave abnormalities and the presence of prominent Q waves. However typical ECG changes are less frequent in elderly patients because of previous baseline age changes.

c. Exercise stress testing/myocardial ischemia—decreased workload tolerance, blood pressure, pulse, and pain levels are indicators but not definitive of myocardial damage.

d. Echocardiogram/abnormal wall motion, thinning of wall post myocardial infarction.

e. Cardiac Catheterization—definitive test for coronary atherosclerosis—may include: examination of right and left sides of the heart, cardiac output studies and coronary angiography. Findings usually demonstrate obstruction of the artery to infarcted area of myocardium, and may show abnormal wall motion or ventricular aneurysm.

f. Ambulatory (Holter) monitoring may be done to pick up "silent ischemia" which is not uncommon in the elderly.

- Management/Treatment

1. Treatment for angina requires physician referral and possible hospitalization. In the elderly person it may begin by identifying and correcting reversible precipitating conditions such as anemia, congestive heart failure, hypertension, and hyperthyroidism which may relieve the angina. Goals of treatment are to control symptoms, improve morbidity and mortality, and enhance quality of life (Fleury, 1992; Gerstenblith & Lakata, 1990).

a. Pharmacologic: nitrates for vasodilation and improved blood flow; beta-blockers to decrease heart rate and oxygen demand; and calcium channel blockers to decrease heart rate, arterial resistance, and increase blood flow. Dose and drug must be individualized for elderly patient and carefully monitored. Precautions are needed for beta-blockers and calcium channel blockers. Note precautions previously listed for these drugs.

Low-dose aspirin (ASA) (325 mg/day) has been effective in reducing risk of M.I. and death following unstable angina. It has also been used to reduce risk of reinfarction following a M.I. (Gerstenblith, 1990).

b. Risk factor reduction related to atherosclerosis such as cessation of smoking, low fat diet, weight reduction, exercise program.

c. Rest to relieve pain

d. Surgical interventions for persistent, uncontrolled pain are: percutaneous transluminal coronary angioplasty (PTCA) or coronary artery bypass graft (CABG)—some controversy regarding use for older patients citing higher mortality and lower success rate than with younger patients. Recent reports (Gerstenblith & Lakata, 1990) indicate low mortality comparable to younger patients.

2. Treatment for myocardial infarction requires physician referral and hospitalization.

Goals of treatment: limit and control damage to the heart muscle; palliative measures to relieve pain, anxiety, dyspnea; and prevent complications. Older patients have a mortality rate twice the rate of younger patients. All patients require immediate hospitalization for definite diagnosis and treatment.

a. Current therapy emphasizes the use of early thrombolytic agents in limiting myocardial damage and improving survival. Early thrombolysis appears to benefit patients up to the age of 75 after which benefit decreases and risk of cerebral hemorrhage increases. Older individuals' higher prevalence of hypertension as well as cerebral vascular accidents are contraindications for thrombolysis.

b. Other medications: nitrates; calcium channel blockers; anticoagulants including aspirin; beta blockers; antiarrhythmics; vasodilators; sympathomimetic drugs (to stimulate the sympathetic nervous system if necessary); analgesics and tranquilizers for pain and anxiety; stool softeners and laxatives (more often in the elderly); and diuretics.

c. Early detection and treatment of complications

d. Stress management

e. Risk factor reduction

f. Cardiac rehabilitation

- Nursing Considerations: Apply to both angina and myocardial infarction. Nursing goals are concerned with relieving symptoms especially pain and dyspnea during the acute phase; assisting the patient to achieve medical goals of treatment; preventing complications; and teaching patient and family about coronary artery disease and risk reduction.

  The amount of hands on care will depend on the severity of the symptoms and the extent of myocardial damage. With transient stable angina and no documented damage the patient may be at home with essentially self care and primary need being education and periodic assurance that he is doing things correctly in regard to risk reduction and life style management. With myocardial infarction patients are admitted to special care or coronary care units for a period of time for close monitoring.

  1. Symptom relief especially with M.I. pain important in early treatment—may involve administration of narcotics and/or tranquilizers for anxiety, administration of oxygen, rest and other comfort measures.
  2. Encourage patient and family to express fears and concerns ask questions, participate in plan of care as much as possible. Older individuals may have more difficulty adjusting to the hospital environment and may become temporarily confused.
  3. Cardiac monitoring to assess heart rate and rhythms and detect early arrhythmias.
  4. Administer cardiac medications as ordered and evaluate effectiveness—observe for side effects; Beta blockers are sometimes used for their secondary preventive effects and may be helpful for patients at increased risk for recurrent M.I. (Gerstenblith, 1990)
  5. If thrombolytic therapy is used, keep in mind increased risk of bleeding or stroke in the older patient
  6. Observe for signs of complications especially decreased cardiac output: decreased blood pressure, decreased pulse, decreased urinary output, decreased level of consciousness; increased restlessness, changes in vital signs

7. Be aware of increased potential for complications in the older person because of preexisting conditions but that does not preclude treatment.

8. After acute phase is over a plan of education for patient and family should be implemented to include:

    a. Disease process and basic cardiac function
    b. Risk factors and how to modify them
    c. Medication instruction and how to take a pulse
    d. Coping behaviors and stress reduction
    e. Life style changes such as diet, exercise, cessation of smoking

    Older patients should also be taught healthy behaviors. Current approaches encourage a similar plan for older and younger patients. Modifications in treatment and management should be individualized to the specific patient and not based on age *per se.* Older people are capable of and do make changes and have shown benefit from a relatively aggressive therapeutic regime.

Congestive Heart Failure (CHF)

- Definition: "Heart failure is the inability of the heart to supply the body and the heart muscle itself with adequate circulatory volume and pressure" (Parker-Cohen, Richardson, & Haak, 1990, p. 963).
- Etiology: There are many causes of heart failure, most of which fit into four major categories: impediments to forward ejection, impaired cardiac filling, volume overload, and myocardial failure. The two most common in the elderly are: hypertension, impeding forward ejection and coronary artery disease (CAD) leading to myocardial failure (Wei, 1990). Degenerative valvular disease is another frequent cause of CHF. Fever, infection, and anemia can put the elderly person with borderline heart failure into decompensation. Heart failure can be acute or chronic and may occur on the right or left side of the heart initially but eventually affects both sides. Acute heart failure comes on suddenly and may follow an acute myocardial infarction or cardiac arrest. Chronic heart failure is the end result of long strain on a damaged chamber of the heart which has enlarged over time but is no longer able to compensate. Left sided failure initially causes congestion in the lungs and right sided failure causes congestion

in the systemic circulation, most evident in the liver and the lower extremities but eventually in either case, both sides fail. CHF occurs as a result of systolic or diastolic dysfunction or both. Congestive heart failure also activates the renin-angiotensin-aldosterone system causing salt and water retention, arteriolar vasoconstriction, and an increase in cardiac afterload resistance. Sodium retention is a prominent feature in the pathology of CHF.

- Incidence: Heart failure is one of the most common cardiac conditions in the older adult. It increases exponentially with age after the 6th decade. The prevalence and incidence are so marked in the older age group that it is estimated that 75% of ambulatory patients with CHF are 60 years or over (Gerstenblith & Lakata, 1990).
- Signs and Symptoms
  1. Left side
     a. Anxiety, restlessness
     b. Shortness of breath, dyspnea
     c. Orthopnea, paroxysmal nocturnal dyspnea
     d. Cough, hemoptysis
     e. Tachycardia, palpitations
     f. Basilar rales, bronchial wheezes
     g. Fatigue, decreased exercise tolerance
     h. Weight gain
     i. Cyanosis or pallor
  2. Right side
     a. Anorexia, nausea
     b. Weight gain
     c. Nocturia, oliguria
     d. Dependent peripheral edema
     e. Weakness
  3. Atypical, nonspecific signs and symptoms related to mental/neurological status may be common in the elderly:
     a. Somnolence

b. Confusion

c. Disorientation

d. Dizziness

e. Syncope

These may be combined with some of the common symptoms such as weakness and fatigue. Some typical symptoms of CHF may be obscured in the elderly. For example, rales may be more often due to pulmonary disease and ankle edema to venous stasis or prolonged sitting rather than right heart failure. Dyspnea may be absent.

- Differential Diagnosis
  1. Chronic Obstructive Pulmonary Disease
  2. Asthma
  3. Pulmonary Embolus
  4. Renal or Liver Dysfunction with edema
- Physical Findings (Dzurinko, 1991; Celentano, 1991).
  1. General appearance in the elderly person may be unremarkable, or demonstrated as fatigue, extremely anxious, short of breath, restless or showing mental status changes.
  2. Cardiovascular
     a. Abnormal heart sounds: murmers, S_3, S_4 gallop
     b. Jugular venous distention especially at 90 degree position
  3. Integumentary
     a. Cyanotic lips or pallor
     b. Cold clammy skin
     c. Edema: sacral, dependent, or ascites
  4. Respiratory
     a. Productive cough, hemoptysis
     b. Wheezes, rales (crackles)

5. Musculoskeletal
    a. Obvious fatigue on slight exertion
6. Neurological
    a. Anxiety, restlessness
    b. Confusion, lethargy
    c. Memory lapse
7. Other
    a. Periorbital edema and slight hemorrhages in fundus
    b. Abdominal pain
    c. Positive hepatojugular reflux

- Diagnostic Evaluation/Findings (Dzurinko, 1991; Celentano, 1991)
    1. Not specific to diagnosis of CHF itself but can give data on causes and severity.
    2. Blood studies: CBC, hematocrit, hemoglobin/anemia, electrolytes, BUN, creatinine/fluid shifts and renal function
    3. Liver function tests/decreased liver function & congestion
    4. Urinalysis/proteinuria & elevated specific gravity/renal function
    5. Chest X-ray/enlarged cardiac silhouette and increased pulmonary vein markings
    6. Electrocardiogram/ arrhythmias
    7. Echocardiogram/heart chamber size, wall thickness, valve abnormalities

- Management/Treatment
    1. Physician referral, may or may not require hospitalization depending on severity of failure. Chronic heart failure is non-reversible; it can be managed and overall physical status improved but heart damage is permanent and the patient requires long term follow-up. Goals are: to decrease workload of the heart; to improve cardiac function; and to prevent complications.
    2. Non-pharmacological medical treatment:
        a. Balance of rest and activity to promote optimum relief to overworked heart; bedrest for acute pulmonary edema and failure.

b. Dietary restriction of sodium and fluids

c. ECG monitoring for arrhythmias

d. Hemodynamic monitoring (Swann-Ganz catheter), if necessary, usually in acute care unit

e. Monitoring of lab values

f. Oxygen for relief of dyspnea

3. Pharmacological

Medication administration depends on whether the dysfunction is diastolic or systolic; need to individualize therapy (Wei, 1990).

a. For diastolic dysfunction when systolic function is preserved:

(1) Calcium antagonists

(2) Beta-adrenergic blockers

b. Systolic dysfunction:

(1) Digitalis (digoxin) carefully monitored, check digoxin levels at regular intervals.

(2) Vasodilators.

(3) Diuretics.

There is some concern regarding long term digitalis therapy in elderly patients, especially if in normal sinus rhythm (Wei, 1990; Gerstenblith & Lakata, 1990) considering high incidence of digitalis toxicity in this population.

3. Surgical Intervention

Surgical treatment is not common in the elderly CHF patient but could include the following (Celentano, 1991):

a. Left ventricular assist device

b. Valve replacement/repair

c. Coronary artery bypass graft

d. Heart transplantation (rarely)

- Nursing Considerations

Goals of nursing care are to relieve symptoms and prevent complications in acute CHF, and to provide for long term management and control in chronic CHF.

1. Acute CHF
   a. Monitor ECG rhythm to detect arrhythmias.
   b. Bed rest initially with increased activity as tolerated to decrease demands on the heart.
   c. Provide assistance with ADLs as needed.
   d. Administer medications as ordered, observe effects both therapeutic and untoward.
   e. Special attention to digoxin levels, toxicity common problem in elderly with symptoms of fatigue, headache, altered mental status, confusion, blurred vision, altered heart rate, anorexia, nausea and vomiting
   f. Fluid intake and output measurements
   g. Daily weights
   h. Oxygen therapy as necessary
   i. Monitor lab values to determine fluid and electrolyte balance.
   j. Maintain calm, reassuring environment.
   k. Explain all procedures, care and patient status to patient and family.
2. Chronic CHF
   a. Patient/family education plan (Havens & Weaver, 1992) about CHF involving the patient/family in the development. Include in teaching:
      (1) CHF, what it is, how it develops.
      (2) Signs and symptoms to report, e.g., shortness of breath, dyspnea, chest pain, sudden unexplained weight gain, increased weakness, cough, increased urination at night, confusion, or other mental symptoms occurring suddenly.

(3) Medications, purpose, schedule, dosage and pertinent side effects as well as expected effects

(4) Individualized activity plan

(5) Dietary instructions and consultation as needed for sodium restriction and individualized acceptable diet plan.

(6) Need for follow-up medical care to health care provider on regular basis and when unexpected changes occur.

(7) Assess need for home care services with patient and family, especially important if patient living alone.

Arrhythmias

- Definition: Arrhythmias or dysrhythmias as they are sometimes called, are alterations in heart rate and rhythm which may range from occasional skipped beats or fast beats of no clinical significance to severe disturbances that can interfere with heart pumping function resulting in heart failure and death. Arrhythmias may be classified according to rate and rhythm and location of the abnormality (Johns, 1992; Fleg, 1990).

    1. Tachycardia, a fast heart beat, refers to a rate over 100 beats per minute (bpm) and may occur in the atrial and ventricular areas. Other terms used to describe extremely fast rates are atrial flutter with an atrial rate of 250–350 bpm and a variable ventricular rate over 100, and atrial fibrillation with atrial rates of 300–600 bpm and ventricular rates of 100–160.
    2. Ectopic beats are contractions originating from a focus outside the normal conduction system in the heart.
    3. Bradycardia refers to a slow heart rate, less than 60 bpm.
    4. Heart block refers to a partial or complete failure of the conduction system to carry the impulse from the pacemaker to the cardiac muscle.

- Etiology: Arrhythmias may be caused either by an abnormality in the pacemaker impulse generation or an abnormality in the conduction of the impulses through the heart. Age related changes, including a loss of cells in the pacemaker node and the conduction Bundle of His, plus increased deposits of adipose and fibrous tissue in the heart, are contributing factors to the development of arrhythmias in the aged. The increased frequency of cardiac pathology in older individuals is another reason for their greater susceptibility to rhythm disturbances of the heart (Johnson, Adams & Bigely, 1992; Fleg, 1990).

In addition to causes arising from the heart itself there are other factors which may precipitate arrhythmias in elderly persons. Some of the most common are drug effects or toxicity, especially digitalis; emotional crisis, stress, fluid and electrolyte imbalance, cellular hypoxia, thyroid disease or other acute or chronic disease states, and ingestion of alcohol, coffee, tea and tobacco (Johns, 1992).

- Incidence: There is an increased incidence of all types of arrhythmias in older people. However, the clinical significance and severity of these conditions in the elderly person are more related to the presence and severity of underlying heart disease than to the arrhythmia itself or to age *per se.* Four arrhythmias which commonly occur in older people and may have serious consequences are:

    1. Atrial fibrillation, one of the most common arrhythmias found in elderly persons, occurs in about 8% of all persons over 65 and in 10 to 15% of those who are hospitalized. It is a disorganization of the atrial activity without effective atria contractions. Fibrillatory waves occur at rates of 300 to 600 bpm. This condition may be acute or chronic but is more often chronic in the aged population.
    2. Heart block is a condition in which there is some disruption of the impulse conduction at the AV node resulting in changes in ventricular contractions. Heart block may be partial or complete.
    3. Adams-Stokes or Stokes-Adams syndrome is a syncopal attack (fainting or black-out attack) caused by low cardiac output with decreased blood supply to the brain. This condition may result from a number of abnormal cardiac rhythms such as complete heart block, severe tachycardia or bradycardia and ventricular fibrillation.
    4. Sick sinus syndrome (SSS) is a common conduction disorder that includes a variety of rhythm disturbances and may be termed "the bradycardia-tachycardia" syndrome. This syndrome is associated with a variety of cardiac diseases (Johnson et al., 1992).

- Signs and Symptoms: In the case of some mild asymptomatic arrhythmias there are no obvious clinical manifestations. In more acute cases the following may be present in varying degrees (Johns, 1992).

    1. Irregular heart rate and rhythm

2. Extreme restlessness
3. Pallor, shortness of breath
4. Diaphoresis
5. Cold, clammy skin
6. Nausea and vomiting
7. Dizziness, syncope
8. Decreased level of consciousness
9. Chest pain, palpitations
10. Claudication
11. Weakness, and fatigue
12. Numbness, tingling in arms
13. Feeling of impending doom

- Differential Diagnosis: Since an arrhythmia in an elderly person is frequently an indication of underlying heart disease this should be a primary consideration, especially acute myocardial infarction or congestive heart failure. Other etiologies such as electrolyte imbalances, drug toxicity, thyroid disease, pulmonary disease, hypo or hyperthermia, infections and other chronic or acute conditions should be considered.
- Physical Findings
    1. Older persons may present with little or no obvious findings or may show signs of acute distress.
    2. Abnormal heart rate and rhythm, measured by pulse palpation and auscultation of chest; type depends on type of arrhythmia.
- Diagnostic Evaluation/Findings: In addition to a thorough history to determine preexisting cardiac conditions or other common etiologic factors there are four diagnostic tests which can be utilized (Johns, 1992).
    1. Continuous ECG monitoring during hospitalization
    2. Electrophysiology test (invasive) identifies the mechanisms of arrhythmias and effectiveness of antiarrhythmic drugs. It requires inserting electrode catheters transvenously to the right side of the heart and electrically stimulating areas of the atrium and ventricle to

induce arrhythmias. It is a high risk procedure and rather uncomfortable for the patient. Emotional support and close nursing observations are very important.

3. The Holter monitor is a device worn by ambulatory patients which records heart rhythm for 24 hours. It notes rhythm changes during various activities and evaluates drug effects. It can be used for inpatients or outpatients.
4. Exercise treadmill testing measures the heart's response to exercise, identifies exercise induced arrhythmias and evaluates drug therapy. Findings of various tests of heart rhythm are based on assessment of five characteristics: rate, rhythm, P wave, PR interval and QRS complex.

- Management/Treatment: All patients require careful observation and continuous cardiac monitoring and supportive care until a diagnosis is made (Johns, 1992; Johnson et al., 1992; Fleg, 1990).
  1. Atrial fibrillation—The goal of treatment is to reduce and maintain the ventricular rate at 60–90 bpm. Persons with untreated fast atrial fibrillation may require emergency direct current cardioversion. Medications used to reduce the ventricular rate are digoxin, quinidine, verapamil, procainamide and propranolol alone, or in combination. The underlying cause of the arrhythmia needs to be identified and treated such as thyrotoxicosis, which may present atypically with cardiac symptoms in the older patient.
  2. Second degree heart block type II often progresses to third degree block and does not have a good prognosis. A temporary pacemaker or drugs such as atropine or isoproterenol may be used until a permanent pacemaker can be installed. Third degree heart block is treated in the same manner.
  3. Acute Stokes-Adams syndrome carries a serious threat of sudden death with severe syncopal attacks and may require CPR, and electrical defibrillation followed by installation of a permanent pacemaker.
  4. Elderly persons with sick sinus syndrome (SSS) although manifesting clinical symptoms of syncope, dizziness, confusion, fatigue, palpitations and other cardiac symptoms do fairly well. A permanent pacemaker is usually recommended to control symptoms and to prevent injuries due to falls.

- Nursing Considerations: Asymptomatic patients without serious cardiac disease usually do not require treatment. General considerations for symptomatic patients with arrhythmias include maintaining a calm quiet environment and providing reassurance especially for patients who have had syncopal attacks or other severe symptoms.
    1. Specific assessment of rhythm disturbances is done by frequent observation and recording of apical and radial pulses and ECG strips from hospital telemetry or outpatient Holter monitors.
    2. Nurses should be aware of the frequent occurrence of drug toxicity with antiarrhythmic drugs especially digoxin. Serum digoxin levels are often higher in older individuals and the drug is active for a longer period than in younger persons. Signs of digoxin toxicity are bradycardia, heart block, tachyarrhythmias, gastrointestinal symptoms such as nausea and vomiting, altered mental status, confusion, headache and blurred vision. Generally doses greater than 0.125 mg per day are not recommended (Gerstenblith & Lakatta, 1990).
    3. Pacemakers—Attention is needed to prevent complication of infection, hematomas at insertion site, pneumothorax, pacemaker failure and perforation of the atrial or ventricular septum by the pacing wire. Nursing measures are:
        a. Provision of IV antibiotics, check insertion site for infection or hematoma
        b. Assessment of chest X-rays for lead placement
        c. Continuous ECG monitoring for pacemaker
        d. Check body temperature for elevation
        e. Bedrest with minimal arm and shoulder movement for 24 hours to prevent displacement of leads.
    4. Patient/client education should include causes or precipitating factors for the specific arrhythmia and need for prompt treatment; possible side effects and toxicity of prescribed drugs; pacemaker information (Johns, 1992). Recommendations for patients with pacemakers are:
        a. Carry pacemaker card at all times in accessible place e.g., wallet or purse
        b. Follow-up care with provider for pacemaker function checks and ECG evaluation

c. Keep incision dry for 1 week after insertion; inspect site for redness, swelling, discharge

d. Learn to take pulse and record

e. Avoid direct blows or injury to pacemaker site and close proximity to high energy generators or magnets (MRI scanners)

f. Microwaves are safe

g. Travel is safe (small pacemaker doesn't set off airport alarm)

Peripheral Vascular Disease

- Definition: Peripheral vascular disease usually refers to conditions affecting the lower extremities in which there is an abnormal narrowing or dilatation of the veins and/or arteries. Common conditions affecting the elderly are: arterial occlusive diseases, acute and chronic including intermittent claudication; and venous diseases, thrombophlebitis and insufficiency.
- Etiology
  1. Arterial occlusive disease is caused by atherosclerosis which has been described as a process occurring in the arterial wall as a reaction to injury to the inner lining of the blood vessel. Predisposing risk factors have been identified as smoking, obesity, hyperlipidemia, hypertension, diabetes mellitus, and a positive family history (Bright & Georgi, 1992; Thiele & Strandness, 1990).
  2. Venous diseases result from obstruction such as a thrombus or inflammation (thrombophlebitis), or incompetent valves. Risk factors are: complication of surgery especially orthopedic surgery; obesity; occupations requiring prolonged standing or sitting, immobility; pregnancy; trauma; tight fitting garments placing pressure on the veins; and family history.
- Incidence
  1. Arterial peripheral disease is a very common condition in old age affecting men between 50–70 years of age with increasing frequency as they age and women after menopause.
  2. Venous peripheral disease in the form of acute venous thrombus occurs in 20 to 30% of all surgical patients and occurs in 50% of elderly surgical patients. It carries a high risk of pulmonary embolism

which is the cause of 140,000 fatalities annually (Bright & Georgi, 1992). Seven million Americans have chronic venous insufficiency with over 500,000 having stasis ulcers (Celentano, 1991).

- Signs and Symptoms

  1. Arterial disease

     Sometimes described as a series of six Ps (Johnson, et al., 1992; Thiele & Strandness, 1990):

     a. Pain, acute, sudden, severe; intermittent claudication is a classic symptom of arterial occlusion in the lower extremities with pain brought on with exercise and relieved with rest
     b. Pallor, when limb elevated and red when dependent
     c. Paresthesia, possible
     d. Pulselessness or diminished, weak pulse in distal extremity
     e. Paralysis results when there is total occlusion
     f. Polar (limb cold to touch)
     g. In addition there may be skin changes with fine texture, shiny and dry; painful ulcer formation on or between toes, upper surface of the foot or over bony prominences such as metatarsal heads.
     h. Hair loss distal to occlusion and thick brittle nails

  2. Venous disease

     a. Little or no pain, if no inflammation, may have dull ache, sensation of heaviness or tenderness along an inflamed vein.
     b. Brawny (reddish-brown skin color); cyanotic if dependent
     c. Skin: stasis dermatitis, veins visible, mottled skin
     d. Limb warm to touch
     e. Stasis ulcers, usually ankle area, mildly painful
     f. Edema present, may be from foot to calf

- Differential Diagnosis

  1. Arterial disease

     a. Thrombophlebitis

b. Diabetic peripheral neuritis

c. Acute trauma

d. Osteoarthritis of the lumbosacral spine or lower extremity joints

2. Venous Disease

a. Lymphatic disease

b. Acute trauma

c. Arterial disease

d. Peripheral neuritis

- Physical Findings (Bright & Georgi, 1992; Celentano, 1991).

1. Arterial disease

a. Delayed capillary filling time

b. Absent or diminished peripheral pulses

c. Pallor or blanching of extremity when elevated and possible rubor(redness) when dependent

d. Temperature changes; cool on affected side, warm on unaffected side (note condition could be bilateral—especially in older patients with bilateral disease and both extremities would be cool to touch).

e. Non-healing or slow-healing painful leg/foot ulcer

f. Gangrene of toes in advanced cases

2. Venous disease

a. Edema of affected leg when dependent with edema decreased when leg elevated—both legs measured and compared for difference of more than 1 cm circumference above ankle

b. Brawny skin color

c. Stasis dermatitis around ankle and lower leg, scaly peeling crusty skin encircles ankle.

d. Veins may be prominent.

e. Skin temperature normal or warm if inflammation present

f. Stasis ulcers may be present in lower third of leg with mild pain relieved by elevation.

g. Peripheral pulses present

- Diagnostic Evaluation/Findings (Bright & Georgi, 1992; Celentano, 1991; Friedman, 1990).

1. Arterial disease

a. Doppler ultrasound/reduced pressures in affected limb (never use as only test in elderly as calcified, stiff arteries can give false high readings).

b. Plethysmography measures blood volume changes and graphs flow along the extremity/identify amount of obstruction.

c. Ankle-brachial-index (ABI, ankle pressure divided by brachial pressure) should be the same or close to 1—less than 1 indicates obstruction and less than .5 indicates severe obstruction.

d. Stress testing on a treadmill/functional ability shows lesions not revealed at rest.

e. Arteriography—invasive test more often used for preoperative data on vessel condition above and below lesion, not really needed for initial diagnosis.

f. CT scan visualizes arterial wall/assess for post-op complications of graft infection, occlusion etc. and screens for abdominal aneurysms.

2. Venous disease

a. Doppler ultrasound/venous obstruction and venous reflux

b. Plethysmography/volume changes indicate decreased flow with thrombosis.

c. Ambulatory-venous-pressure (AVP) measurement/resting and exercise pressures, identify occlusion if no drop in pressure with exercise.

d. Manual compression and retrograde filling tests help assess competency of veins.

e. MRI (magnetic resonance imaging)/detect deep-vein thrombosis from iliac veins to leg veins.

f. Venography/evidence of obstruction, insufficiency, extent of collateral circulation, reflux

g. B/mode venous imaging new technique/visualizes vein's size, compressibility, flow, valve function, presence of thrombus.

- Management/Treatment

1. Arterial disease (Friedman, 1990; Thiele & Strandness, 1990)

Most elderly people with arterial occlusive disease and intermittent claudication are successfully managed with conservative treatment and never need surgery. The severity of the disease determines the treatment. There are three general groups of patients: asymptomatic, those with intermittent claudication only, and those with significant arterial occlusion with or without claudication.

a. Asymptomatic (feet perfused adequately through collateral circulation) treatment is focused primarily on preventive foot care:

(1) Avoid extremes of heat or cold, avoid heating pads or ice paks to extremities

(2) Legs should be positioned level when sleeping and not crossed when sitting.

(3) Skin care should be meticulous, feet washed with mild soap, and warm water, lanolin or cold cream for dry skin—feet inspected carefully every week in a good light for any cracks, cuts, color changes and reported to health care provider immediately.

(4) Toe nails need special attention by podiatrist or skillful family caregiver—cut straight across, avoid cutting too short

(5) Corns and calluses treated by podiatrist.

(6) Shoes and socks should be comfortable and well-fitting, avoid going barefoot.

(7) If foot injury sustained seek immediate professional attention—self-medication should be avoided.

(8) Exercise (walk) regularly to improve circulation.

b. Intermittent claudication with adequate blood flow, In addition to foot care, instructions should include:

(1) Stop smoking if they are smokers (This greatly exacerbates the progress of arterial disease).

(2) Weight loss if overweight.

(3) Walk as much as possible—recommendation is walk to point of pain (claudication) then stop, then continue walking. Walking programs like this have resulted in significant improvement of exercise tolerance and symptom relief.

c. Significant disease with severe symptoms may require:

(1) Percutaneous transluminal angioplasty (PTA)

(2) Endarterectomy

(3) Bypass surgery

(4) Amputation in cases of gangrene and non-healing lesions

Decision for surgery based on many factors: general health, lifestyle factors, age, presence of other diseases especially heart, location of lesions.

2. Venous disease (Celentano, 1991; Johnson et al., 1992).

a. Chronic venous insufficiency

(1) Compressive elastic stocking

(2) Leg elevation

(3) Exercise

(4) Skin care to dermatitis (emollients, topical corticosteroids).

(5) Skin care for ulcers: wet to dry dressings, unna paste boot, debridement, topical antibiotics

(6) Surgery in cases of non-healing ulcers for revascularization

b. Superficial thrombophlebitis (Friedman, 1990)

Usually does not lead to pulmonary embolism, may be treated at home or outpatient basis.

(1) Below the knee: warm soaks, decreased ambulation, nonsteroidal antiinflammatory agent (aspirin), process self

limiting, clears up in 5–10 days with no residual findings.

(2) Lower thigh: Short course of heparin—discontinued after inflammation subsides.

c. Deep vein thrombophlebitis (Friedman, 1990; Celentano, 1991)

(1) Above the knee; hospitalization, anticoagulation with heparin/coumadin, coumadin continued 2–6 months, bed rest, discontinue estrogens.

(2) Below the knee: hospitalization or out-patient treatment, rest, local heat, anticoagualtion based on risk factors, analgesics, elevated affected limb, discontinue estrogens.

- Nursing Considerations (Havens & Weaver, 1992)

1. Goals of nursing care are: to relieve symptoms, improve tissue perfusion and prevent complications, and protect the affected extremity from further damage.

a. Relief of symptoms and improvement of tissue perfusion:

(1) Position the extremity correctly depending on whether it is arterial disease or venous disease; a dependent position may improve circulation and relieve pain in arterial disease; elevating legs may relieve discomfort in venous disease

(2) Provide analgesics as necessary.

(3) Encourage progressive exercise program as planned.

(4) Follow guidelines for skin and foot care as outlined in the medical management.

(5) Attention to smoking cessation if necessary

b. Protection of extremity from further damage:

(1) Follow nursing care plan regarding positioning, skin and foot care, general medical regime while patient hospitalized.

(2) Begin teaching plan as soon as possible, involve patient and family in developing plan to include:

(a) Importance of good hygiene, skin and foot care

(b) Assessment of discomfort and disability for reversible causes and correction—sometimes elderly people accept discomfort and disability as expected age changes and do not report symptoms

(c) An explanation of the disease process, signs and symptoms of altered tissue perfusion (cold, mottled extremity, swelling, absence of pulses).

(d) Teaching patient and family how to inspect the extremity and check pulses.

(e) Discussion of proper clothing and well-fitting shoes and stockings.

(f) Instruction on reporting changes, ulcerations, injuries etc.

(g) Emphasis on importance of follow-up care as these are chronic conditions which need continued monitoring.

(h) Encouragement of a daily schedule with balanced rest and activity.

Questions

1. In primary hypertension the etiology is:
   a. Due to renal and hormonal disease
   b. Genetic in origin
   c. A heterogenous process
   d. Due to type A personality
   e. Due to drugs, chemicals, foods

2. Primary hypertension accounts for:
   a. 80–90% of all hypertension
   b. 10–20% of all hypertension
   c. 50–60% of all hypertension
   d. Unknown % of all hypertension

3. The most dominant form of hypertension in the elderly population is:
   a. Severe hypertension
   b. Moderate hypertension
   c. Very severe hypertension
   d. Isolated systolic hypertension
   e. Mild hypertension

4. The following statement is *not* true of hypertension in the elderly population in the United States:
   a. There is a higher morbidity and mortality rate in untreated persons.
   b. Treatment should be based primarily on age
   c. Treatment is similar to that of younger individuals
   d. Elderly individuals have a good response to treatment

5. Hypertension may be described as:
   a. Affecting 10–20% of people over 65 years
   b. Asymptomatic in early stages
   c. More prevalent in older men than older women
   d. Not usually diagnosed on routine examination

6. Isolated systolic hypertension may be defined as systolic blood pressure of— when the diastolic is less than 90mm/Hg:
   a. Equal to or greater than 140mm/Hg

b. Equal to or greater than 150mm/Hg
c. Equal to or greater than 160mm/Hg
d. Equal to or greater than 170mm/Hg

7. Stage 2 (moderate) hypertension may be defined as:

a. SBP of 140-159mm/Hg & DBP of 90-99mm/Hg
b. SBP of 180-209mm/Hg & DBP of 110-119mm/Hg
c. SBP of 130-139mm/Hg & DBP of 85-89mm/Hg
d. SBP of 160-179mm/Hg & DBP of 100-109mm/Hg

8. The following age-related factors are associated with hypertension except for:

a. Weight gain
b. Increased sodium intake
c. Increased peripheral vascular resistance
d. Decreased bone mass

9. The following statement is not true of hypertension in the elderly:

a. Systolic BP rises after age 65 more in women than in men
b. Hypertension among elderly has no relationship to aging
c. Diastolic pressure rises with age until age 60
d. Systolic pressure may continue to rise after age 60.

10. Life style modifications for hypertension in the elderly consists of:

a. Weight reduction, salt and alcohol restriction, moderate exercise program, and stress reduction
b. Weight reduction, vitamin supplements, exercise program, and stress reduction
c. High carbohydrate, low salt diet; exercise
d. Life style modifications will not help true hypertension

11. Pharmacological therapy for hypertension in the elderly is based on:

a. Structured step method using diuretics first and gradually introducing other drugs as necessary
b. Selection of drugs based on patient's age, weight, and cost
c. Selection of drugs based on existing medical conditions, possible drug interactions and side effects, age, and cost
d. None of the above

12. Due to altered responses in older people which of the following common clinical manifestations of an M.I. may be absent?

    a. Weakness
    b. Chest pain
    c. Nausea/vomiting
    d. Dizziness

13. Angina pain differs from that of M.I. in the following way:

    a. Substernal location
    b. Squeezing, heavy sensation
    c. Not due to change in coronary arteries
    d. Relieved by rest or nitroglycerine

14. Risk factors for coronary artery disease include all of the following *but:*

    a. Hypertension
    b. Smoking
    c. Hyperlipidemia
    d. Hypoglycemia
    e. Family history

15. The following statement regarding cardiovascular disease in the elderly is *true:*

    a. There is a low incidence of M.I. in the elderly
    b. A major risk factor for coronary artery disease is hypertension
    c. Women have a lower incidence of M.I. after menopause
    d. Anginal pain is always seen with myocardial ischemia

16. Which of the following is least helpful in diagnosing a myocardial infarction?

    a. Serum enzymes
    b. Electrocardiagram
    c. History
    d. Chest X-ray

17. Which of the following statements is *not* true concerning coronary artery disease (CAD)?

    a. Deaths due to CAD have been on the decline for several years
    b. CAD is the leading cause of death in the United States
    c. Over 80% of the cases of CAD are in the over age 65 group
    d. Thrombolytic treatment is recommended for the over age 75 group

18. The elderly person with a myocardial infarction may not have the typical pain of coronary occlusion because of all but the following:

    a. Limited physical activity
    b. No damage to the heart muscle
    c. Diminished pain sensation
    d. Failure to recognize the pain

19. Elderly persons with myocardial infarctions may not be diagnosed accurately because:

    a. It doesn't occur as often in this age group
    b. It is not as serious a condition for older people
    c. Symptoms may be vague and atypical
    d. They have no symptoms

20. The most definitive finding in angina pectoris is:

    a. Serum enzyme levels
    b. Chest X-ray findings
    c. Chest pain relieved by rest or nitroglycerine
    d. Electrocardiographic findings

21. The most definitive diagnostic test for myocardial infarction is:

    a. Serum enzyme levels
    b. Chest X-ray
    c. Severe, squeezing pain
    d. Electrocardiographic findings
    e. Echocardiographic findings

22. Management for patients with myocardial infarctions includes all but:

    a. Hospitalization in early period
    b. Bed rest and pain relief
    c. Medications to increase perfusion to heart muscle and limit damage
    d. Cardiac monitoring to detect arrhythmias
    e. Early aerobic activity

23. Frequent causes of congestive heart failure in the elderly are;

    a. Coronary artery disease, hypertension, and degenerative valvular disease
    b. Congenital heart disease, fractured hip, and arthritis
    c. Weight loss, hypotension, and gastric disturbances
    d. None of the above

24. The following statements about congestive heart failure are true *except:*

    a. 75% of ambulatory patients with CHF are over age 60
    b. It increases exponentially with age after the 6th decade
    c. Left sided failure initially affects the systemic circulation
    d. Fever, anemia, and infection may precipitate CHF in the elderly person.

25. Pharmacological treatment for congestive heart failure includes the following:

    a. Diuretics
    b. Vasodilators
    c. Digoxin
    d. Nitrates
    e. All of the above

26. Which of the following are signs and symptoms of CHF in the elderly person?

    a. Bradycardia
    b. Tachycardia
    c. Cheyne-Stokes respirations
    d. Diminished sensation

27. Which of the following drugs has been questioned in the long term management of elderly persons with CHF due to high toxicity?

    a. Nitrates
    b. Beta-blockers
    c. Digoxin
    d. Diuretics

28. Right sided heart failure initially causes all the following signs and symptoms except:

    a. Anorexia, nausea
    b. Weight gain
    c. Dependent edema
    d. Dyspnea
    e. Weakness

29. Left sided heart failure initially causes all the following signs and symptoms except:

    a. Dyspnea, breathlessness
    b. Dependent edema

c. Fatigue
d. Anxiety
e. Weight gain

30. The most common factor in the etiology of peripheral arterial occlusive disease is:

    a. Trauma
    b. Congenital
    c. Infection
    d. Atherosclerosis

31. Frequent risk factors for peripheral arterial disease include all of the following except:

    a. Smoking
    b. Diabetes
    c. Obesity
    d. Hypolipidemia

32. Functional disability and symptoms in peripheral vascular disease are related to which of the following conditions?

    a. Cardiac status
    b. Amount of vessel occlusion
    c. Amount of collateral circulation
    d. All of the above

33. Arterial occlusive disease of the lower extremity would manifest all the following except:

    a. Brawny color
    b. Pale color
    c. Cool temperature
    d. Weak or absent pulse

34. Management of intermittent claudication includes recommendations for a walking program which is described as:

    a. Continuous brisk walking to the point of pain and then stopping
    b. Slow walking for short intervals without pain
    c. Walking to the point of pain, stopping, then walking again
    d. Walking briskly, then slowly, then briskly but not to point of pain

35. If calf pain which was once relieved after a short rest is now present, even at rest, it is probably due to:

    a. Neuritis
    b. Development of collateral circulation
    c. Progression of occlusion
    d. Non-pathological changes

36. Cramping pain in the leg at rest due to arterial disease may be relieved by having the patient:

    a. Dangle leg over the side of the bed
    b. Use cold or warm applications
    c. Elevate foot on pillows
    d. Keep leg horizontal and massage

37. The major complication of peripheral arterial occlusion (ischemia) is:

    a. Skin breakdown
    b. Pain and discomfort
    c. Ulceration
    d. Gangrene

38. Which of the following tests measures blood volume changes?

    a. Plethysmography
    b. Venous imaging
    c. Magnetic resonance imaging (MRI)
    d. Ambulatory venous pressure measurement

39. Incidence of venous thrombosis in surgical patients is:

    a. 10–15%
    b. 20–30%
    c. 30–40%
    d. 40–50%

40. Incidence of venous thrombosis in elderly surgical patients is:

    a. 20%
    b. 40%
    c. 50%
    d. None of the above

41. Risk factors for venous insufficiency and thrombosis in elderly patients include all but:

    a. Surgery
    b. Obesity
    c. Immobility
    d. Diet
    e. Trauma

42. The severity of an arrhythmia in an older person is determined primarily by:

    a. Preexisting age changes
    b. Location in the conduction system
    c. Presence of ectopic beats
    d. Existing cardiac disease

43. An age related change which contributes to the development of arrhythmias in elderly people is:

    a. Loss of cells in the conduction system
    b. Decrease in fibrous tissue in the heart
    c. Increased number of cells in the Bundle of His
    d. Decreased heart size

44. A rate of 300–600 bpm is characteristic of which common arrhythmia in older people?

    a. Heart Block, type II
    b. Stokes-Adams Syndrome
    c. Atrial Fibrillation
    d. Sick Sinus Syndrome

45. The following statement about the incidence of arrhythmias in the older population is true.

    a. The incidence of arrhythmias is about the same in the older population as in the younger population.
    b. There is an increased incidence of arrhythmias in the older population.
    c. There is a decreased incidence of arrhythmias in the older population.
    d. The incidence of arrhythmias in the older population is unrelated to age.

46. A diagnostic test requiring an invasive procedure to diagnose arrhythmias is known as:

a. Continuous ECG monitoring
b. A treadmill test
c. A Holter monitor test
d. An electrophysiology test

47. Pacemakers may be used to treat all of the following arrhythmias except:

a. Second degree heart block
b. Acute Stokes-Adams Syndrome
c. Atrial fibrillation
d. Sick Sinus Syndrome

48. A diagnostic test providing 24 hour data on heart rhythms in ambulatory patients utilizes:

a. A Holter monitor
b. A pacemaker
c. A treadmill
d. An internal cardiac catheter

49. Education for patients with pacemakers should include:

a. Keeping the pacemaker card at home in a safe place
b. Avoiding contact with microwave ovens
c. Avoiding airline travel
d. Avoiding contact with magnetic scanners

Answers

1. c
2. a
3. d
4. b
5. b
6. a
7. d
8. d
9. b
10. a
11. c
12. b
13. d
14. d
15. b
16. d
17. d
18. b
19. c
20. c
21. a
22. e
23. a
24. c
25. e
26. b
27. c
28. d
29. b
30. d
31. d
32. d
33. a
34. c
35. c
36. a
37. d
38. a
39. b
40. c
41. d
42. d
43. a
44. c
45. b
46. d
47. c
48. a
49. d

Bibliography

Allman, R. (1989). Basic evaluation of older persons with hypertension. *Clinics in Geriatric Medicine, 5*(4), 717–732.

Applegate, W. (1990). Hypertension. In W. Hazzard, R. Andres, E. Bierman, & J. Blass (Eds.), *Principles of geriatric medicine and gerontology* (2nd ed.) (pp. 485–497). New York: McGraw-Hill.

Baxendale, L. M. (1992). Pathophysiology of coronary artery disease. *Nursing Clinics of North America, 27*(1), 143–152.

Bierman, E. L. (1990). Congestive heart failure. In W. Hazzard, R. Andres, E. Bierman, & J. Blass (Eds.), *Principles of geriatric medicine and gerontology* (2nd ed.) (pp. 458–465). New York: McGraw-Hill.

Bright, L. D., & Georgi, S. (1992). Peripheral vascular disease: Is it arterial or venous? *American Journal of Nursing, 92*(9), 34–47.

Carethers, M., & Blanchette, P. (1989). Pathophysiology of hypertension. *Clinics in Geriatric Medicine, 5*(4), 657–674.

Celentano, D. (1991). Cardiovascular problems. In V. Millonig (Ed.), *The adult nurse practitioner certification review guide* (pp. 38–71). Potomac, MD.: Health Leadership Associates.

Dzurinko, C. L. (1991). Congestive heart failure. In D. K. Newman & D. J. Smith (Eds.), *Geriatric care plans* (pp. 70–85). Springhouse, Pa.: Springhouse Co.

Fleg, J. (1990). Arrhythmias and conduction disorders. In W. Abrams, R. Berkow & A. Fletcher (Eds.), *Merck manual of geriatrics.* (pp. 370–380), Rahway, N.J.: Merck & Co.

Flack, J., Woolley, A., Esunge, P., & Grimm, R. (1992). A rational approach to hypertension treatment in the older patient. *Geriatrics, 47*(11), 24–38.

Fleury, J. (1992). Long term management of the patient with stable angina. *Nursing Clinics of North America, 27*(1), 205–220.

Friedman, S. A. (1990). Peripheral vascular diseases. In W. Abrams, R. Berkow, & A. Fletcher (Eds.), *Merck manual of geriatrics* (pp. 386–413). Rahway, N.J.: Merck, Sharp & Dohme Research Laboratories.

Frohlich, E. D. (1990). Hypertension. In W. Abrams, R. Berkow, & A. Fletcher (Eds.), *Merck manual of geriatrics* (pp. 336–348). Rahway, N.J.: Merck, Sharp & Dohme Research Laboratories.

Gerstenblith, G. (1990). Coronary artery disease. In W. Abrams, R. Berkow, & A.

Fletcher (Eds.), *Merck manual of geriatrics* (pp. 353–358). Rahway, N.J.: Merck, Sharp & Dohme Research Laboratories.

Gerstenblith, G., & Lakatta, E. (1990). Disorders of the heart. In W. Hazzard, R. Andres, E. Bierman, & J. Blass (Eds.), *Principles of geriatric medicine and gerontology* (2nd. ed.) (pp. 466–475). New York: McGraw-Hill.

Havens, L. L., & Weaver, J. W. (1992). Cardiovascular system. In M. Hogstel (Ed.), *Clinical manual of gerontological nursing* (pp. 70–90). St. Louis: Mosby Yearbook.

Hurst, J. W., Schlant, R. C., Rockley, C. E., Sonnenblick, E. H., & Wenger, N. K. (1990). *The Heart, arteries and veins* (7th. ed.). New York: McGraw-Hill.

Johns, C. (1992). Nursing role in management of dysrhythmias. In S. Lewis and I. Collier (Eds.), *Medical-Surgical nursing: Assessment and management of clinical problems* (3rd ed.) (pp. 849–887). St Louis: Mosby Year Book.

Johnson, J., Adams, K., & Bigely, M. B. (1992). Cardiovascular function. In M. Burke & M. Walsh (Eds.), *Gerontological nursing: Care of the frail elderly* (pp. 198–222). St. Louis: Mosby Year Book.

Lazar, E., Lazar, J., & Frishman, W. (1992). Angina pectoris and silent ischemia in the elderly: A management update. *Geriatrics 47*(7), 24–36.

National Center for Health Statistics: Monthly Vital Statistics Report: Births, Marriages, Divorces, and Deaths for November, 1989. Washington Department of Health and Human Services 1990, DHH Publication N. (PHS) 90–1120.

National Heart, Lung, and Blood Institute (1993). The Fifth Report of the *Joint National Committee on Detection, Evaluation, and Treatment of High Blood Pressure*, U.S. Department of Health and Human Services, NIH Publication No. 93-1088, January 1993, Bethesda, MD.: National Institutes of Health.

Parker-Cohen, P., Richardson, S., & Haak, S. (1990). In K. McCance & S. Huether (Eds.), *Pathophysiology: The biologic basis for disease in adults and children* (pp. 916–991). St. Louis: C.V. Mosby.

Rossi, L., & Leary, E. (1992). Evaluating the patient with coronary artery disease. *Nursing Clinics of North America, 27*(1), 171–188.

Thiele, B. L., & Strandness, D. E. (1990). Peripheral vascular disease. In W. Hazzard, R. Andres, E. Bierman, & J. Blass (Eds.), *Principles of geriatric medicine and gerontology* (2nd ed.) (pp.476–484). New York: McGraw-Hill.

Underhill, S. L., Woods, S. L., Froelicher, E. S., & Halpenny, C. J. (1989). *Cardiac nursing* (2nd ed.). Philadelphia: J. B. Lippincott.

Wei, J. Y. (1990). Heart failure (HF). In W. Abrams, R. Birkow, & A. Fletcher (Eds.), *Merck manual of geriatrics* (pp. 380–386). Rahway, N.J.: Merck & Co.

Woo, M. A. (1992). Clinical management of the patient with acute myocardial infarction. *Nursing Clinics of North America, 27*(1), 189–203.

GASTROINTESTINAL DISORDERS

Pamela Cacchione

Hiatal Hernia

- Definition: Protrusion of an upper portion of stomach through an opening in the diaphragm.
- Etiology: Weakening of the esophagogastric juncture or trauma. Risk factors include smoking, alcohol abuse, lumbar kyphosis in which there is a widening of the diaphragm; obesity, ascites, tumors, forced recumbent position.
- Incidence: 50% of all elderly 65 years and older have hiatal hernias, most are asymptomatic; especially common in obese older women.
- Signs and Symptoms: Can be severe or mild, intermittent or constant
  1. Dysphagia
  2. Indigestion; heartburn occurring 30 to 60 minutes following a meal
  3. Substernal pain due to reflux; worsens lying down
  4. Feeling of abdominal fullness
  5. Belching, regurgitation, bitter taste in mouth
- Differential Diagnosis
  1. Coronary heart disease
  2. Esophageal spasm
  3. Gallbladder disease
  4. Gastritis
  5. Peptic ulcer
  6. Malignant disease of esophagus or stomach
- Physical Findings: Absent without diagnostic tests
- Diagnostic Evaluation/Findings
  1. Barium swallow
  2. Endoscopy with biopsy to assess for malignancy
  3. Referral to gastroenterologist if severe
  4. Potential complications include esophageal reflux, pulmonary aspiration and esophagitis

- Management/Treatment
  1. Diet modification: small, frequent, bland meals
  2. Antacids as needed
  3. H_2 receptor inhibitor, where acid reflux is problem (cimetidine, ranitidine, famotidine)
  4. Relaxation techniques
  5. Blocks under the head of the bed or elevate head of bed 4-6 inches
  6. Occasionally surgical repair required
- Nursing Considerations
  1. Patient education regarding
     a. Dietary modifications
        (1) Weight reduction, if indicated
        (2) Avoid bedtime snacking
        (3) Small, frequent, bland meals
        (4) Avoid recumbent position for 45-60 minutes following meals
        (5) Avoid spicy, acid foods, alcohol, tobacco
     b. Mild exercise after meals
     c. Avoid use of girdles and corsets
  2. Head of bed elevated on 6 to 8 inch blocks
  3. Avoid feeding patient in bed (recumbent position)

Peptic Ulcer Disease

- Definition: Ulceration of the gastrointestinal mucosa, including the stomach, duodenum, and (less commonly) the distal esophagus and jejunum.
- Etiology: Exact cause unknown; contributing factors include
  1. Altered gastric acid and serum gastrin levels
  2. Smoking and alcohol use
  3. Regular use of moderate to large doses of aspirin, nonsteroidal anti-inflammatory drugs, and steroids

4. Genetic predisposition
5. Psychosomatic factors (e.g. chronic anxiety, severe stress)

- Incidence: Any elderly person experiencing a major body insult, medical or psychogenic, is at risk for ulcer development particularly if preexistent atrophic gastritis is present. Gastric ulcers are more common than duodenal in the elderly and are more often fatal.
- Signs and Symptoms: Epigastric pain is not a prominent feature in the derly
  1. Poorly localized upper gastrointestinal pain
  2. Decreased appetite
  3. Decreased general energy level
  4. Stools may be positive for occult blood
  5. Weight loss
  6. Pain may begin two hours after eating and may awaken at night
  7. Pain usually relieved by food or antacids
  8. Vomiting, may be positive for blood
  9. Systemic response to blood loss may be dominant indicator i.e., fatigue, dyspnea secondary to blood loss, and/or anemia induced heart failure.
- Differential Diagnosis
  1. Gastric cancer
  2. Cardiovascular disease
  3. Hiatal hernia
  4. Small bowel obstruction
  5. Gastrointestinal bleeding from another source
- Physical Findings
  1. Epigastric tenderness
  2. Emesis or stools may be positive for blood

Table 1
MEDICATIONS FOR THE GASTROINTESTINAL SYSTEM

H_2 Receptor Antagonists
Cimetidine/Tagamet
Dosage = 300 mg, orally, q.i.d. initially, then 400 mg at bedtime
Considerations: May cause confusion, multiple doses recommended, multiple drug interactions
Ranitidine/Zantac
Dosage = 150 mg, orally, at bedtime to 150 mg, orally, b.i.d.
Considerations: May cause confusion in the elderly, some drug interactions.
Famotidine/Pepsid
Dosage = 40 mg, orally, at bedtime (× 4–8 weeks) then 20 mg, orally, every day
Considerations: Less expensive, few drug interactions
Gastric Acid Pump Inhibitor
Omeprazole/Prilosec
Dosage = 60 mg, orally, daily
Considerations: Often causes GI upset/diarrhea, potential drug interactions with valium, dilantin, and coumadin
GI Protectant
Sucralfate/Carafate
Dosage = 1 gm, orally, q.i.d. 1 hour before meals and at bedtime
Considerations: Causes constipation, decreases action of dilantin, tetracycline, and fat soluble vitamins

- Diagnostic Evaluation/Findings
    1. CBC and chemistry panel; may demonstrate a low Hct and signs of dehydration
    2. Referral to a gastroenterologist
    3. Barium swallow may demonstrate an ulcer in the lining of the mucosa of the stomach or duodenum.
    4. Endoscopy with biopsy may demonstrate a reddened inflamed erosive area which often requires biopsy to rule out malignancy.
    5. Stools and emesis may test positive for blood
- Management/Treatment: Aggressive therapy is important due to high incidence of complications i.e., hemorrhage, perforation or obstruction.
    1. Referral if no improvement of symptoms in four weeks, bleeding, or signs of peritonitis.
    2. One of the following medications
        a. Antacids: Alternate aluminum and magnesium containing products every four hours to be given after meals. Be aware of sodium content of antacids in order to avoid sodium overload.
        b. H_2 receptor inhibitor, may cause confusion in the elderly (See Table 1)

(1) Ranitidine/Zantac

(2) Cimetidine/Tagamet

(3) Famotidine/Pepsid

c. Gastric acid pump inhibitor

(1) Omeprazole/Prilosec

d. Protectant; safer in elderly due to low side effect profile

(1) Sulcralfate/Carafate

3. Gastric irradiation
4. Transfuse anemic patients who have gastrointestinal bleeding
5. Iron supplements for six weeks, for patients who have gastrointestinal bleeding with anemia
6. Remove aggravating factors.

   a. Discontinue aspirin containing products and nonsteroidal anti-inflammatory drugs.

   b. Eliminate or reduce alcohol and caffeine use, and smoking.

7. Follow up

   a. Four weeks assess for improvement of symptoms, evidence of gastrointestinal bleeding or side effects of medications

   b. Schedule repeat endoscopy or barium swallow at 6 to 12 weeks, depending on symptoms and size of original ulcer.

- Nursing Considerations

1. Patient and family education to include

   a. Report any increase in pain, blood in stools, continued weight loss, or weakness and dizziness.

   b. Medication use, including dosages and side effects

   c. Diet modifications to include

      (1) Small, frequent, bland meals

      (2) Avoid foods that cause pain.

      (3) Avoid caffeine, alcohol, and spicy foods.

Bowel Obstruction

- Definition: A blockage of intestine which may be a simple obstruction or strangulated.
- Etiology
  1. Mechanical causes: Adhesions and hernias are most common; other mechanical causes include ulcers, peritonitis, gallstones, tumors, or bed rest.
  2. Systemic causes: Low potassium levels, myocardial infarction, infection, or surgery
  3. Medication related causes: Anticholinergics, narcotics, or diuretics
- Incidence: Common in frail elderly and elderly with previous bowel surgery
- Signs and Symptoms
  1. Rapid onset of abdominal cramps
  2. Projectile vomiting; seen in early small bowel obstruction and much later in colonic obstruction.
  3. Abdominal distention increasing over time
  4. Decreased or absent bowel sounds
  5. Constipation
- Differential Diagnosis
  1. Gastrointestinal tumor or ulcer
  2. Acute appendicitis
  3. Acute cholecystitis
  4. Diverticulitis
  5. Pancreatitis
- Physical Findings
  1. Abdominal distention more pronounced in upper abdominal area.
  2. Abdominal tenderness may be absent unless strangulation present.
  3. Decreased or absent bowel sounds unless cramping is present then may be high pitched bowel sounds.

4. Fecal impaction may be present.

- Diagnostic Evaluation/Findings
  1. Abdominal examination to evaluate for surgical scars, hernias, masses, tenderness; auscultate for bowel sounds. Perform rectal and vaginal exams.
  2. CBC, blood chemistry panel and urinalysis to evaluate for infection, dehydration, or hypokalemia.
  3. Determine baseline urine output, degree of hydration and respiratory status.
  4. Flat plate X-ray of the abdomen will demonstrate distension of the loops of the small bowel, may also depict fecal impaction, if present.
- Management/Treatment
  1. NPO or clear liquids as tolerated, may require intravenous hydration if not able to take clear liquids.
  2. Nasogastric tube to intermittent suction, especially in the presence of emesis.
  3. Referral to gastroenterologist or surgeon, most require surgery.
- Nursing Considerations
  1. Explain all procedures, disease process and treatment plan to patient and family
  2. Monitor for change in patient's condition

Chronic Cholecystitis

- Definition: Chronic inflammation of the gallbladder; almost always associated with gallstone formation.
- Etiology:
  1. Most frequently due to migration of a calculus into the common duct (90-95% of all cases).
  2. Risk factors: Changing from a high fat to an extreme low fat diet, family history and a high fat diet

- Incidence: It is estimated that 10% of adults in the U.S. have cholelithiasis. The management of cholelithiasis in the elderly is evolving. Many patients do experience progressive symptoms and cholecystectomy is necessary (Fay & Lance, 1992)
- Signs and Symptoms
    1. Cramping pain in right upper quadrant (RUQ) or epigastrium, possibly radiating to back, adjacent to right scapula (biliary colic).
    2. Low grade fever
    3. Fat intolerance
    4. Heartburn/indigestion
    5. Flatulence
    6. Tenderness in RUQ is not always present
    7. May present with obstructive jaundice
- Differential Diagnosis
    1. Acute cholecystitis
    2. Cardiovascular disease
    3. Hepatitis
    4. Pancreatic cancer
    5. Cholecystitis with pancreatitis
- Physical Findings
    1. Jaundice
    2. Tenderness in RUQ and epigastric area may be present
    3. Low grade fever and leukocytosis
- Diagnostic Evaluation/Findings
    1. CBC, blood chemistry panel; may have elevated white blood cell count, and elevated BUN and Creatinine due to dehydration.
    2. Bilirubin and liver function tests will be elevated especially if bile duct obstructed
    3. Amylase and lipase may be elevated if pancreas is involved.

4. Ultrasound of liver area; if stones are present usually visualized in over 95% of the cases.
5. Radioisotope scans using dyes (HIDA scans) will also visualize gall stones
6. Endoscopic retrograde cholangiopancreatography (ERCP) and Transhepatic Cholangiography (THC) are used when common duct involvement is suspected. These can be used to extract the gallstones when possible.

- Management/Treatment
  1. Medications:
     a. Antibiotics: Second and third generation cephalosporins
     b. Antispasmodics
  2. Pain management
  3. Referral to a gastroenterologist
  4. Removal of gallstone by extracorporeal shock wave lithotriptor (ESWL), cholesterol solvents, oral drugs that dissolve stones, and endoscopic sphincterotomy.
  5. Surgical options:
     a. Elective cholecystectomy is advised especially if less than 70 years old with recurrent disease.
     b. Surgery to remove gallstones, pus, bile, and/or provide drainage
     c. Endoscopic cholecystectomy
  6. Diabetics require aggressive management because perforation is common in this population.

- Nursing Considerations
  1. Patient education regarding
     a. Disease process, course, outcomes
     b. Medication dosages and side effects
     c. Dietary changes
        (1) Bland food in small amounts

(2) Low fat

(3) High fiber

2. Encourage weight loss, but advise against very low fat meals and/or supplements; these can precipitate gallstones.
3. Refer to dietician as indicated
4. Preoperative teaching regarding postoperative care
5. Follow up annually, if surgery not indicated
6. Advise to seek medical attention promptly for acute episodes

Chronic Pancreatitis

- Definition: Progressive inflammation of pancreas which leads to permanent structural damage of the pancreatic tissue.
- Etiology: Greater than 50% of chronic pancreatitis is due to alcoholism; can also be a result of trauma, idiopathic causes, or familial pancreatitis. Repeated episodes of acute pancreatitis will also lead to chronic pancreatitis.
- Incidence: Low incidence in elderly because most alcoholic patients with this complication will not survive to old age.
- Signs and Symptoms
    1. Atypical presentation; absence of pain or pain in the lower abdomen
    2. Steatorrhea is often presenting symptom
    3. Diabetes mellitus due to pancreatic insufficiency
    4. Pain in the epigastric area which is worse after meals and alcohol consumption.
    5. Anorexia
- Differential Diagnosis
    1. Cholecystitis
    2. Gastric ulcer
    3. Cardiovascular disease
    4. Pancreatic cancer

5. Acute pancreatitis
6. Vascular disease; mesenteric thrombosis or embolism

- Physical Findings
  1. Epigastric tenderness
  2. Mild jaundice in severe cases
  3. Steatorrhea
  4. Weight loss
- Diagnostic Evaluation/Findings
  1. CBC, and blood chemistry panel will demonstrate leukocytosis, hypocalcemia, hyperglycemia and a low hematocrit (if bleeding is present).
  2. Lipase levels are elevated
  3. Amylase levels will be elevated initially then may return to normal. Urine amylase levels will be elevated.
  4. Abdominal CAT Scan is best method for evaluating the pancreas
  5. Abdominal x-ray may show a sentinel loop of gas filled jejunum in left upper quadrant.
  6. Seventy two hour stool for fat collection demonstrates poor pancreatic exocrine function with high levels of fat in stool.
  7. Endoscopic retrograde cholangiopancreatography (ERCP) is helpful to rule out traumatic injury of pancreatic duct. However it is not commonly used due to the risk of exacerbation of pancreatitis.
- Management/Treatment
  1. Supportive care: Nasogastric suction for exacerbations, NPO, Total Parenteral Nutrition (TPN) and fluid replacement as necessary.
  2. Pain management
  3. Pancreatic enzyme replacement therapy
     a. Pancrease: 3 capsules with each meal
     b. Viokase: 6 to 8 tablets with each meal
     c. Cotazym: 6 to 8 capsules with each meal
  4. Maintain gastric pH above 4 with antacid or H_2 receptor inhibitor

5. Eliminate alcohol consumption
6. Low fat diet to help reduce pancreatic secretions

- Nursing Considerations
  1. Diet modification with special emphasis on elimination of alcohol and caffeine
  2. Instruct patient on dosages of medications and possible side effects.
  3. Instruct patient to notify primary care provider for exacerbations of symptoms.
  4. Manage endocrine insufficiency; Initiate dietary and insulin therapy for diabetes mellitus secondary to pancreatic insufficiency.

Acute Pancreatitis

- Definition: Inflammation of pancreas which can range from a mild self-limiting condition to a fatal acute hemorrhagic pancreatitis
- Etiology: Major causes are alcohol consumption, gallstones, and postoperative inflammation. Pancreatitis due to gallstones is the most common form in the elderly. Other causes of acute pancreatitis include drugs, hyperlipidemia, trauma, and pancreatic cancer.
- Incidence: Acute pancreatitis is an uncommon first presentation condition in the elderly.
- Signs and Symptoms
  1. Epigastric pain or tenderness which lasts for hours and may radiate to the back.
  2. Hyperamylasemia
  3. Nausea and vomiting
  4. Fever
  5. Severe cases: shock, respiratory distress, renal failure, pericarditis, hypocalcemia, leukocytosis and fever
  6. Jaundice
  7. Mental confusion
- Differential Diagnosis
  1. Cholecystitis

2. Gastric ulcer
3. Pancreatic cancer
4. Cardiovascular disease
5. Vascular disease: Mesenteric thrombosis or embolism

- Physical Findings
  1. Epigastric tenderness
  2. Mild jaundice in severe cases
  3. Sepsis presentation
- Diagnostic Evaluation/Findings
  1. CBC, and blood chemistry panel will demonstrate leukocytosis, hypocalcemia, hyperglycemia and a low hematocrit if bleeding is present
  2. Lipase levels are elevated
  3. Amylase levels initially elevated, then may return to normal; urine amylase levels will be elevated.
  4. Abdominal CAT Scan is the best method for evaluating the pancreas
  5. Abdominal x-ray may show a sentinel loop of gas filled jejunum in the left upper quadrant.
  6. Abdominal ultrasound is helpful except in cases of paralytic ileus or obesity
  7. Endoscopic retrograde cholangiopancreatography (ERCP) is helpful to rule out traumatic injury of pancreatic duct. However, it is not commonly used due to the risk of exacerbation of pancreatitis.
- Management/Treatment
  1. Supportive care: Nasogastric suction, NPO, Total Parenteral Nutrition (TPN) and fluid replacement as necessary.
  2. Pain management
  3. Eliminate alcohol consumption
  4. Ongoing evaluation for patients who do not respond to treatment

- Nursing Considerations
    1. Diet modification with special emphasis on elimination of alcohol
    2. Instruct patient on dosages of medications and possible side effects
    3. Instruct patient to notify primary care provider for exacerbation of symptoms.

Constipation

- Definition: A change in bowel habits with diminished frequency of stools associated with increased difficulty in passing stools. There are three types of constipation in the elderly: hypertonic, hypotonic and habit.
    1. Hypertonic: Characterized by hard, dry stools and occasionally lower abdominal pain.
    2. Hypotonic: Characterized by soft putty like stool in the rectum; colon is full of feces and impactions are common.
    3. Habit: Characterized by altered bowel pattern related to poor eating habits.
- Etiology
    1. Hypertonic: Decreased transit of bowel contents resulting in increased reabsorption of water.
    2. Hypotonic: Most commonly due to a decrease in intestinal motility. May be the result of diabetes, hypokalemia, bed rest and medications.
    3. Habit constipation: Primarily due to poor eating habits, ignoring or preventing the urge to defecate, or, particularly, a diet devoid of bulk.
- Incidence: Is extremely common in the elderly
- Signs and Symptoms
    1. Hard infrequent stools or soft putty like stools
    2. Increase in hemorrhoidal complaints
    3. Complaints of abdominal bloating
    4. Fecal incontinence
    5. Fecal impaction

- Differential Diagnosis
  1. Colon cancer
  2. Bowel obstruction
  3. Diverticulosis
  4. Depression
  5. Hypothyroidism
- Physical Findings
  1. Distended abdomen
  2. Fecal impaction
  3. Decreased bowel sounds
  4. Stool may be palpated on abdominal examination of thin patients
- Diagnostic Evaluation/Findings
  1. Thorough history and physical examination to determine underlying cause
  2. Abdominal series, barium enema, colonoscopy or sigmoidoscopy and anorectal manometry to determine suspected causes
  3. Stool for occult blood
  4. Rectal examination
  5. History of past laxative use
- Management/Treatment
  1. High fiber diet, add bran to foods
  2. Increase fluids to 2,000 cc per day
  3. Increase physical activity
  4. Regular toileting times
  5. Cathartics
     a. Stool softeners to soften and lubricate fecal mass
        (1) Docusate sodium/Colace
     b. Bulk-forming agents to increase fecal bulk and retain fluid in bowel lumen

(1) Bran

(2) Psyllium hydrophilic mucilloid/metamucil

c. Saline and osmotic solutions to cause retention of fluid in intestinal lumen.

(1) Magnesium Hydroxide/Milk of magnesia

(1) Magnesium citrate

d. Stimulants to increase peristalsis

(1) Cascara

(2) Bisacodyl/Dulcolax

(3) Senna/Senokot

(4) Lactulose/Chronulac Syrup

(5) Phenolphthalein/Ex Lax

e. Suppositories; cause mucosal irritation

(1) Glycerine and Sodium Stearate/Glycerin

(2) Bisacodyl/Dulcolax

f. Enemas; act by either irritating the colon or by lubricating the colon and softening the feces.

(1) Soap suds enema acts as an irritant

(2) Fleets/Sodium biphosphate, sodium phosphate; softens the feces

(3) Mineral oil; lubricates and softens feces

- Nursing Considerations

1. Evaluate patient's feelings/beliefs regarding normal bowel patterns.
2. Screen patient for depression
3. Patient education regarding

a. High fiber diet

b. Adequate fluid intake

c. Routine toileting times

d. Increase in exercise

e. Need for record of frequency and amount of feces

Hemorrhoids

- Definition: Dilated varicose veins of the anus or rectum; either external or internal. Internal hemorrhoids arise above the internal sphincter with an outer mucous membrane. External hemorrhoids arise outside the external sphincter.
- Etiology: Develop when the flow of blood through the veins of the hemorrhoidal plexus is impaired; caused by many factors including pregnancy, prolonged constipation, heavy lifting, prolonged standing or sitting, congestive heart failure, and portal hypertension. Internal hemorrhoids often lead to the formation of external hemorrhoids.
- Incidence: Common in the elderly due to increased straining during constipation, and venous insufficiency.
- Signs and Symptoms
  1. Internal hemorrhoids
     a. May be asymptomatic
     b. Bright red rectal bleeding may occur
     c. Pain may be present if prolapse or strangulation occurs
     d. Pain on defecation
  2. External hemorrhoids
     a. May be asymptomatic
     b. Pain if thrombus occurs
     c. Bright red bleeding noted on stool or toilet tissue
     d. Pain on defecation
- Differential Diagnosis
  1. Rectal cancer
  2. Colon cancer

- Physical Findings
  1. External hemorrhoids may be visible on visual inspection of anus; almost always signify presence of internal hemorrhoids
  2. Soft masses may be palpable on rectal examination
  3. Rectal bleeding on rectal examination
- Diagnostic Evaluation/Findings
  1. Proctoscopy; will visualize the internal hemorrhoids
  2. Sigmoidoscopy; to rule out rectal and distal colon cancer
  3. Colonoscopy; is indicated to rule out colon cancer
- Management/Treatment
  1. Mild hemorrhoidal disease
     a. Soft diet
     b. Bulk producing laxative i.e., psyllium hydrophilic mucilloid
     c. Avoid straining to defecate
     d. Avoid lifting heavy objects
     e. Hemorrhoidal creams or suppositories, e.g. Anusol or Preparation H to decrease pain and shrink tissues
  2. More severe hemorrhoidal disease (rectal bleeding and pain present)
     a. Soft diet
     b. Bulk producing laxative
     c. Avoid straining either with bowel movements or lifting
     d. Sitz baths
     e. Hemorrhoidectomy
     f. Sclerotherapy
     g. Cryosurgery and laser therapy
  3. Thrombosed external hemorrhoid characterized by sudden onset of severe perianal pain
     a. Local anesthetic injections
     b. Evacuation of the thrombus

- Nursing Considerations
  1. Assessment to determine underlying causes
  2. Visual inspection for presence of external hemorrhoids; digital examination for presence of internal hemorrhoids
  3. Patient education regarding:
     a. Diet modifications
     b. Medications
     c. Use of sitz baths
     d. Proper lifting techniques
     e. Need for follow up when bleeding and pain occur

Diverticular Disease

- Definition
  1. Diverticulosis: Outpouching of the mucous membrane lining of the bowel through a defect in the muscle layer; often asymptomatic.
  2. Diverticulitis: Inflammatory condition which involves one or more of diverticula and is usually symptomatic.
- Etiology: No known cause, but strong association with diets deficient in dietary fiber
- Incidence: Increase with age; 50% prevalence after age 70; women more prone than men
- Signs and Symptoms
  1. Change in bowel habits
  2. Diarrhea alternating with constipation or both
  3. Blood in stool
  4. If diverticulitis develops, flatus, low grade fever and leukocytosis may be present
- Differential Diagnosis
  1. Colonic bleeding
  2. Colon cancer

3. Appendicitis
4. Intestinal obstruction

- Physical Findings
  1. Majority with diverticulosis have no symptoms; some may have abdominal pain in left lower quadrant
  2. Diverticulitis presents with abdominal pain over involved area; tender left lower quadrant mass may be felt on palpation of abdomen
- Diagnostic Evaluation/Findings
  1. CBC, SMA 7; elevated white count, signs of dehydration
  2. Barium enema; out-pouching in sigmoid colon
  3. Abdominal CAT scan or laparotomy should be done to rule out appendicitis if tenderness is present in right lower quadrant
  4. Abdominal flat plate; distention of the bowel at infected site
  5. Anoscope may reveal distal diverticula
  6. Sigmoidoscopy may reveal distal diverticula
  7. Arteriography may be required if patient is actively bleeding
- Management/Treatment
  1. Diverticular Disease
     a. Diet high in fiber
  2. Diverticulitis
     a. Liquid diet and oral antibiotics
     b. Referral and hospitalization for high fever, leukocytosis, severe pain or bleeding
     c. Intravenous antibiotics if an abscess or peritonitis is suspected
     d. Monitor intake and output
     e. Local heat application
     f. Referral to surgery (20% require surgery)
     g. After acute phase, increase fiber in diet. Consider addition of bran or psyllium hydrophilic mucilloid

- Nursing Considerations
  1. Patient education regarding
     a. High fiber diet
     b. Adequate fluid intake
     c. Need for follow up with any of the following:
        (1) abdominal pain
        (2) fever
        (3) bloody stools
        (4) constipation

Colorectal Cancer

- Definition: Malignant lesions in the colon or rectum
- Etiology: Causes remain unclear; risk factors include history of colonic polyps, breast or female genital tract cancer, chronic inflammatory bowel disorders, positive family history, chronic parasitic infections; high fat, low fiber, high-caloric diet is strong environmental factor.
- Incidence: Second most common cancer in western world, more common in higher socioeconomic groups; most prevalent over the age of 50, peaks in the eighth decade.
- Signs and Symptoms: Vary by their location:
  1. Right sided colon cancer
     a. Usually asymptomatic
     b. Vague or crampy colicky abdominal pain
     c. Unexplained weight loss
     d. Anemia, secondary to gastrointestinal bleeding, may be first presenting symptom
  2. Left sided colon cancer
     a. Alternating constipation with diarrhea
     b. Change in stool caliber (narrow, ribbon-like)
     c. Lower abdominal pain

    d. Rectal bleeding
    e. Sensation of incomplete evacuation

3. Rectal cancer
    a. Tenesmus
    b. Rectal bleeding
    c. Mucous discharge

- Differential Diagnosis
    1. Diverticular disease
    2. Lymphoma
- Physical Findings
    1. Palpable mass primarily in right colon
    2. Lymphadenopathy
    3. Rectal mass found on rectal exam
    4. Stools positive for occult blood
- Diagnostic Evaluation/Findings
    1. Barium enema x-ray; air contrast preferable to single contrast, may see an apple core lesion or mass
    2. Colonoscopy; may allow for biopsy of lesion found by barium enema
    3. Fiberoptic sigmoidoscope; may find distal tumors
    4. Testing of stools for occult blood; cancers detected with this technique are usually early stage and have a high cure rate.
    5. Carcinoembryonic antigen (CEA) test often performed, although not specific for colon cancer; normal level of CEA does not exclude possibility of malignancy.
    6. CBC can demonstrate an anemia (normochromic, normocytic)
- Management/Treatment:
    1. Referral for surgical excision or resection depending upon the depth of invasion of tumor

2. Patients with metastatic lesions, noted at the time of diagnosis, have a poor prognosis. Palliative treatment is then indicated.
3. Patients with a resection often require a temporary colostomy.

- Nursing Considerations
  1. Screening for colon cancer
     a. Test stools for occult blood annually
     b. Digital rectal examination annually
     c. Sigmoidoscopy every 3-5 years after age 50
  2. Monitor for signs of dehydration during colon preps
  3. Instruct patient on possibility of a colostomy after procedure and begin patient teaching on care of colostomy preoperatively
  4. Encourage patient and family to ventilate feelings regarding the diagnosis
  5. Make referrals to pastoral care or mental health liaison as indicated
  7. Refer to community agencies for assistance after discharge; i.e., American Cancer Society, Ostomy Association.

Appendicitis

- Definition: Infection and inflammation of the appendix
- Etiology: Obstruction of appendix by stricture, inflammation, or hardened feces.
- Incidence: In patients over age 65 the incidence is 20/100,000. Because of its atypical presentation in the elderly, there is a higher risk of perforation.
- Signs and Symptoms
  1. Atypical presentation in the elderly; the pain begins in the right lower quadrant and may not be severe until perforation occurs.
  2. Nausea and vomiting
  3. Rebound tenderness in lower quadrants
  4. Fever and leukocytosis; fever may be absent

5. Constipation
6. Anorexia

- Differential Diagnosis
  1. Diverticulitis
  2. Colon cancer
- Physical Findings
  1. Rebound tenderness
  2. Positive psoas sign
  3. Rectal tenderness
  4. Tenderness in both right and left lower quadrants
- Diagnostic Evaluation/Findings
  1. CBC with differential; leukocytosis
  2. Psoas sign
  3. Marked tenderness on rectal exam
- Management/Treatment
  1. Referral for surgery consult
  2. Antibiotics prior to surgery and for 48 hours post operatively, if no perforation
  3. Appendectomy
- Nursing Considerations
  1. Patient education regarding
     a. Postoperative care
     b. Medication (analgesics and/or antibiotics), dosages and side effects

Questions

1. On your routine yearly exam of a 76 year old male, which of the following procedures should be done?
   a. Barium x-ray
   b. Test stool for occult blood
   c. Anoscope
   d. Colonoscopy

2. Your patient presents with right upper quadrant pain that worsens after eating fatty foods. What lab tests would you order prior to referring this patient to a gastroenterologist?
   a. CBC, blood chemistry, amylase and liver function tests
   b. CBC, blood chemistry, flat plate of the abdomen
   c. CBC, blood chemistry, Bilirubin, and liver function tests
   d. CBC, blood chemistry, stool for ova and parasites

3. What is the order of physical assessment of the abdomen?
   a. Inspect, palpate, percuss, and auscultate
   b. Inspect, auscultate, percuss, then palpate
   c. Inspect, percuss, auscultate, then palpate
   d. None of the above

4. A hiatal hernia presents with the following symptoms:
   a. Chest pain, diarrhea and vomiting
   b. Indigestion, belching, and flatus
   c. Dysphagia, substernal pain due to reflux
   d. Headaches, belching and chest pain

5. All of the following are important to teach patients with hiatal hernias except:
   a. Weight reduction if they are obese
   b. To place blocks under the head of their bed
   c. Not to lie down until at least one hour after meals
   d. To increase fiber in the diet

6. Peptic ulcer disease is treated by any of the following with the exception of:
   a. Bran or other bulk forming agents
   b. Antacids

c. GI protectants
d. H_2 receptor antagonists

7. Bowel obstruction can be caused by all the following except:

   a. Adhesions, hernias
   b. Infections
   c. High fiber diets
   d. Medications

8. An 82 year old female presents with the following symptoms: abdominal distension, constipation and vomiting. What other information would be *least* helpful?

   a. History of prior abdominal surgery
   b. A list of medications
   c. Dietary intake of potassium
   d. Presence of fever

9. Which of the following would be an appropriate work up of cholecystitis?

   a. CBC, Chemistry panel and Upper GI
   b. CBC, Liver Function Tests, and Ultrasound of liver area
   c. Chemistry panel, bilirubin levels, and a colonoscopy
   d. ERCP, abdominal ultrasound and a barium swallow

10. Constipation is a symptom of all of the following except:

   a. Cholecystitis
   b. Colon cancer
   c. Depression
   d. Small bowel obstruction

11. What information is least important to discern in patients who are complaining of constipation?

   a. Dietary intake of fiber and fluids
   b. Family history of constipation
   c. Activity history and list of medications
   d. Toileting routine

12. What are the physical findings in patients with diverticulitis?
    a. Right upper quadrant tenderness
    b. Left lower quadrant tenderness
    c. Generalized abdominal tenderness
    d. Rebound tenderness

13. What is the recommended screening for colon cancer?
    a. Rectal exams every 2 years, colonoscopy and CEA levels every 3-5 years after age 50
    b. Stools for occult blood yearly, and colonoscopy every 5 years after age 50
    c. Stools for occult blood and rectal exam yearly and sigmoidoscopy every 3-5 years
    d. Colonoscopy every five years, sigmoidoscopy every three years and CEA levels yearly

14. What is the atypical presentation of appendicitis in the elderly?
    a. RLQ pain that is not severe until perforation occurs
    b. Sharp epigastric pain that radiates to the RLQ
    c. Sharp LLQ pain that radiates to the epigastric area
    d. An acute abdomen and high fever

15. An atypical presentation for chronic pancreatitis includes:
    a. Absence of pain or pain in lower abdomen
    b. Pain only in RUQ
    c. Pain in the epigastric area that radiates to LUQ
    d. Sharp pain LUQ

16. Management of chronic pancreatitis includes:
    a. Diet high in fat
    b. Abstinence from alcohol
    c. High carbohydrate diet
    d. None of the above

17. Which is not a common type of constipation in the elderly
    a. Hypertonic
    b. Hypotonic
    c. Hypospasmodic
    d. Habit

18. An elderly patient presents with the following symptoms: poorly localized upper gastrointestinal pain, weakness, abdominal pain that awakens him at night and black stools. What is the most likely diagnosis?

    a. Diverticulitis
    b. Peptic ulcer disease
    c. Appendicitis
    d. Acute pancreatitis

19. An elderly patient presents with the following symptoms: fever, leukocytosis, LLQ pain, diarrhea alternating with constipation. Which is the most likely diagnosis?

    a. Appendicitis
    b. Chronic cholecystitis
    c. Angiodysplasia
    d. Diverticulitis

20. Your elderly 83 year old female patient is complaining of an aggravation of her diverticulitis. Which of the following is not part of the management regimen?

    a. Liquid diet
    b. Dulcolax suppositories
    c. Oral antibiotics
    d. Local heat application

21. What are the most common symptoms of rectal cancer?

    a. GI bleeding and cramping abdominal pain
    b. Diarrhea alternating with constipation and rectal bleeding
    c. Rectal pain and pain radiating to the umbilicus
    d. Mucous like rectal discharge and rectal bleeding

22. You suspect that a recent stressor, due to an aggravation of your patient's asthma, and a change in his medications has caused his suspected gastric ulcer. Which medication is the probable cause?

    a. Solucortef 200 mg, intravenously, every six hours
    b. Theodur 300 mg, orally, every twelve hours
    c. Brethine 2.5 mg, orally, every eight hours
    d. Alupent 0.65 mg, 2 puffs t.i.d.

23. Treatment of internal hemorrhoids include all of the following except?
    a. Psyllium hydrophilic mucilloid
    b. Instructions on proper lifting techniques
    c. Hemorrhoidectomy
    d. Rectal lavage

Answers

1. b
2. c
3. b
4. c
5. d
6. a
7. c
8. c
9. b
10. a
11. b
12. b
13. c
14. a
15. a
16. b
17. c
18. b
19. d
20. b
21. d
22. a
23. d

Refrences

Abrams, W., Berkow, R. (1990). *The Merck manual of geriatrics.* New Jersey: Merck Sharp and Dohme Research Laboratories.

American Cancer Society (1992). *Cancer facts and figures-1992.* Georgia: Author.

Burk, J.E. (1992). In W. Greenberger & K. Frame (Eds.), *Lippincott's review series medical-surgical nursing.* New York: J. B. Lippincott.

Carnevali, D., & Patrick, D. (1993). *Nursing management for the elderly.* Philadelphia: J. B. Lippincott.

Fay, D. E., & Lance, P. (1992). Disorders of the alimentary tract. In E. Calkins, A. Ford, & P. Katz (Eds.), *Practice of geriatrics* (2nd ed.). Philadelphia: W. B. Saunders.

Reichel, W. (1989). *Clinical aspects of aging.* Baltimore: Williams and Wilkins.

Salerno, M. (1991). Gastrointestinal problems. In V.L. Millonig (Ed.), *The adult nurse practitioner certification review guide.* Potomac, MD: Health Leadership Associates.

Renal Disorders

Debbie G. Kramer

Urinary Incontinence

- Definition: Urinary Incontinence (UI)—the involuntary loss of urine which results in a social and/or hygienic problem. Types of UI are as follows:
    1. Stress incontinence—loss of urine when coughing, sneezing, laughing, or other physical activity which increases intra-abdominal pressure
    2. Urge incontinence—loss of urine from inability to delay voiding long enough to reach the toilet
    3. Overflow incontinence—loss of urine associated with overdistension of the bladder
    4. Functional incontinence—loss of urine associated with the physical and/or cognitive inability to reach the toilet
    5. Mixed incontinence—loss of urine from more than one of the types previously defined
- Etiology
    1. Stress incontinence—most common causes are an incompetent urethra as well as weakening of the bladder neck and pelvic floor musculature; atrophic vaginitis or trauma during gynecological/urological surgery
    2. Urge incontinence—due to involuntary detrusor muscle contraction known as detrusor hyperreflexia; associated with disorders of lower genitourinary tract such as tumors, uterine prolapse and stones; disorders of the central nervous system such as stroke, dementia, hypertrophy or carcinoma of prostate; fecal impaction
    3. Overflow incontinence—most common causes are an anatomic obstruction of the bladder outlet such as prostate and urethral stricture; atonic/hypotonic bladder with inadequate contraction of the detrusor muscle; therefore bladder remains chronically full in medical conditions such as diabetes mellitus, spinal cord injury, and with anticholinergic medications
    4. Functional incontinence—due to impaired mobility such as in arthritis, gait disorders; impaired mental status such as in dementia, depression; environmental factors such as in physical barriers, lack of caregiver assistance

5. Mixed incontinence—due to a combination of two or more factors previously noted

- Incidence: Affects approximately 10 million Americans, mostly elderly, in community and institutional settings; estimated 15 to 30 percent for community dwelling older persons and more than 50 percent of nursing facility residents; prevalence rates are higher in women than men, estimated annual cost of $10 billion; many individuals do not seek assistance due to embarrassment and myth that incontinence is a normal part of aging.
- Signs and Symptoms
    1. Stress incontinence—loss of urine when coughing, laughing or other physical activity; more common in women
    2. Urge incontinence—loss of urine following sensation of urgency to void; usually moderate to large volumes of urine loss
    3. Overflow incontinence—loss of urine in frequent, small amounts; loss of sensation of bladder fullness; incomplete emptying
    4. Functional incontinence—inability to toilet appropriately due to impaired mobility; lack of awareness of desire to void
    5. Mixed incontinence—due to a combination of signs and symptoms noted above
- Differential Diagnosis: Includes identifying if acute vs. persistent urinary incontinence
    1. Acute UI—recent onset following acute medical or surgical conditions, immobility, initiation of new medications, such as diuretics, tricyclic antidepressants, anticholinergics, and antiparkinsonian drugs.
    2. Persistent UI—stress, urge, overflow, functional and mixed UI
    3. Urinary tract infection
- Physical Findings—client may be asymptomatic
    1. General
        a. Edema—may contribute to nocturia and nocturnal UI
        b. Gait abnormalities—inability to toilet oneself

2. Mental Status
    a. Decreased cognitive function—delirium, dementia, Parkinson's disease
    b. Mood and affect changes
3. Abdominal exam
    a. Presence of masses
    b. Bladder distension—evacuation disorder
4. Genital exam
    a. Foreskin irritation
    b. Glans penis irritation
5. Pelvic exam
    a. Perineal skin irritation
    b. Decreased perineal sensation
    c. Pelvic floor laxity (cystocele, rectocele, uterine prolapse)
    d. Pelvic mass
    e. Decreased perivaginal muscle tone (contraction of muscles around examining finger)
    f. Atrophic vaginitis
    g. Vaginal discharge
    h. Decreased external anal sphincter tone
6. Rectal exam
    a. Decreased perineal sensation
    b. Decreased sphincter tone
    c. Fecal impaction
    d. Rectal mass
    e. Prostatic enlargement—the size of the prostate on digital rectal examination does not imply or exclude obstruction

- Diagnostic Evaluation/Findings
    1. Provocative stress testing—conducted if stress UI suspected; may be conducted in standing or lithotomy position; have client feel bladder

fullness; place small pad over urethral area; ask client to forcefully cough three times; observe for leakage of urine which confirms stress UI

2. Normal voiding—conducted on all clients
   a. Voiding difficulty (hesitancy, strain, intermittent stream); may indicate obstruction or bladder contractility problem (urge or overflow UI)
   b. Have client void in private facility or bedside commode
   c. Measure voided amount
3. Post-void residual (PVR) volume
   a. Determined by catheterization or pelvic ultrasound within 5–10 minutes following voiding
      (1) PVR less than 50cc—adequate bladder emptying
      (2) PVR greater than 200cc—inadequate bladder emptying
   b. If difficulty passing catheter—obstruction may be present
   c. If PVR is elevated, obstruction or a bladder contractility problem may be present (urge or overflow UI)
4. Voiding records—ask client to complete record of number and pattern of incontinent accidents (frequency, volume and condition for each episode)
   a. Stress UI—accidents occur when coughing, sneezing, laughing, or during physical activity; typically small amounts of urine loss
   b. Urge UI—accidents occur when immediate urge to void occurs with immediate urine loss; typically moderate to large amounts of urine loss
   c. Overflow UI—accidents occur frequently; frequent voiding; typically small amounts of urine loss frequently or continuously
   d. Functional UI—accidents occur due to inability or unwillingness of client to toilet appropriately; large amounts of urine loss
   e. Mixed UI—accidents occur in a variety of incidences noted above

The following are used to detect associated and contributing conditions such as renal disease, cancer, stones and infection.

5. Urinalysis and culture
6. Blood tests
   a. BUN/creatinine
   b. Glucose
   c. Prostate-specific antigen (PSA)

- Management/Treatment
  1. Behavioral management
     a. Bladder training/retraining (urge UI)
        (1) Education of client regarding normal and abnormal functioning of the lower urinary tract incorporating a variety of instructional methods
        (2) Scheduled voiding—adjusting the interval between mandatory voidings, such as every two hours, gradually increasing the interval, and training the client to consciously delay voiding while utilizing relaxation techniques and positive reinforcement
     b. Habit training
        (1) Scheduled toileting/timed voiding on a planned time schedule
        (2) Coordinate with client's regular voiding patterns
        (3) Learn bladder pattern, alter voiding to avoid accidents
     c. Prompted voiding (for cognitively and mobility impaired clients to teach to discriminate continence status)
        (1) Monitor—check continence status on regular basis
        (2) Prompt—request client void
        (3) Praise—positive reinforcement
     d. Pelvic muscle exercises, known as Kegel exercises (stress UI)
        (1) Improve urethral resistance by exercising the pubococcygeus muscle

(2) Strengthen the voluntary periurethral and pelvic muscles

(a) Contract perivaginal and anal sphincter as if to control urination or defecation

(b) Do not contract abdominal, buttocks or inner thigh muscles

(3) Give written instructions

(a) Sustain contraction for up to 10 seconds

(b) Relax muscles for 10 seconds

(c) Repeat 30–80 times per day

(d) Continue for a minimum of six weeks

e. Vaginal cones—used intravaginally to strengthen the pelvic muscles

f. Biofeedback—(stress and urge UI)

(1) Use of mechanical instruments to train clients to contract pelvic floor muscles and relax the bladder

(2) Used in conjunction with other forms of behavioral therapies

(3) Limited by knowledge/skill of health care provider and invasive techniques necessary (bladder and/or rectal probe)

g. Electrical stimulation

(1) Stimulation of pelvic muscles and organs as well as nerve supply

(2) Used for bladder and urethral dysfunction

(3) Advanced training is required

2. Pharmacological management

a. Stress Incontinence—drugs used to cause muscle contraction in the bladder neck, bladder base and proximal urethra, thereby increasing bladder outlet resistant

(1) Phenylpropanolamine—alpha-adrenergic agonist agent

(a) Used to treat sphincter insufficiency

        (b) Side effects include anxiety, insomnia, respiratory difficulty, headache, and cardiac arrhythmias

        (c) All side effects occur more commonly in the elderly

    (2) Estrogen therapy—females only

        (a) May restore urethral mucosal coaptation and increase vascularity, tone and increase bladder outlet resistance

        (b) Can be used orally, vaginally, or by transdermal method

        (c) Contraindicated in clients with undiagnosed vaginal bleeding, cancer of the breast, uterus; active liver disease, thromboembolic disorders

        (d) Side effects include headaches, breast tenderness, fluid retention, nausea

        (e) Beneficial effects may include decreased risk of heart disease and osteoporosis

        (f) Benefit to urge UI documented

    (3) Combined alpha-adrenergic agonist and estrogen therapy—limited studies at present

b. Urge incontinence—drugs used to treat storage disorders and increase bladder capacity

    (1) Propantheline—anticholinergic agent

        (a) Blocks contraction of the normal bladder

        (b) Inexpensive; widely used—avoid in elderly with dementia

        (c) Side effects include xerostomia, blurred vision, constipation and dizziness; can cause urinary retention, confusion and increased intraocular pressure

    (2) Oxybutynin—anticholinergic

        (a) Direct smooth muscle relaxant

(b) Side effects include dry skin, blurred vision, nausea, constipation and marked xerostomia which are dose dependent

(3) Calcium channel blockers—detrusor muscle contraction blocker; not recommended for general use

(4) Tricyclic agents

(a) Found statistically significant for nocturnal incontinence

(b) Side effects include fatigue, xerostomia, dizziness, blurred vision, insomnia and urinary retention

(c) Associated with increased risk of falling and hip fracture

(5) Dicyclomine hydrochloride—anticholinergic agent

(a) Smooth muscle relaxant properties

(b) Shown effective in research studies to control detrusor overactivity

(c) Side effects include xerostomia, blurred vision, constipation and dizziness; can cause urinary retention

c. Mixed UI

Imipramine

(a) A tricyclic antidepressant which blocks the uptake of norepinephrine and has anticholinergic properties

(b) Useful in nocturnal incontinence, clinical experience suggests benefit for mixed urge and stress UI

(c) Side effects include impaired myocardial contractility and postural hypotension; anticholinergic side effects may occur

3. Surgical Treatment

a. Only after all other therapies have been unsuccessful

b. Referral made to specialists

c. Type of treatment is dependent on type of incontinence

(1) Stress—bladder neck suspension

(2) Urge—removal of obstructing pathological lesions

(3) Overflow—removal of anatomic obstruction such as benign prostatic hypertrophy (BPH), urethral stricture and prostatic cancer

d. Various other surgical and non-surgical interventions

(1) Intermittent self-catheterization

(2) Indwelling catheters

(3) Suprapubic catheters

(4) External collection devices such as condom catheters

(5) Penile clamps

(6) Pessaries

(7) Absorbent pads and undergarments

- Nursing Considerations

1. Education

a. Public awareness that UI is not a consequence of aging; is manageable if not treatable

b. Patient education of all treatment options available

2. Nursing intervention

a. Stress UI

(1) Maintain fluid balance

(2) Regulate voiding patterns utilizing voiding records

(3) Prevent skin breakdown

(4) Observe for drug side effects

(5) Close management to monitor change

(6) Evaluate need for pads

(7) Institute behavioral therapies

b. Urge UI—as above and include:
   (1) Limit fluid intake in evenings to reduce nocturnal incontinence
   (2) Condom catheters may be useful in non-responsive male clients

c. Overflow—as above and include:
   (1) Perform Crede maneuver (apply external pressure over the symphysis pubis)
   (2) Perform Valsalva maneuver
   (3) Monitor for fecal impaction
   (4) Maintain good bowel habits

d. Functional—as above and include:
   (1) Provide physical assistance and guidance (wheelchairs, bedside commodes, appropriate clothing to toilet easily, accessible facilities)
   (2) Provide staff training and management

Cystitis

- Definition: Cystitis is an inflammation of the bladder wall; may result from poor perineal hygiene, sexual intercourse or surgical procedures and instrumentation
- Etiology: The cause of cystitis is a bacteria generally due to an ascending infection from the bladder; most common organism in women is *Escherichia coli*; most common organism in men is Proteus species
- Incidence: The prevalence of urinary tract infections (UTI) increase with age; most common type of infection in the elderly; individuals with diabetes, neurogenic bladders or in a debilitated state are also at high risk; the elderly may be asymptomatic
- Signs and Symptoms
  1. Dysuria and burning on urination
  2. Urgency and frequency of urination

3. Nocturia
4. Hematuria
5. Suprapubic pain

- Differential Diagnosis
    1. Vaginitis
    2. Sexually transmitted diseases
    3. Urethritis
    4. Prostatitis
    5. Pyelonephritis
    6. Abdominal disease
    7. Reinfection
- Physical Findings
    1. Normal temperature or low grade fever up to 101° F
    2. Suprapubic tenderness
    3. No flank pain
    4. Foul smelling urine; possibly gross hematuria
    5. Incontinence
- Diagnostic Evaluation/Findings
    1. Clean catch urine specimen
        a. Urinalysis—presence of white blood cells, red blood cells and bacteria
        b. Culture and sensitivity—bacteriuria greater than 100,000 bacteria/cu mm
- Management/Treatment
    1. Antibiotic therapy specific to organism for seven to ten days
        a. Trimethoprim—sulfamethoxazole double strength b.i.d.
        b. Amoxicillin 250 or 500 mg t.i.d.
        c. Erythromycin 250 to 500 mg q.i.d. (for clients allergic to penicillin)

   d. Nitrofurantoin 50 mg q.i.d.
   e. Sulfisoxazole 1 gram q.i.d.
2. Repeat urinalysis and culture following completion of medication to ensure cure

- Nursing Considerations
  1. Increase fluid intake (as long as no medical contraindications) to decrease concentration of urine and irritation
  2. Avoid alcohol and caffeine if bladder spasm present
  3. Teach medication protocol; instruct to complete entire regimen even though symptoms may subside within 72 hours
  4. Explain disease course; more common in females because of close proximity of urinary, vaginal and rectal openings; need for good perineal care
  5. Encourage juices that acidify urine such as cranberry and prune juice
  6. Recommend cotton underwear and loose-fitting clothes
  7. Avoid bubble baths and perfumed products

Acute Pyelonephritis

- Definition: Acute pyelonephritis is an infection of the renal parenchyma and the renal pelvis
- Etiology: Usually the result of an ascending infection; usually bacterial (the most common *Escherichia coli*) but may be secondary to metabolic diseases, renal disease, urinary obstruction and trauma
- Incidence: Eight to ten percent of clients with symptomatic UTIs have pyelonephritis. It occurs more frequently in debilitated, hospitalized or diabetic clients
- Signs and Symptoms
  1. Fever of 101° F to 104° F
  2. Chills
  3. Flank, back, or abdominal pain (unilateral or bilateral)
  4. Nausea, vomiting

5. Frequency of urination
6. Dysuria
7. Malaise
8. Incontinence
9. Mental confusion

- Differential Diagnosis
    1. Cystitis
    2. Prostatitis
    3. Renal pelvis or ureteral stones
    4. Other causes of back pain
- Physical Findings
    1. Fever of 101° F to 104° F
    2. Tenderness over flank or costovertebral region
    3. Foul smelling urine; possibly gross hematuria, proteinuria
    4. Incontinence
- Diagnostic Evaluation/Findings
    1. Clean catch urine specimen
        a. Urinalysis—pyuria, WBC casts, bacteriuria, hematuria
        b. Immunofluorescence of antibody-coated bacteria—differentiates cystitis from pyelonephritis
    2. Serum creatinine/BUN—elevated
    3. Ultrasound—renal pelvis or ureteral obstruction
    4. Blood cultures—if clinical condition deteriorates
- Management/Treatment
    1. Referral to a specialist for treatment
    2. Antibiotic therapy to cover all important gram-negative uropathogens; minimum 10 days
        a. May successfully treat community-acquired infections as an outpatient with second-generation cephalosporin

   b. In clients with hospital-acquired infections, a third-generation cephalosporin or an aminoglycoside is preferred

3. Urinary analgesic such as phenazopyridine hydrochloride as needed for dysuria

- Nursing Considerations
  1. If treated as an outpatient, maintain regular telephone contact during acute phase
  2. Increase fluid intake up to two to three liters per day to decrease concentration of urine
  3. Teach proper medication regimen—include importance of completing full course of therapy
  4. Teach methods to prevent reinfection, good personal hygiene, emptying bladder regularly to avoid overdistension
  5. Monitor other major health problems closely
  6. Explain severity of acute pyelonephritis with repeated infections; end-state renal failure may result
  7. Screen urine routinely for reoccurrences

Prostatitis

- Definition: Inflammation of the prostate gland; may have recent history of catheterization, gastrointestinal, genitourinary or upper respiratory infection
- Etiology: Result of bacterial infection; often caused by *Escherichia coli*, but Klebsiella, Enterobacter and *Proteus mirabilis* are also common pathogens; prostatitis contributes to the recurrence of UTI in men
- Incidence: In men less than 50 years of age, prostatitis is rare; incidence increases with advancing age; prostate may become chronically inflamed from microcalculi; any condition which obstructs urinary flow can predispose to infection
- Signs and Symptoms
  1. Dysuria
  2. Urgency
  3. Frequency

4. Nocturia
5. Malaise
6. Chills
7. Fever
8. Suprapubic, perineal, lower back, rectal pain

- Differential Diagnosis
  1. Benign prostatic hypertrophy
  2. Prostatic cancer
  3. Back pain from other causes
  4. UTI
- Physical Findings
  1. Digital rectal exam—prostate may be normal, enlarged; in acute prostatitis, prostatic massage is contraindicated
  2. Tender or boggy
  3. Fever 100° F or higher
- Diagnostic Evaluation/Findings
  1. Urine specimen
     a. Urinalysis—presence of WBC; possibly RBC
     b. Urine culture—identify causative organism
  2. CBC
  3. Bacterial count of prostatic secretions
- Management/Treatment: Antibiotic therapy for two to twelve weeks; commonly used drugs include trimethoprim—sulfamethoxazole, doxycycline, and erythromycin
- Nursing Considerations
  1. Explain medication regimen; purpose of length of course of therapy; symptoms should subside within seven days
  2. Nutrition:
     a. Increase fluid intake to two to three liters per day

   b. Avoid food/fluid irritants such as coffee, tea, alcohol, spicy foods and nuts

3. Instruct on sitz baths to promote muscle relaxation
4. Bedrest may be necessary during acute phase
5. Refer to specialist if recurrent

Benign Prostatic Hypertrophy (BPH)

- Definition: Benign prostatic hypertrophy is the enlargement of the prostate gland; common in men over age 50, the prostate increases its fibromuscular stroma and encroaches on the urethra, obstructing the urine flow
- Etiology: Unclear; associated with decreased testicular hormones; as prostate enlarges, a change in the urinary pattern of elimination occurs; the bladder initially compensates but eventually becomes non-compliant and hypotonic
- Incidence: The disease is associated with aging; majority of older men have some degree of BPH
- Signs and Symptoms
  1. Difficulty initiating stream, hesitancy
  2. Decreased force of stream
  3. Urgency
  4. Post void dribbling
  5. Frequency
  6. Nocturia
  7. Retention
  8. Sensation of full bladder immediately after voiding
  9. Incontinence
- Differential Diagnosis
  1. Prostatic cancer
  2. Other causes of abnormal bladder emptying—diabetes mellitus, medications

- Physical Findings
  1. Digital rectal exam—enlarged prostate, possibly nodular
  2. Abdominal exam—palpate bladder for overdistension
- Diagnostic Evaluation/Findings
  1. Urinalysis—if infection is suspected
  2. Blood Studies
     a. Creatinine and BUN
     b. Serum acid phosphatase—seen in prostatic carcinoma with bone metastasis
     c. Prostate specific antigen (PSA)—a serine protease produced by both benign and malignant prostatic epithelium
  3. Ultrasound
- Management/Treatment
  1. Dependent on severity
  2. Evaluate medication usage; avoid diuretics, anticholinergics and anti-arrhythmic agents
  3. Refer to specialist for evaluation for prostatectomy; type dependent on size of gland and client status
- Nursing Considerations
  1. Observe for signs of urinary retention
  2. Evaluate for bladder distention
  3. Client verbalizes understanding of BPH; is aware when to report symptoms
  4. Teach client that impotency is not a complication of surgery
  5. Avoid caffeine and alcohol to decrease bladder irritation

Prostate Cancer

- Definition: Cancer is a malignant growth; it may spread to surrounding tissue and metastasize to other areas of the body
- Etiology: Cancer of the prostate arises primarily in the peripheral zone; may spread to involve other areas; when it occupies the greater part of

the gland, it may infiltrate the sphincter, and metastasize to the bones of the pelvis, spine or femur; most prostatic cancers are adenocarcinomas

- Incidence: Prostatic cancer is the second most common cause of cancer death in men over 75 years of age; cancer is present in 10–12 percent of men in the 60s; between 20–40 percent in men over age 70; up to 70 percent of men over 80 years of age have prostatic cancer although most are not clinically apparent; the prognosis is dependent on the stage of the cancer when detected; incidence of prostate cancer is 50% greater in African-Americans than whites and relatively uncommon on Orientals
- Signs and Symptoms
  1. May be asymptomatic
  2. May have subtle urinary symptoms in early stages
  3. In advanced stages
     a. Impotency
     b. Symptoms of urethral obstruction
        (1) Frequency
        (2) Dysuria
        (3) Hesitancy, delay of stream
        (4) Hematuria
     c. Back pain
     d. Weakness
- Differential Diagnosis
  1. Benign prostatic hypertrophy
  2. Prostatitis
- Physical Findings
  1. Digital rectal exam
     a. Firm prostatic nodules
     b. Indurated irregular prostate
  2. Urinary retention with bladder distension
  3. Unexplained weight loss

- Diagnostic Evaluation/Findings
  1. Blood tests
     a. Serum acid phosphatase—seen in prostatic carcinoma with bone metastasis
     b. Prostate-specific antigen (PSA)—a serine protease produced by both benign and malignant prostatic epithelium; rate of change in serial PSA levels may be a clinical marker for the development of prostate cancer; normal level of PSA is less than 4.0 ng/mL; values greater than 10 ng/mL are suggestive of neoplasm
     c. CBC—detect anemia
  2. Chest x-ray
  3. Bone scan—20 percent of clients presenting with prostate cancer have a positive bone scan
  4. Computerized tomography (CT) and nuclear magnetic resonance (NMR) imaging are used to identify pelvic lymph node involvement
- Management/Treatment

  Dependent on clinical presentation and stage of cancer when detected
  1. Referral to specialist for:
     a. Prostatectomy—radical perineal, retropubic or transcoccygeal
     b. Hormonal manipulation (delayed until evidence of disease progression)
        (1) Orchiectomy
        (2) Leuprolide—blocks release of FSH and LH and decreases testosterone production
        (3) Antiandrogens
     c. Radiotherapy
  2. Pain management with long-acting oral morphine compounds
  3. Other new drug therapies being investigated
     a. Diphosphonates—for bony metastases
     b. Estracyt—estrogen and alkylating agent combination for metastatic disease

    c. Prednimustine—chlorambucil and prednisolone combination

4. With failure of above options, some clients may benefit from chemotherapy

- Nursing Considerations
    1. Educate the client and family
        a. Treatment options, complications
        b. Physiological and psychological effects of treatments
        c. Effect on bony metastases; risk of falls, fractures
    2. Refer to support group or counselor
    3. Refer to hospice for pain management at home
    4. Teach relaxation techniques

Renal Failure

- Definition: Significant decrease in renal function occurs in normal aging. Renal failure is the impairment of renal function; the kidneys are unable to concentrate and excrete urine, maintain fluid and electrolyte and acid-base balance, or filter nitrogenous wastes. The glomerular filtration rate declines beginning in mid-life and by age 70 the blood urea nitrogen (BUN) nearly doubles. There are two classifications of renal failure:
    1. Acute renal failure (ARF)—the clinical condition associated with abrupt, steadily increasing azotemia with dramatic reduction in urine output (<500 ml/day) usually caused by poor perfusion, obstruction or infection
    2. Chronic renal failure (CRF)—the clinical condition associated with persistent alteration in and insufficiency of renal function with decreased renal blood flow
- Etiology
    1. Acute renal failure—ARF occurs in the elderly because of significant events such as marked volume depletion from hypotension, major surgery or procedures, and indiscrimant use of antibiotics. The elderly may have pre-existing moderately decreased renal function which increases the risk
    2. Chronic renal failure—CRF is caused by renal disease and other

age-dependent illnesses and chronic diseases such as BPH, chronic glomerulonephritis, urinary tract obstruction, hypertension, diabetes mellitus, heart failure, volume depletion, connective tissue disorders, or multiple myeloma

- Incidence
  1. Acute renal failure—seen more frequently in the elderly; recent research suggests age has a significant impact on the outcome of acute renal failure; up to 50 percent of hospitalizations for acute renal failure are for clients over the age of 70
  2. Chronic renal failure—seen more frequently in the elderly; pre-existing diseases may complicate renal disease
- Signs and Symptoms
  1. Acute renal failure
     a. Fatigue, drowsiness
     b. Nausea, vomiting
     c. Scant urine output
     d. Flank pain
  2. Chronic renal failure
     a. Asymptomatic
     b. Fatigue, drowsiness
     c. Anorexia
     d. Nausea, vomiting
     e. Pruritis
     f. Mental status changes
     g. Uremic frost—crystallized perspiration on the skin
- Differential Diagnosis: Obstruction due to prostatism, tumor, kidney stones; acute tubular necrosis
- Physical Findings
  1. Acute renal failure
     a. Decreased skin turgor
     b. Low jugular venous pressure

c. Postural tachycardia

d. Hypotension

e. Flank pain

2. Chronic renal failure

a. Fluid accumulation resulting in:

(1) Hypertension

(2) Peripheral edema

(3) Pulmonary edema

b. Pericarditis

c. Confusion, coma

- Diagnostic Evaluation/Findings

1. Acute renal failure

a. Blood work

(1) Plasma creatinine concentration—recent increase of at least 0.5 mg/dl if the baseline level is ≤3.0 mg/dl, or at least 1.0 mg/dl if baseline level is >3.0 mg/dl

(2) Blood urea nitrogen (BUN)/plasma creatinine ratio-greater than 20:1

(3) Serum potassium, chloride, phosphate, magnesium-elevated

(4) Serum sodium, calcium, bicarbonate-decreased

(5) Arterial blood gases—acidosis

b. Urinalysis—hyaline casts may be seen

2. Chronic renal failure

a. Blood work

(1) Blood chemistries

(a) Potassium > 6.0 meq/l

(b) BUN > 70–80 mg/dl

(c) Creatinine > 6 ml/dl—may fail to rise as high in elderly due to decreased muscle mass

(d) Calcium—decreased

(2) Hematocrit—normochromic, normocytic anemia

(3) Arterial blood gases—metabolic acidosis

b. Urinalysis—proteinuria, hematuria, white and red blood cells, and casts

- Management/Treatment

1. Acute renal failure

a. Refer to specialist to rule out urinary obstruction (from conditions such as BPH, prostatic carcinoma or gynecological malignancy); consider dialysis and monitor status

b. Treat underlying cause

c. Re-evaluate medication regimen to limit drugs excreted by the kidneys

d. Fluid restriction—600 ml/day

e. Limit sodium and potassium intake

f. Daily weights—ARF client loses about 1 lb. of body mass/day due to catabolism

2. Chronic renal failure

a. Identify reversible cause

b. Control hypertension

c. Re-evaluate medication regimen to limit drugs excreted by kidneys; adjust dose and dosing schedule of medications—especially digoxin

d. Treat anemia

(1) Evaluate serum iron and ferritin

(2) Do not rely on RBC indices

(3) Give iron supplements

e. Nutritional status

(1) Monitor protein, sodium and potassium to maintain nitrogen balance; moderate protein and salt restriction; strict restrictions often unnecessary

(2) Monitor fluid balance

f. Refer to specialist; consider if renal transplant or dialysis candidate; currently renal transplant is generally not considered in clients >60 years of age

- Nursing Considerations
  1. Explain to client the importance of taking only prescribed medication, some over-the-counter medications can cause further renal damage if excreted by the kidneys
  2. Monitor weight daily and record; notify of weight gain
  3. Nutritional education
     a. Client should be referred to a dietician for counseling
     b. Avoid salt substitutes, high in potassium
     c. Watch fluid restrictions to prevent hypervolemia
  4. Teach the client the early signs of fluid imbalance
  5. Encourage use of moisturizing lotions for the skin if pruritis exists
  6. Discuss renal failure and how it progresses
  7. Review implications for renal dialysis

Questions

1. Mr. Jones, age 80, can no longer get to the toilet before becoming incontinent. He has:

   a. Stress incontinence
   b. Urge incontinence
   c. Overflow incontinence
   d. Functional incontinence

2. Mr. Brown, age 90, lives in a nursing home. He is mildly demented and spends most of his day in a wheelchair near the nurse's station. The most likely cause of his incontinence is:

   a. Mixed incontinence
   b. Urge incontinence
   c. Overflow incontinence
   d. Functional incontinence

3. Mrs. Hamilton is 72 years old and lives at home with her younger sister. Mrs. Hamilton has episodes of urinary incontinence when laughing and when hurrying to the bathroom. She exhibits signs of:

   a. Stress incontinence
   b. Mixed stress and urge incontinence
   c. Mixed stress and functional incontinence
   d. Overflow incontinence

4. Mrs. Hamilton has not spoken to anyone about her incontinence. This is probably due to:
   a. The myth that incontinence is a normal change of aging
   b. Fear that she may have a serious problem
   c. The fact that there is no treatment
   d. The cause is unknown

5. Stress incontinence can be caused by weakening of the pelvic floor musculature as well as:

   a. A chronically full bladder
   b. Outlet obstruction
   c. An incompetent urethra
   d. An obstructed ureter

6. When the detrusor muscle is unable to contract sufficiently to have complete bladder emptying, it is likely to result in:

   a. Overflow incontinence
   b. Functional incontinence
   c. Mixed incontinence
   d. Urge incontinence

7. In addressing the acute onset of urinary incontinence, the evaluation of the client's medication regimen is reviewed. All of the following medications may affect urinary incontinence except:

   a. Anticholinergics
   b. Diuretics
   c. Antidepressants
   d. Aminoglycosides

8. When assessing an incontinent client, it is important to evaluate the client's functional status because of:

   a. The ability to toilet oneself appropriately
   b. Physiological changes
   c. The complete bladder emptying
   d. Obstructive disorders

9. A post void residual (PVR) urine is determined by:

   a. An MRI
   b. A CT scan of the pelvis
   c. A pelvic ultrasound
   d. Observing the voiding pattern

10. Bladder training and retraining, a behavioral method to treat urge incontinence, uses:

   a. Voiding upon request
   b. Scheduled voiding with adjusted intervals between voidings
   c. Prompted voiding
   d. Rigid sequential voiding schedule

11. Kegel exercises:

   a. Improve abdominal muscles
   b. Strengthen the pubococcygeus muscle

c. Decrease urethral resistance
d. Relax the anal sphincter

12. Biofeedback is useful for:

    a. Mixed stress and urge incontinence
    b. Functional incontinence alone
    c. Mixed functional and overflow incontinence
    d. Urge incontinence alone

13. Alpha-adrenergic agonist agents are used to treat sphincter insufficiency in stress incontinence. Side effects include all of the following except:

    a. Respiratory difficulty
    b. Cardiac arrhythmias
    c. Gastric irritation
    d. Anxiety

14. Estrogen therapy may be used for stress incontinence. It is contraindicated in women with the following condition:

    a. Thromboembolic disease
    b. Hypertension
    c. Diabetes
    d. Ulcerative colitis

15. The most common organism responsible for cystitis in women is:

    a. Proteus
    b. Chlamydia
    c. *Escherichia coli*
    d. Enterobacter

16. Mr. Johnson, a 62 year old gentleman, presents to the clinic complaining of dysuria, urgency, suprapubic pain and incontinence. The urinalysis reveals the presence of white blood cells, red blood cells and bacteria. You suspect:

    a. Cystitis
    b. Pyelonephritis
    c. Benign prostatic hypertrophy
    d. Prostatitis

17. After you establish a diagnosis, you learn Mr. Johnson is allergic to penicillin. You decide to treat him with:

    a. Trimethoprim
    b. Amoxicillin
    c. Sulfamethoxazole
    d. Erythromycin

18. A 75 year old man comes to see you at the clinic for nonspecific complaints of weakness and fatigue. He has a past history of coronary artery disease with a triple vessel bypass five years ago. He is currently on no medications. The physical examination reveals a blood pressure of 110/70. Skin turgor is normal and he has no signs of edema. He then comments that he has not voided since yesterday. On his last visit you drew blood work showing a BUN and creatinine of 18/1.6. You repeat it today and the results are 50/2.2. The urinalysis is normal. The hematocrit is unchanged at 39%. You suspect:

    a. Acute pyelonephritis
    b. Acute renal failure
    c. Urinary obstruction
    d. Prostate cancer

19. You are discussing BPH with your client. While assessing his knowledge, he relates the following information to you. He is correct in all of his statements *except:*

    a. "The UTIs may be caused by my large prostate."
    b. "I need to be examined twice a year for the rest of my life to detect cancer."
    c. "If I need surgery, I should not have a problem with impotency."
    d. "BPH is very common in older men."

20. A 72 year old woman complains of frequency, urgency and dysuria for two days. She also has suprapubic tenderness and a mild fever. You suspect cystitis. Your initial step is to:

    a. Start client on antibiotic therapy
    b. Refer to a specialist
    c. Obtain a clean-catch urinalysis, culture and sensitivity
    d. Schedule a cystoscopy

21. Nursing considerations for client education for cystitis include:
    a. Avoid combining alcohol and caffeine
    b. Limit fluid intake to 500 cc per day
    c. Recommend nylon underwear
    d. Avoid bubble baths and perfumed products

22. Mr. Garcia is a 68 year old gentleman who you follow for hypertension, diabetes mellitus and emphysema. He complains today of nausea, vomiting, fever and flank pain. On physical exam you confirm a temperature elevation of 102° F and costovertebral tenderness. The urinalysis and blood chemistries suggest acute pyelonephritis. You order a renal ultrasound to identify:
    a. Prostatic lesion
    b. Ureteral obstruction
    c. Vaginal prolapse
    d. Overdistension of the bladder

23. After placing Mr. Garcia on appropriate antibiotic therapy, you explain the following important interventions:
    a. Kegel exercises
    b. Limit fluid intake
    c. Attempt to void less frequently
    d. Screen urine routinely to identify recurrent infections

24. If Mr. Garcia starts having recurrent symptoms of frequency, urgency, hesitancy and nocturia, your next step is:
    a. Start another course of antibiotic therapy
    b. Schedule a prostatic biopsy
    c. Schedule a cystoscopy
    d. Refer him to a specialist

25. Prostatic enlargement begins at:
    a. Puberty
    b. About 40 years of age
    c. About 50 years of age
    d. About 70 years of age

26. Mrs. Adams, a client with chronic renal failure is being discharged. Your instructions are:

a. Take aspirin for fever
b. Use salt substitutes to decrease sodium intake
c. Drink eight glasses of water a day to prevent dehydration
d. Report significant weight gain

27. A client presenting with acute renal failure exhibits which of the following symptoms:

    a. Fatigue and scant urine output
    b. Pruritis and hypotension
    c. Anorexia and fever
    d. Distended bladder

28. When the kidneys are unable to concentrate urine, maintain electrolyte balance and filter waste, this describes:

    a. Renal failure
    b. Benign prostatic hypertrophy
    c. Prostate cancer
    d. Urinary tract infection

29. A client presents to clinic to see you. Upon examination, you find he has an enlarged prostate and an overdistended bladder. Your most likely diagnosis is:

    a. Benign prostatic hypertrophy
    b. Prostate cancer
    c. Prostatitis
    d. Overflow incontinence

30. The client's PSA 6 months ago was 4 ng/ml. The client returns for a follow-up visit stating: "My pants are too baggy." When prompted for more information, he admits to having trouble urinating. You redraw the PSA with the following result: 78 ng/ml. The most likely diagnosis is:

    a. Renal failure
    b. Urinary retention
    c. Prostate cancer
    d. Prostatitis

31. What symptoms would you find in *advanced* prostate cancer?

    a. Hematuria
    b. Fever

c. Suprapubic pain
d. Polyuria

32. Frequently, clients with UI are asymptomatic except for their incontinence. However, during the examination, previously undiagnosed findings may be noted. Which of the following physical findings may contribute to UI:

    a. Orthostatic hypotension
    b. Edema
    c. Testicular enlargement
    d. Dehydration

Answers

1. b	12. a	23. d
2. d	13. c	24. d
3. b	14. a	25. c
4. a	15. c	26. d
5. c	16. a	27. a
6. a	17. d	28. a
7. d	18. b	29. a
8. a	19. b	30. c
9. c	20. c	31. a
10. b	21. d	32. b
11. b	22. b	

Bibliography

Abrams, W. B., & Berkow, R. (Eds.). (1990). *The Merck manual of geriatrics.* Rahway, NJ: Merck Sharp & Dohme Research Laboratories.

Brocklehurst, J. C., & Tallis, R. C. (Eds.). (1992). *Textbook of geriatric medicine and gerontology* (4th ed.). New York: Churchill Livingstone.

Burgio, K. L., & Engel, B. T. (1990). Biofeedback-assisted behavioral training for elderly men and women. *Journal of the American Geriatrics Society,* 38(3), 338–340.

Eaton, N. (1988). *Urinary incontinence in adults.* National Institutes of Health Consensus Development Conference Consensus Statement, 7(5), 1–32.

Carter, H. B., Pearson, J. D., Metter, E. J., Brant, L. J., Chan, D. W., Andres, R., Fozard, J. L., & Walsh, P. C. (1992). Longitudinal evaluation of prostate-specific antigen levels in men with and without prostate disease. *Journal of the American Medical Association,* 267(16), 2215–2220.

Eliopoulos, C. (1993). *Gerontological nursing.* Philadelphia: J. B. Lippincott.

Hogstel, M. O. (Ed.). (1992). *Clinical manual of gerontological nursing.* St. Louis: Mosby Year Book.

International Continence Society Committee for the Standardization of Terminology of the Lower Urinary Tract Function. (1990). *British Journal of Obstetrics and Gynaecology,* Suppl. 6, 1–16.

Kane, R. L., Ouslander, J. G., & Abrass, I. B. (1989). *Essentials of clinical geriatrics.* New York: McGraw-Hill Information Services Company.

McDowell, B. J., & Burgio, K. L. (1990). Urinary incontinence. In A. S. Staab, & M. F. Lyles (Eds.), *Manual of geriatric nursing* (pp. 432–476). Glenview, IL: Scott, Foresman and Company.

Nursing93 drug handbook. (1993). Springhouse, PA: Springhouse Corporation.

Resnick, N. M. (1988). Urinary incontinence-A treatable disorder. In J. W. Rowe, & R. W. Besdine (Eds.), *Geriatric medicine* (pp. 246–265). Boston: Little, Brown and Company.

Rose, B. D., & Black, R. M. (1988). *Manual of clinical problems in nephrology.* Boston: Little Brown and Company.

Rowe, J. W. (1988). Renal system. In J. W. Rowe, & R. W. Besdine (Eds.), *Geriatric medicine* (pp. 231–245). Boston: Little, Brown and Company.

Siroky, M. B., & Krane, R. J. (Eds.). (1990). *Manual of urology.* Boston: Little, Brown and Company.

Urinary Incontinence Guideline Panel. *Urinary Incontinence in Adults: Clinical Practice Guideline.* AHCPR Pub. No. 92-0038. Rockville, MD: Agency for Health Care Policy and Research, Public Health Service, U.S. Department of Health and Human Services. March 1992.

Musculoskeletal Disorders

Maren Stewart Mayhew

Osteoporosis

- Definition: Loss of bone mineral and matrix leading to decreased density of bone that results in decreased strength of the bones and impaired skeletal function.
- Etiology:
  1. Primary Osteoporosis: The etiology of primary osteoporosis is not known. However, certain risk factors have been identified. The disease process differs somewhat between men and women. Women have an accelerated bone loss at menopause and for the next five years. Men lose more bone from the femoral neck than the vertebrae, while women lose bone at the same rate from both sites. The disease is often called postmenopausal osteoporosis in females and senile osteoporosis in males. Identified risk factors include:
     a. In women
        (1). Estrogen depletion
        (2). History of anorexia nervosa
     b. In men
        (1). Alcoholism
        (2). Testosterone depletion
     c. In both sexes
        (1). Age
        (2). Genetic—family history, caucasian race
        (3). Low body weight, small frame
        (4). Sedentary lifestyle, bed rest
        (5). Low dietary intake of calcium
        (6). Limited exposure to sunlight
        (7). Smoking, alcohol, caffeine
  2. Secondary osteoporosis has many causes including:
     a. Hyperparathyroidism
     b. Cushing's disease
     c. Multiple myeloma

d. Hyperthyroidism

e. Malabsorption

f. Chronic renal failure

g. Medications including corticosteroids and anticonvulsants

- Incidence: One of the most important disorders associated with aging. Common, 30% of women over 60 and 15% of men over 60 have clinical osteoporosis.
- Signs & Symptoms: The diagnosis of osteoporosis is by exclusion. X-rays are not sensitive until the osteoporosis is advanced. Signs & symptoms include:
  1. Loss of height
  2. Kyphosis
  3. Low back pain
  4. Hip, wrist, vertebral fractures
- Differential Diagnosis
  1. Secondary osteoporosis
  2. Osteomalacia
  3. Paget's disease of bone
  4. Malignancy
- Physical Findings: Physical examination will be normal unless a fracture has occurred.
- Diagnostic Evaluation/Findings
  1. Routine x-ray evaluation for fractures, will show osteoporosis only if advanced
  2. Dual-photon absorptiometry is more sensitive but not generally available
- Management/Treatment
  1. Prevention is the first step of treatment
     a. Diet
        (1) Calcium 1000–1500 mg per day

(2) Protein intake not to exceed 20% of total calories

(3) Adequate vitamin C and D, RDA vitamin C 60 mg, vitamin D 5 μg (200 IU)

b. Exercise—regular weight bearing

c. Stop smoking

d. Decrease alcohol & caffeine intake

2. Estrogen replacement therapy (ERT)

a. Start as soon as possible after menopause

b. Is an individual decision for each patient

c. Benefits

(1) Maintains bone mass

(2) Decreases risk of osteoporosis

(3) Decreases risk of coronary artery disease

d. Risks/adverse reactions

(1) Endometrial cancer unless progesterone given

(2) Unknown effect upon risk of breast cancer

(3) Edema, cramping, bloating

(4) May increase frequency of vascular headaches

e. Contraindications

(1) Unexplained vaginal bleeding

(2) Breast or uterine cancer, or history of

(3) Thrombotic disorders, thrombophlebitis or history of

(4) Active liver disease, hepatitis

- Nursing Considerations: Many life style changes will deceased the risk of osteoporosis. The nurse is in a good position to counsel patients to avoid the risks of osteoporosis.

1. Patient education

a. Women on ERT need regular follow-up to include:

(1) Annual mammogram

(2) Annual pelvic exam

b. Nutrition to include adequate calcium

(1) Dairy products, e.g., 1 oz. cheddar cheese = 204 mg; 1 cup skim milk = 302 mg; 1 cup low-fat yogurt = 415 mg.

(2) Calcium supplements: calcium carbonate absorbed best

c. Exercise—regular weight bearing

Osteoarthritis (OA)

- Definition: A slowly progressive, monarticular (or less common, polyarticular) disorder occurring late in life that is characterized clinically by pain, deformity, and limitation of motion and pathologically by focal erosive lesions, cartilage destruction, subchondral sclerosis, cyst formation, and large osteophytes at the joint.
- Etiology: Unknown; has been classified into idiopathic (primary) and secondary forms, depending on the absence or presence of some clearly evident underlying local or systemic etiological factors; classification may at times be artificial. Increasing consensus that osteoarthritis is not a single disorder but rather a heterogeneous group of disorders which most likely results from a complex interplay of several factors, all of which end in a stereotypical final common pathway of joint damage.
- Incidence: Most common arthritis; found in over 85% of adults over age 50 (Staab & Lyles, 1990)
- Signs and Symptoms
    1. Joint pain worse with movement and relieved by rest
    2. Stiffness of short duration (less than 15 min) after inactivity, or in the morning
    3. Pain described as aching, poorly localized
- Differential Diagnosis
    1. Osteoporosis
    2. Gout

- Physical Findings
  1. Decreased range of motion (ROM) of affected joints
  2. Crepitus (grating sensation) on ROM
  3. Little or no inflammation
  4. Joints most often affected:
     a. Hands
     b. Knee
     c. Hips
     d. Foot
     e. Spine
     f. Bony enlargement often seen in distal interphalangeal (Heberden's nodes); proximal interphalangeal (Bouchard's nodes)
- Diagnostic Evaluation/Findings
  1. Erythrocyte sedimentation rate (ESR) normal
  2. Characteristic changes visible by x-ray of joint
     a. Joint space narrowing
     b. Subchondral bony sclerosis
     c. Marginal osteophyte formation
     d. Cyst formation
- Management/Treatment
  1. Nonpharmacologic
     a. Weight reduction if arthritis is of weight bearing joints
     b. Exercise—individual exercise prescription
     c. Physical therapy
     d. Protection of joint from overuse
     e. Moist heat
     f. Ice
     g. Proper posture/body mechanics

h. Assistive devices (cane, walker)
i. Splints

2. Pharmacologic
   a. Aspirin (ASA)
   b. Nonsteroidal anti-inflammatory drugs (NSAIDs)
   c. Acetaminophen for pain, if no acute inflammation
   d. Intra-articular steroids
3. Surgery—hip and knee replacement

- Nursing Considerations
  1. Patient education
     a. Side effects of NSAIDs
        (1) GI bleed
        (2) Hepatotoxicity
        (3) Exacerbate congestive heart failure (CHF)
        (4) Confusion
        (5) Acute renal failure
     b. Individualized exercise program
        (1) Protect weight bearing joints
        (2) Swimming or water exercise
        (3) Rest after exercise

Rheumatoid Arthritis (RA)

- Definition: Systemic chronic inflammatory disease of corrective tissue that commonly manifests as a joint disorder
- Etiology: Unknown; prevailing theory is arthritogenic agents stimulate immune responses in genetically predisposed individuals (Staab & Lyles, 1990)
- Incidence: After age 55, 2–3% of population will have rheumatoid arthritis

- Signs and Symptoms
  1. Highly variable course with acute exacerbations and remissions
  2. Constitutional symptoms—fatigue, malaise, myalgias, weight loss
  3. Morning stiffness lasting 30 minutes to 2 hours
- Differential Diagnosis
  1. Osteoarthritis
  2. Gout
  3. Polymyalgia rheumatica (PMR)
  4. Systemic lupus erythematosus (SLE)
- Physical Findings
  1. Bilateral symmetrical inflammation of joints
  2. Swelling, tenderness and loss of function of joints
  3. Joints most often affected:
     a. Hands—proximal interphalangeal, metacarpal
     b. Wrists
     c. Knees
     d. Foot—metatarsal
  4. Rheumatoid nodules—subcutaneous nodules over bony prominences
  5. Late complications
     a. Limited ROM of affected joints
     b. Contractures of joints including:
        (1) Ulnar deviation of hands
        (2) Swan neck deformity
        (3) Boutonniere deformity
  6. Extra-articular complications
     a. Sjogren's syndrome—dry eyes and mouth
     b. Pleural effusion
     c. Pericarditis

   d. Diffuse distal neuropathy
   e. Vasculitis

- Diagnostic Evaluation/Findings
  1. X-ray shows characteristic pattern
     a. Soft tissue swelling in early phases
     b. Joint space narrowing, bone erosion, and subluxations in later stages
     c. Evidence of osteoporosis frequently seen in advanced RA
  2. Elevated sedimentation rate during acute inflammation
  3. Mild anemia not due to iron deficiency
  4. Serum rheumatoid factor usually (not always) positive
- Management/Treatment
  1. Nonpharmacological similar to osteoporosis
  2. Rest
     a. Local rest for acute inflammation of joint
     b. Adequate general rest
  3. Individualized exercise program
  4. Pharmacological
     a. ASA (can cause GI distress, hearing loss)
     b. NSAIDs
  5. Refer to rheumatologist
- Nursing Considerations
  1. Patient education
     a. Exercise
     b. Medications
  2. Multidisciplinary management
     a. Physical therapy (PT)
     b. Social work
     c. Occupational therapy (OT)

3. Management plan for all aspects of patient's life

Gout

- Definition: Deposition of needle-shaped crystals of monosodium urate in the joints with resultant inflammatory response
- Etiology
  1. Genetic predisposition
  2. Precipitating factors
     a. Ingestion of:
        (1) Diuretics
        (2) Food with high purine content
        (3) Alcohol
     b. Emotional upset
     c. Minor trauma
     d. Surgery
- Incidence—275 per 100,000 per year
- Signs and Symptoms
  1. Acute—sudden onset of acute inflammation of single joint of extremity (most often large toe)—pain, tenderness, redness, swelling, and warmth
  2. Chronic—joint pain in several joints
- Differential Diagnosis
  1. Acute—septic arthritis
  2. Chronic—osteoarthritis, rheumatoid arthritis
- Physical Findings
  1. Acute inflammation of single joint, usually peripheral
  2. Tophi around previously affected joints

- Diagnostic Evaluation/Findings
  1. Aspirate joint fluid—crystals seen, on microscopic examination in acute gout
  2. X-ray shows characteristic lesions in chronic gout—Tophus formation
  3. Twenty-four hour urine to evaluate uric acid production
- Management/Treatment
  1. Acute gout
     a. NSAID—Indomethacin (Indocin) 50 mg po 3–4 times/day, OR
     b. Colchicine 0.5 mg orally every hour until improvement, GI distress, or maximum dose of 6 mg
     c. Rest affected joint
     d. Increase fluid intake
     e. Diet low in purines
     f. Avoid alcohol
     g. Pain medication may be necessary
  2. Chronic gout
     a. Diet low in purines
     b. Avoid alcohol
     c. Allopurinol
        (1) Not used in acute gout
        (2) Dose 100–300 mg/day
        (3) Has life threatening side effects
            (a) Hypersensitivity syndrome
            (b) Bone marrow depression
- Nursing Considerations
  1. Patient education
     a. Avoid foods high in purines
        (1) Organ meats

(2) Shell fish

(3) Preserved fish (anchovies, sardines)

b. Avoid alcohol

c. How to take medications

(1) Acute gout

(2) Chronic gout

d. Rest affected joint

Falls

- Definition: To drop, collapse under influence of gravity from lack of structural support
- Etiology: Multifactorial
  1. Environmental hazards
  2. Sensory impairment
  3. Altered posture with shift in center of gravity
  4. Decreased strength caused by muscle atrophy and/or deconditioning
  5. Slowed neurological reaction time
  6. CNS—stroke, Parkinsons, TIA, seizure, peripheral neuropathy
  7. Cognitive—dementia with impaired judgment
  8. Musculoskeletal—osteoporosis, OA, RA, foot problems
  9. Metabolic—electrolyte imbalance, dehydration, diabetes mellitus (DM)
  10. Drugs—especially those that cause orthostatic hypotension
  11. Alcohol
- Incidence
  1. Of patients over age 65, 30% fall each year
  2. Accidents are the sixth leading cause of death in persons over 65
- Signs and Symptoms: Patient often will not volunteer information, nurse will have to ask about falls

- Differential Diagnosis
  1. Dizziness
  2. Syncope
  3. TIA
  4. Seizure
- Physical Findings
  1. Injuries from fall
     a. Fractures
     b. Bruises; lacerations
  2. Cause of fall may be evident during physical examination
     a. Eyes
        (1) Impaired vision
        (2) Visual field defects
     b. Ears
        (1) Decreased hearing
        (2) Vestibular dysfunction
     c. Cardiac
        (1) Arrhythmia
        (2) Orthostatic hypotension
     d. Musculoskeletal
        (1) Muscle weakness
        (2) Impaired gait
        (3) Foot abnormalities
        (4) Arthritis
     e. Neurological
        (1) Mental status—impaired judgment
        (2) Peripheral neuropathy
        (3) Decreased position sense

(4) Impaired balance

(5) Positive Romberg present

- Diagnostic Evaluation/Findings
  1. Workup based on physical findings
  2. Home safety evaluation
- Management/Treatment
  1. Identify risk factors
  2. Modify environment
  3. Treat existing medical conditions
- Nursing Considerations
  1. Conduct home safety evaluation to identify remediable risk factors
     a. Good lighting
     b. Good shoes
     c. Remove obstacles in paths
        (1) Rugs
        (2) Electrical wires
        (3) Telephone cords
  2. Counsel patient regarding fear of falling—fear of injury and embarrassment
  3. Counsel to avoid consequent decrease in activity
  4. Foot care
     a. Proper foot gear
     b. Care of toenails
     c. Corns, callouses, bunion, hammer toe—refer to podiatry

Fractures

- Definition: A break in a bone
- Etiology
  1. Osteoporosis

2. Unsteady gait
3. Falls

- Incidence: Over 200,000 hip fractures occur per year
- Signs and symptoms
  1. Hip
     a. Leg shortened
     b. Externally rotated
     c. Pain with weight bearing
  2. Distal radius (wrist)
     a. Fall with outstretched hand
     b. Pain, swelling, bruising of wrist
  3. Vertebral compression fracture
     a. Precipitated by sneezing, twisting, or no precipitant
     b. Acute back pain lasting 6–8 weeks
- Differential Diagnosis: None
- Physical Findings: See signs and symptoms
- Diagnostic Evaluation/Findings
  1. X-ray of joint
  2. May need to repeat X-ray if initially negative
- Management/Treatment
  1. Intertrochanteric surgery—pin
     a. Complications—bleeding, instability, deformity
  2. Femoral neck surgery—prosthesis
     a. Complications—avascular necrosis, infection
  3. Complications of surgery, hospitalization
     a. Deep vein thrombosis, pulmonary embolism
     b. Pressure ulcers
     c. Foley catheter UTI

   d. Constipation, impaction
   e. Confusion
4. Distal radius—cast until X-ray reveals fracture is healed
5. Vertebral compression fx—symptomatic treatment

- Nursing Considerations
  1. Rehabilitation after hip fracture a multidisciplinary effort
  2. Discharge planning to prevent
     a. Impaired mobility
     b. Social isolation

Questions

1. Which of the following is a risk factor for osteoporosis?
    a. Cigarette smoking
    b. Large body frame
    c. Black race
    d. Exercise

2. A 95 year old caucasian woman weighs 87 pounds. She has severe kyphosis. She complains of sudden onset of back pain. The most likely diagnosis is:
    a. Osteoarthritis
    b. Paget's disease of the bone
    c. Vertebral compression fracture secondary to osteoporosis
    d. Spinal tumor

3. Mrs. S. is a 65 year old white female. Her mother had severe osteoporosis. To prevent osteoporosis she should:
    a. Take calcium 500 mg per day
    b. Increase her protein intake
    c. Get regular weight bearing exercise
    d. Drink two glasses of wine with dinner

4. Mrs. S. is considering estrogen replacement therapy (ERT). An absolute contraindication would be:
    a. Family history gall bladder disease
    b. Unexplained vaginal bleeding.
    c. Past history migraine headaches
    d. Family history breast cancer

5. Mrs. S. elects to take ERT. Her nurse should teach her all except:
    a. She no longer needs to take calcium supplements
    b. She should have her blood pressure checked periodically
    c. She should have an annual mammogram
    d. She should get regular exercise

6. A common side effect of NSAIDs is:
    a. Hypertension
    b. Ataxia

c. Aplastic anemia
d. GI bleed

7. Gout can be precipitated by what category of medications?

   a. Antidepressants
   b. NSAIDs
   c. Seizure medications
   d. Diuretics

8. Which drug is NOT used in acute gout?

   a. NSAIDs
   b. Colchicine
   c. Allopurinol
   d. Pain med

9. Which of the following is NOT a characteristic of osteoarthritis?

   a. Slowly progressive course
   b. Bilateral symmetrical involvement
   c. Pain in joints
   d. Deformity of joints

10. Mrs. L., age 69, complains of a vague aching in her left knee, made worse when she walks, better when she rests. She has no morning stiffness. The most likely diagnosis is:

    a. Osteoarthritis
    b. Rheumatoid arthritis
    c. Gout
    d. Osteoporosis

11. You would consider giving Mrs. L. the following program except:

    a. Weight reduction
    b. Exercise program
    c. Nonsteroidal anti-inflammatory medication
    d. Allopurinol

12. A good exercise program for Mrs. L might be any of the following except:

    a. Walking
    b. Swimming

c. Jogging
d. Exercise bicycling

13. The most common arthritis in the elderly is:

    a. Rheumatoid arthritis
    b. Gout
    c. Osteoporosis
    d. Osteoarthritis

14. Risk factors for osteoporosis include all of the following except:

    a. Obesity
    b. Sedentary lifestyle
    c. Age
    d. Alcohol

15. Which of the following diseases has systemic constitutional symptoms?

    a. Osteoarthritis
    b. Rheumatoid arthritis
    c. Osteoporosis
    d. Gout

16. Which of the following foods is NOT high in purine?

    a. Organ meats
    b. Shell fish
    c. Cheese
    d. Preserved fish

17. Mrs. Y has bilateral acute inflammation of her wrists. She has morning stiffness lasting about two hours. The most likely diagnosis is:

    a. Osteoarthritis
    b. Rheumatoid arthritis
    c. Gout
    d. Osteoporosis

18. For Mrs. Y's initial workup you would order all the following except:

    a. CBC
    b. ESR

c. Rheumatoid factor
d. Serum albumin

19. Patient education for a patient with gout includes all of the following except:

    a. Decrease fluid intake
    b. Diet low in purine
    c. Avoid alcohol
    d. Rest affected joint

20. Risk factors for falls include all of the following except:

    a. Dementia
    b. Peripheral neuropathy
    c. Peptic ulcer disease
    d. Dehydration

21. In evaluating a patient who fell, it is important to include all of the following EXCEPT:

    a. Assess patient for injuries
    b. Identify the one single cause of the fall
    c. Evaluate home safety
    d. Workup for existing medical conditions

Answers

1. a
2. c
3. c
4. b
5. a
6. d
7. d
8. c
9. b
10. a
11. d
12. c
13. d
14. a
15. b
16. c
17. b
18. d
19. a
20. c
21. b

Bibliography

Burke, M. M., & Walsh, M. B. (1992). *Gerontologic nursing: Care of the frail elderly.* Baltimore, MD: Mosby Year Book.

Collo, M. B., Johnson, J. L., Finch, W. R., & Felicetta, J. V. (1991). Evaluating arthritic complaints. *Nurse Practitioner, 16* (2), 9–20.

Craven, R., & Dietsch, K. (1993). Musculoskeletal problems. In D. L. Carnevali & M. Patrick (Eds.), *Nursing management for the elderly* (3rd ed.). Philadelphia: J. B. Lippincott.

Grady, D., Cummings, S. R., Petitti, D., Rubin, S. M., & Audet, A. M. (1992). Guidelines for counseling postmenopausal women about preventive hormone therapy. *Annals of Internal Medicine, 117,* 1038–1041.

Grady, D., Rubin, S. M., Petitti, D. B., Fox, C. S., Black, D., Ettinger, B., Ernster, V. L., & Cummings, S. R. (1992). Hormone therapy to prevent disease and prolong life in postmenopausal women. *Annals of Internal Medicine, 117,* 1016–1036.

Guccione, A. A. (1989). Understanding arthritis in the elderly. *Focus on Geriatric Care and Rehabilitation, 3*(1), 1–8.

Hazzard, W. R., Andres, R., Bierman, E. L., & Blass, J. P. (1990). *Principles of geriatric medicine and gerontology.* New York: McGraw-Hill.

Reid, I. R., Ames, R. W., Evans, M. C., Gamble, G. D., & Sharpe, S. J. (1993). Effect of calcium supplementation on bone loss in postmenopausal women. *New England Journal of Medicine, 328,* 460–464.

Riggs, B. L., & Melton, L. J. (1992). The prevention and treatment of osteoporosis. *New England Journal of Medicine, 327* (9), 620–627.

Schulman, B. K., & Acquaviva, T. (1987). Falls in the elderly. *Nurse Practitioner, 12*(11), 30–37.

Schumacher, H. R. (1988). *Primer on the rheumatic diseases* (9th ed.). Atlanta, GA: Arthritis Foundation.

Staab, A. S., & Lyles, M. F. (1990). *Manual of geriatric nursing.* Glenview, IL: Scott, Foresman/Little Brown Higher Education.

Swartz, D. P. (Ed.). (1992). *Hormone replacement therapy.* Baltimore, MD: Williams & Wilkins.

Neurological Disorders

Maren Stewart Mayhew

Transient Ischemic Attack (TIA)

- Definition: Brief episode of focal neurologic dysfunction caused by ischemia that resolves completely without any residual deficit within 24 hours.
- Etiology: The two main causes of interrupted blood flow to the brain are:
    1. Recurrent embolism usually secondary to heart disease
    2. Cerebrovascular insufficiency (atherosclerosis of major neck vessels)
- Incidence: Important precursor to stroke; one third of those who have TIA will have a stroke within 5 years. Carotid TIAs are more frequent than vertebrobasilar and carry a worse prognosis. TIAs are also a warning sign for myocardial infarction.
- Signs and Symptoms
    1. Carotid
        a. Monocular blindness
        b. Contralateral weakness and sensory symptoms
        c. Often localized to hand or face
        d. Speech disturbance
    2. Vertebrobasilar—must have one of first four:
        a. Vertigo
        b. Dysarthria
        c. Diplopia
        d. Bilateral paresthesias
        e. Dizziness
        f. Ataxia
        g. Visual blurring
- Differential Diagnosis
    1. Seizure
    2. Syncope
    3. Migraine

4. Hypoglycemia
5. Brain tumor

- Physical Findings
    1. Variable focal neurological deficit at the time of the TIA
    2. Neurological exam usually normal between TIAs
    3. Look for:
        a. Atherosclerotic changes in fundi
        b. Hypertension
        c. Carotid bruit
        d. Arrhythmia
- Diagnostic Evaluation/Findings
    1. Initial TIA—refer to physician for probable hospitalization
    2. Workup to include as needed:
        a. History and physical examinations
        b. Urinalysis
        c. CBC, glucose, BUN, lipids, prothrombin time (PT), partial thromboplastin time (PTT)
        d. Chest x-ray
        e. EKG—look for atrial fibrillation as a cause of emboli
        f. EEG—to rule out seizures
        g. Doppler flow studies—to evaluate blood flow
        h. CT scan
- Management/Treatment
    1. Management of risk factors for stroke (hypertension, diabetes, and coronary artery disease)
    2. Recurrent embolism—anticoagulate with warfarin
    3. Cerebrovascular insufficiency
        a. Aspirin 650 mg po bid; if unable to tolerate consider ticlopidine (Ticlid) 250 mg, orally b.i.d.

b. Consider carotid endarterectomy if internal carotid artery stenosis is significant

- Nursing Education
  1. Patient education
     a. Risk factor reduction
     b. Medication dosage and side effects, e.g., aspirin may cause GI bleeding, hearing loss
     c. Anticoagulation
        (1) Watch for bruising, bleeding
        (2) Need for frequent monitoring of blood studies
  2. Allow patient to verbalize feelings related to prognosis

Stroke

- Definition: Also known as cerebrovascular accident (CVA); dysfunctions in sensory, perceptual, communication, or motor function as the result of impaired blood flow to an area of the brain. May be sudden and massive in onset or slowly develop over a period of time.
- Etiology: Strokes are classified as either due to ischemia (80% of strokes; includes thrombosis, embolism, and decreased perfusion) or hemorrhage (20% of strokes; includes subarachnoid and intracerebral)
  1. Thrombosis - Obstruction of blood flow due to local occlusive process within the blood vessel; usually atherosclerosis; most common cause
  2. Embolism - Material formed proximally, lodges in a vessel and blocks blood flow; majority of emboli originate in the inside layer of the heart with plaques or tissue breaking off.
  3. Decreased systemic perfusion - Decreased blood flow to brain due to low systemic perfusion pressure; usually caused by cardiac pump failure (as in myocardial infarction or arrhythmia) or systemic hypotension (as in hypovolemia secondary to blood loss).
  4. Subarachnoid hemorrhage - Blood leaks out of vascular bed onto

brain's surface and is disseminated quickly via the spinal fluid pathways into the spaces around the brain; usually from aneurysms or arteriovenous malformations (AVMs); can be sudden and rapid or slowly progressing.

5. Intracerebral hemorrhage - Bleeding directly into brain substance; usually caused by hypertension, with leakage of blood from arterioles damaged by the high blood pressure. Can also be caused by anticoagulation, trauma, AVMs.
6. Risk factors for thrombosis:
   a. History of TIA
   b. Carotid bruit
   c. Coronary artery disease (CAD)
   d. Diabetes mellitus (DM)
   e. Hypertension
   f. Hypercholesterolemia
   g. Cigarette smoking
   h. Alcohol consumption
   i. Family history
7. Risk factors for embolism
   a. Heart valve disease
   b. Endocarditis
   c. Atrial fibrillation
   d. Family history
8. Risk factors for hemorrhage:
   a. Hypertension
   b. Alcoholism

- Incidence
  1. More than 500,000 strokes annually; 150,000 die from stroke each year; there are 2 million stroke survivors.
  2. Third leading cause of death in adult Americans; a significant cause of both short and long term disability

- Signs and symptoms - Depend on the mechanism, the location, and the severity of the stroke.
  1. Seven common localization patterns of strokes are:
     a. Left hemisphere lesion - Aphasia, right-limb weakness, right-limb sensory loss, right visual field defect, poor right conjugate gaze, difficulty reading, writing, and calculating.
     b. Right hemisphere lesion - Neglect of the left visual space, difficulty drawing and copying, left visual-field defect, left-limb motor weakness, left-limb sensory loss, poor left conjugate gaze.
     c. Left posterior cerebral artery (PCA) lesion - right visual-field defect, difficulty reading with retained writing ability, difficulty naming colors and objects presented visually, good repetition of spoken language, occasional numbness of right limbs.
     d. Right PCA lesion - Left visual-field defect, often with neglect, occasional left-limb sensory loss.
     e. Vertebrobasilar territory infarction - Dizziness, diplopia, blindness or dim vision, bilateral motor or sensory findings, ataxia, vomiting, headache
     f. Pure motor stroke - Weakness of face, arm and leg on one side of the body without abnormalities of higher cortical function, sensory or visual dysfunction, or reduced level of consciousness
     g. Pure sensory stroke - Numbness or decreased sensation of face, arm, and leg on one side of the body, without weakness, or higher cortical function abnormalities.
  2. Historical features may help differentiate the mechanism of the stroke.
     a. Prior cerebrovascular symptoms
     b. Activity at onset
     c. Early course of development of the deficit
     d. Accompanying symptoms
  3. A Subarachnoid stroke is accompanied by a headache; may also have:

a. Vomiting
b. Decreased level of consciousness
c. Onset while awake
d. Seizures

- Differential Diagnosis
  1. Brain tumor
  2. Intoxication
  3. Traumatic injury with subdural hematoma
  4. TIA
  5. Seizure disorders
  6. Arteritis
  7. Global metabolic insult (hypoxemia, encephalopathy)
- Physical Findings - Periodic physical examinations completed over the course of the stroke should include
  1. Eyes - Examine:
     a. Vision for blindness or dim vision
     b. Visual field for defects
     c. Extraocular movements for conjugate gaze defects
     d. Fundi for:
        (1) Hypertensive retinopathy
        (2) Arteriosclerotic changes
        (3) Hemorrhages
        (4) Papilledema
  2. Cardiovascular system - Assess for any cardiac signs of coronary artery disease, congestive heart failure, valve disease - Examine:
     a. Heart for heart sounds, murmurs, rhythm
     b. Lungs for adventitious sounds
     c. Peripheral pulses, including carotid, femoral and pedal pulses for strength of pulse, presence of bruits

   d. Extremities for signs of peripheral vascular disease, edema

3. Neurological system - Examine:
   a. Mental status
      (1) Level of consciousness
      (2) Memory
      (3) Language - ability to speak, read, write
      (4) Visuospatial function
   b. Cranial nerve function
   c. Motor function
      (1) Test each limb for proximal and distal strength and sensation; coordination of upper and lower extremities
   d. Gait - Observe for weakness, ataxia
   e. Reflexes - Elicit Babinski
4. Common Findings:
   a. Hemiparesis/hemiplegia
   b. Vision impairments
   c. Aphasia may be:
      (1) Receptive - Difficulty understanding speech or writing
      (2) Expressive - Difficulty expressing thoughts
      (3) Global - Both receptive and expressive
   d. Dysarthria - Difficulty speaking
   e. Dysphagia - Difficulty swallowing
   f. Vertigo
   g. Sensory impairment - Usually unilateral
      (1) Decreased superficial pain
      (2) Decreased proprioception (position sense)
      (3) Deep pain is not impaired
   h. Loss of perception of body and environment on one side
   i. Gait or balance disturbances

j. Apraxia - Inability to carry out purposeful movements

k. Emotional lability

l. Memory deficits

m. Cranial nerve signs

n. Loss of consciousness

- Diagnostic Evaluation/Findings

1. Screening blood tests

   a. Complete blood count (CBC)

   b. Prothrombin time (PT)

   c. Partial thromboplastin time (PTT)

   d. Erythrocyte sedimentation rate (ESR)

   e. Blood chemistries including glucose

2. Imaging

   a. CT scan (without contrast) within the first 24 hours to differentiate between ischemic and hemorrhagic stroke

   b. May also consider magnetic resonance imaging (MRI)

3. Electrocardiogram (EKG) if suspect arrhythmia or myocardial infarction (MI)

4. Lumbar puncture if suspect subarachnoid hemorrhage

5. Echocardiography if suspect embolism

6. Carotid ultrasound if stroke is in carotid territory and patient is potential candidate for surgery

7. Arteriography if patient is being considered for carotid endarterectomy

- Management/Treatment

1. Acute - Hospitalization

   a. Basic emergency measures, maintain airway, prevent aspiration

   b. Monitor cardiovascular status closely; avoid overenthusiastic use of antihypertensives; inadvertent blood pressure reduction may increase area of infarction.

c. Monitor fluid and electrolytes; maintain fluid balance; avoid overload and dehydration

d. Assess gag reflex as an indication of ability to tolerate oral feedings

e. Bedrest, only in initial stages

f. Antithrombotic stockings

g. Osmolar therapy, if indicated, to treat cerebral edema

h. Anticonvulsants for seizure activity

2. Chronic - Rehabilitation (most recovery occurs within the first three to six months), should begin immediately.

   a. Assess and prevent complications of immobility.

   b. Manage nutritional status.

   c. Manage sensory-perceptual alterations.

   d Manage impaired verbal communication.

   e. Manage cognitive problems.

   f. Manage bowel and bladder problems.

   g. Manage psychological and emotional responses.

   h. Assist with plans for long-term rehabilitation.

- Nursing Considerations

  1. Active and passive range of motion

  2. Avoid complications of immobility.

     a. Turning and positioning

     b. Assess skin integrity.

     c. Use elbow and heel protectors.

     d. Use special mattress, footboards, splints, trochanter rolls.

     e. Avoid prolonged periods of hip flexion.

  3. Maintain adequate nutrition.

     a. Assess difficulty swallowing.

     b. Assess and document bowel sounds.

c. Perform daily weights.
d. Assist in selection of high-protein, high-caloric diet.
e. Provide oral hygiene before and after meals.
f. Utilize semi-Fowler's position for feeding and 30 minutes post-feeding.
g. Place food on back of tongue in unaffected side of mouth.

4. Maintain appropriate communication skills.
   a. Assess type of aphasia.
      (1) Expressive
      (2) Receptive
   b. Consult with speech therapy.
   c. Speak clearly, simple words, low voice, if receptive aphasia.
   d. Use flashcards, drawings, gestures for/with communication.
   e. Address frustration over difficulties in communication.
   f. Provide alternative means of communication.
   g. Allow additional time for processing thoughts.
   h. Provide words for practice.
   i. Praise continued efforts.

5. Prevent unilateral neglect related to homonymous hemianopsia/hemiplegia.
   a. Assess effect of unilateral neglect on ability to perform self-care and function safely.
   b. Compensate (initially) by working with patient from unaffected side
   c. Gradually force recognition of affected side by slow integration
   d. Stimulate affected side (touching, rubbing).
   e. Instruct patient to bathe and dress affected side first
   f. Teach patient to inspect position of affected extremities.
   g. Teach patient to inspect affected side of mouth during meals for "pocketing of food"

6. Prevent incontinence
    a. Offer bedpan/urinal every 2 hours
    b. Encourage fluid intake of 3000 cc every 24 hours unless on fluid restriction
    c. Monitor for signs and symptoms of urinary tract infection
    d. Keep perianal area clean and dry
7. Manage sensory-perceptual alterations
    a. Assess alterations
    b. Assess awareness to different stimuli
    c. Encourage verbalization about deprivations
    d. Provide sensory stimulation
    e. Provide and encourage family members to provide touch.
    f. Provide consistent caregivers.
8. Manage cognitive problems
    a. Assess extent of impairment in orientation, memory, attention span, behavioral changes
    b. Reacquaint to time, place, person, circumstances, events
    c. Encourage family members to provide familiar objects, photographs, calendar and clock
    d. Maintain quiet, calm environment.
    e. Approach patient calmly and slowly
    f. Use short sentences, simple words
    g. Provide resocialization
    h. Assist patient and family in grieving process
9. Manage psychological and emotional response
    a. Recognize disturbance in body image, loss of self-esteem, role changes
    b. Encourage patient and family to verbalize fears, concerns, feelings
    c. Accept feelings of fear, rejection, and hostility.

   d. Reassure patient and family that behaviors such as emotional lability, swearing and exposing oneself is the result of brain injury and will eventually improve
   e. Monitor for depression

10. Assist with plans for long-term rehabilitation
   a. Older patients should not be disqualified from rehabilitation programs because of age.
   b. Assess appropriateness for inpatient rehabilitation; there must be potential for regaining functional capacity that will allow a degree of independence.
   c. Instructions in activities of daily living (ADL)
   d. Utilize team approach to rehabilitation.
   e. Assist family in reinforcing strategies taught by rehabilitation team.

Seizures

- Definition: An excessive paroxysmal neuronal discharge in the brain causing a temporary and reversible behavioral alteration
- Etiology: In the elderly
  1. Systemic
     a. Metabolic
        (1) Hyponatremia
        (2) Hypoglycemia, hyperglycemia
        (3) Hypoxia,
        (4) Renal failure
        (5) Hepatic failure
     b. Toxic
        (1) Drugs—especially antidepressants, neuroleptics
        (2) Drug withdrawal—especially barbiturates, benzodiazepines
        (3) Alcohol intoxication or withdrawal

2. Intracranial
    a. CVA
    b. Brain tumor
    c. Head injury
    d. Brain surgery with resultant scar
    e. Epilepsy—rare in the elderly

- Incidence: About the same in elderly as in infants under one year old
- Signs and Symptoms
  1. An eye witness account can be very helpful
  2. Partial—arise from a locus in one cerebral hemisphere
      a. Simple—no loss of consciousness
          (1) Unilateral paresthesia, numbness, tingling
          (2) Jacksonian march movements
          (3) May be preceded by an aura
      b. Complex partial—progress to alteration of consciousness
          (1) May have hallucinations
          (2) Automatisms (repetitive movements)
          (3) Emotional phenomena
          (4) May progress to generalized
  3. Generalized—associated with loss of consciousness
      a. Usually preceded by an aura
      b. Tonic (contraction) then
      c. Clonic (alternating contraction/relaxation)
      d. Bowel or bladder incontinence
      e. Postictal state (may be confused)
- Differential Diagnosis
  1. TIA
  2. Migraine

3. CVA
4. Syncope

- Physical Findings: Nonspecific
- Diagnostic Evaluation/Findings
  1. CT scan
  2. LP
  3. EEG
  4. Blood chemistries, CBC
  5. Metabolic and toxicological screening as indicated
- Management/Treatment
  1. Acute
     a. Protect from injury
     b. Turn head to side to prevent aspiration
  2. Chronic—refer
     a. Drugs—obtain serum levels PRN
        (1) Phenytoin (Dilantin) 100 mg po tid
        (2) Carbamazepine (Tegretol) 100–200 mg qd or bid
     b. Treat precipitating cause
- Nursing Considerations
  1. Patient education
     a. Medication—monitor compliance
     b. Protect from injury

Parkinson's Disease:

- Definition: A degenerative disorder of the basal ganglia and extra pyramidal nervous system. Patients lack normal concentrations of dopamine due to cell loss in the substantia nigra
- Etiology: Unknown; suspected causes include
  1. Viral infections, e.g., encephalitis
  2. Chemical toxicity, e.g., carbon monoxide

3. Cerebrovascular disease
4. Drugs, e.g., phenothiazines, reserpine
5. Structural, e.g., repeated head trauma incidence: The most common neurological disorder after stroke, Alzheimer's disease, and epilepsy. One percent of the population over age 50 has Parkinson's disease.

- Signs and Symptoms: The onset of Parkinson's disease is usually insidious, with the patient complaining of ill defined aches and pains, numbness and tingling. The classic triad of symptoms includes
  1. Tremor - Present in two thirds of patients with Parkinson's disease
     a. Present at rest, decreases with intention and in sleep
     b. Increases with stress and cold weather
  2. Rigidity of muscles - Increased resistance to passive movement throughout entire range of motion (ROM) with rhythmic release of rigidity (called cogwheel rigidity). Occurs primarily in shoulder, neck, face; leads to decreased arm swing with walking, decreased blinking, and decreased facial expression.
  3. Bradykinesia (slowness in movement) and akinesia (difficulty initiating movement); associated with shuffling gait, micrographia (small writing), difficulty getting up from chair, reduced voice volume, and slowness in eating.
- Differential Diagnosis
  1. Progressive supranuclear palsy
  2. Benign essential tremor
- Physical Findings
  1. Gait and postural reflex impairment leads to increased risk of falling.
  2. Mental changes
     a. Passivity
     b. Confusion
     c. Depression - Up to 40% will be depressed, especially early in the disease
     d. Dementia - Increased incidence of dementia late in the disease.
  3. Autonomic symptoms

a. Orthostatic hypotension

b. Urinary retention

c. Constipation

d. Seborrheic dermatitis

- Diagnostic Evaluation/Findings
  1. Clinical diagnosis based on complete history and physical examination
  2. CBC, electrolytes, EEG, CT scan will be normal
- Management/Treatment: Symptomatic, not curative
  1. Pharmacologic
     a. Carbidopa/levodopa (Sinemet), the most effective treatment for the symptoms of Parkinson's disease for most patients
        (1) Initial dose 25 - 100 mg orally t.i.d.
        (2) Increase dose as needed
        (3) Side effects include dyskinesia, nausea, hallucinations, confusion, dizziness.
     b. Selegiline (Eldepryl) use is controversial, but it is suggested that nearly all patients with early to moderate Parkinson's disease should be placed on selegiline in hopes of slowing the progress of the disease
        (1) Dose is 5 mg orally b.i.d.
        (2) May need to decrease dose of Sinemet when adding selegiline
     c. Centrally-acting anticholinergics are used primarily to relieve tremor
        (1) Trihexyphenidyl HCL (Artane) 2 mg orally t.i.d.
        (2) Benztropine mesylate (Cogentin) 0.5 mg orally b.i.d.
     d. Dopamine receptor agonists may be used as adjunct therapy in patients who are taking levodopa, or carbidopa/levodopa.
        (1) Bromocriptine (Parlodel) 5 mg orally t.i.d.
        (2) Pergolide (Permax) 1 mg orally t.i.d.

2. Nonpharmacologic
    a. Exercise program
    b. Physical therapy

- Nursing Considerations
    1. At risk for falls
    2. Emotional support for patient and family
    3. Decrease social isolation
    4. Patient education
        a. Medications
        b. Monitor for adverse reactions
    5. Exercise, ROM
    6. Monitor for skin breakdown
    7. Manage constipation

Benign Essential Tremor

- Definition: Shaking of hands, usually mild in nature
- Etiology: Unknown, although tends to run in families.
- Incidence: A relatively common condition. Incidence rate of 5.5 per 1000
- Signs and Symptoms
    1. Shaking of hands, head, face and voice
    2. Course is variable, may progress with age.
    3. Tremor increases with action, reduced or absent with rest.
    4. Tremor decreases or disappears when patient drinks alcohol.
- Differential Diagnosis: Parkinson's disease
- Physical Findings
    1. Tremor
    2. No rigidity, bradykinesia, balance or gait impairment
- Diagnostic Evaluation/Findings: Usually none indicated

- Management/Treatment
  1. Nonselective beta-adrenergic blocker such as propranolol (Inderal); initial dose 40 mg, orally, b.i.d.
  2. Primidone (Mysoline); a barbiturate derivative; dosage must be individualized; side effects include ataxia and vertigo.
- Nursing Considerations
  1. Patient should be informed that the condition is not Parkinson's disease.
  2. If tremor is troublesome, patient counseled to take medication as needed to function.

Headache

- Definition: A pain or ache in head
- Etiology
  1. Headache with onset in early adulthood has many common causes:
     a. Infections—sinus, upper respiratory infections, influenza
     b. Overindulgence in food, drink, smoking
     c. Muscle contraction
     d. Vascular—migraine, cluster
  2. Most important causes of new onset of headache in the elderly:
     a. Temporal arteritis
     b. Post head injury
     c. Brain tumor
- Incidence: Most people have had headaches during their lives. Older people seldom have new onset of headaches. If so, a careful investigation is warranted.
- Signs and Symptoms
  1. Temporal arteritis
     a. Throbbing or aching
     b. Tenderness over artery

c. May be unilateral or bilateral

d. May have pain in ear, teeth, or occipital area

2. Post head injury

a. Wide variability of symptoms

b. May be vague or may have pain in area of injury

c. May also have insomnia

3. Brain tumor

a. Progressive, intermittent headache

b. Induced by activities that increase intracranial pressure such as coughing, sneezing

c. May be localized

- Differential Diagnosis
  1. Temporal arteritis
  2. Post head injury
  3. Brain tumor
  4. Subdural hematoma
  5. Cerebral aneurysm
- Physical Findings
  1. Temporal arteritis
     a. Vision in one eye may be compromised
     b. Involved artery may be enlarged and rigid
  2. Post head injury
     a. Neurological examination will be normal
     b. Patient may have emotional irritability
     c. May have impaired memory, concentration
  3. Brain tumor
     a. Neurological findings
        (1) Visual abnormalities
        (2) Dysphagia

(3) Dysarthria

(4) Emesis

(5) Unilateral weakness

- Diagnostic Evaluation/Findings
  1. Skull X-ray
  2. CT scan or MRI to rule out subdural hematoma, brain tumor
  3. Biopsy of temporal artery to diagnose temporal arteritis
  4. Chemistry profile
  5. Complete blood count
  6. ESR - elevated in temporal arteritis
- Management/Treatment
  1. Temporal arteritis—Refer immediately for high dose steroid therapy to prevent blindness
  2. Post head injury
     a. Symptomatic treatment
     b. Monitor for progressive neurological signs
  3. Brain tumor—Refer for surgery
- Nursing Considerations
  1. Post head injury headaches can occur without documented head injury
  2. Be alert for changes in patient's usual complaint of headache

Questions

1. The most common mechanism of stroke is:
   a. Thrombosis
   b. Decreased systemic perfusion
   c. Subarachnoid hemorrhage
   d. Intracerebral hemorrhage

2. The differential diagnosis of stroke includes all of the following except:
   a. Brain tumor
   b. Intoxication
   c. TIA
   d. Parkinson's Disease

3. Risk factors for thrombotic stroke include all of the following except:
   a. Diabetes mellitus
   b. Coronary artery disease
   c. Hypertension
   d. Heart valve disease

4. Risk factors for embolic stroke include all of the following except:
   a. Heart valve disease
   b. Endocarditis
   c. Mild hypertension
   d. Atrial fibrillation

5. A patient with a left hemisphere stroke is likely to have all of the following except:
   a. Aphasia
   b. Right limb weakness
   c. Ataxia
   d. Difficulty reading

6. While watching television, Mr. Q has a sudden onset of severe headache accompanied by vomiting and a seizure. He then loses consciousness. The most likely cause of his stroke is:
   a. Subarachnoid hemorrhage

b. Decreased systemic perfusion
c. Embolism
d. Thrombosis

7. Initial workup of a stroke patient includes all of the following except:

a. Complete blood count (CBC)
b. Angioplasty
c. CT scan
d. Erythrocyte sedimentation rate

8. Common causes of seizures in the elderly include all of the following except:

a. Adverse drug reaction
b. Epilepsy
c. Hyponatremia
d. Head Injury

9. Mrs. P has a seizure in which she does not lose consciousness but her right leg, then her right arm jerks. This would be a:

a. Complex partial seizure
b. Syncopal episode
c. Generalized seizure
d. Simple partial seizure

10. Mrs. K complains of a tremor which is not troublesome unless she tries to knit. She denies any other signs and symptoms. The most likely diagnosis is:

a. Parkinson's disease
b. Epilepsy
c. Supranuclear Palsy
d. Benign essential tremor

11. Parkinson's disease can be caused by all of the following except:

a. Infection
b. Drugs
c. Hyperthyroidism
d. Toxic agents

12. Mr J is diagnosed with Parkinson's disease. He is experiencing difficulty with rigidity. Which medication would you be most likely to start:

a. Bromocriptine (Parlodel) 5 mg orally, t.i.d.
b. Sinemet 25-100 mg orally, t.i.d.
c. Trihexyphenidyl (Artane) 2 mg, orally, t.i.d.
d. Pergolide (Permax) 1 mg orally, t.i.d.

13. Mrs. V is diagnosed with benign essential tremor. She is embarrassed to go to lunch with her friends because the tremor causes her to spill food. You would:

a. Counsel her that medications are not necessary
b. Consider Inderal 40 mg orally, b.i.d.
c. Tell her to have a drink of alcohol before she goes out
d. Consider Sinemet 25-100 mg orally, t.i.d.

Answers

1. a
2. d
3. d
4. c
5. c
6. a
7. b
8. b
9. d
10. d
11. c
12. b
13. b

Bibliography

Brass, L. M., Fayad, P. B., & Levine, S. R. (1992). Transient ischemic attack in theelderly: Diagnosis and treatment. *Geriatrics,* 47(5), 36-53.

Bruno, A. (1993). Ischemic stroke, part 1: Early accurate diagnosis. *Geriatrics,* 48(3), 26-34.

Bruno, A. (1993). Ischemic stroke, part 2: Optimal treatment and prevention. *Geriatrics,* 48(3), 37-54.

Caplan, L. R. (1993). *Stroke: A clinical approach* (2nd ed.). Boston: Butterworth-Heinemann.

Hart, G. (1990). Strokes causing left vs right hemiplegia: Different effects and nursing implications. *Geriatric Nursing,* 11(2), 67-70.

Hazzard, W. R., Adres, R., Bierman, E. L., & Blass, J. P. (1990). *Principles of geriatric medicine and gerontology.* New York: McGraw-Hill.

Hobson, R. W., Weiss, D. G., Fields, W. S., Goldstone, J., Moore, W. J., Towne, J. B., & Wright, C. B. (1993). Efficacy of carotid endarterectomy for asymptomatic carotid stenosis. *New England Journal of Medicine,* 328(4), 221-227.

Kane-Carlson, P. A. (1990). Transient ischemic attacks: Clinical features, pathophysiology and management. *Nurse Practitioner,* 15(7), 9-14.

Lewis, S. M., & Collier, I. C. (Eds.). (1992). *Medical-Surgical nursing: Assessment and management of clinical problems* (3rd ed.). St. Louis: Mosby Year Book.

Linde, M. (1993). Parkinson's disease. In D. Carevali & M. Patrick (Eds.). *Nursing management for the elderly* (3rd ed.). Philadelphia: J. B. Lippincott.

Mahler, M. E. (1987). Seizures:Common causes and treatment in the elderly. *Geriatrics,* 42(7), 73-78.

Paulson, G. W. (1993). Management of the patient with newly-diagnosed Parkinson's disease. *Geriatrics,* 48(2), 30-40.

Staab, A. S., & Lyles, M. F. (Eds.). (1990). *Manual of geriatric nursing.* Glenview, IL: Scott, Foresman\Little Brown Higher Education.

Gynecologic Disorders

Anne S. Rosenberg

Postmenopausal Bleeding

- Definition
    1. Episodes of irregular vaginal bleeding or spotting six months or more after last menstrual period
    2. Any vaginal bleeding between episodes of withdrawal bleeding if patient is on Hormone Replacement Therapy (HRT)
- Etiology
    1. Bleeding may originate from one or more sites of genital tract. Most typical is uterine bleeding.
    2. Bleeding from urinary tract and rectum is sometimes mistaken for vaginal bleeding.
    3. Benign causes include: atrophic vaginitis and other infections, trauma, or polyps.
    4. Hormone induced uterine bleeding due to unopposed exogenous and/or endogenous estrogen. May lead to endometrial hyperplasia (certain forms are considered a precancerous condition).
    5. One or more causes may exist; a malignancy must be ruled out before a decision is made regarding treatment.
- Incidence
    1. Malignant or premalignant sources may originate from uterus, ovaries, tubes, cervix, vagina, or vulva. Most common for the postmenopausal group are uterine (25%) and vulvar carcinoma (3–5%). Peak incidence of cervical cancer between ages 45–55.
    2. Of those diagnosed with ovarian cancer, 25% present with vaginal bleeding as symptom.
- Signs and Symptoms
    1. Spontaneous heavy to light bleeding or spotting other than withdrawal bleeding from HRT
    2. Postcoital bleeding
    3. Vaginal and/or vulvar discomfort
    4. Vaginal discharge
    5. Vaginal puritis and burning

- Differential Diagnosis
    1. Vaginal carcinoma
    2. Foreign body induced bleeding
    3. Vaginitis
    4. Trauma
    5. Post-surgical bleeding following a subtotal or total hysterectomy
    6. Cervical carcinoma
    7. Cervical/endometrial polyps
    8. Leiomyoma
    9. Uterine sarcoma
    10. Endometrial carcinoma
    11. Ovarian cancer
    12. Extragenital sources
        a. Blood dyscrasias
        b. Drugs, e.g., Coumadin
        c. Systemic diseases, e.g., liver disease
- Physical Findings—may have one or more of the following:
    1. Atrophic appearance of vaginal epithelium—thin, pale, dry mucosa with no rugation
    2. Vaginal/vulvar lesions/ulcerations
    3. Presence of foreign body
    4. Cervical bleeding
    5. Palpable pelvic mass
    6. Absence or presence of blood in the vaginal vault
    7. May have no abnormal physical finding
- Diagnostic Evaluation/Findings
    1. Papanicolaou smear for detection of cervical carcinoma

2. Wet mounts of vaginal secretions including Normal Saline Solution (NSS) and Potassium Hydroxide (KOH) preperation for evaluation of vaginitis
3. Endometrial biopsy for detection of endometrial hyperplasia of carcinoma
4. Vulvar biopsy if indicated
5. Use of pelvic ultrasound to rule out possible mass

- Management/Treatment
  1. Thorough history and physical
  2. Refer to gynecologist for evaluation of vaginal bleeding in order to rule out malignancy
  3. Once malignancy is ruled out, consider use of systemic HRT or topical estrogen creme for treatment of atrophic vaginal epithelium
- Nursing Considerations
  1. Patient education
     a. Importance of medical and possible surgical evaluation of bleeding
     b. Physiologic changes of genitalia after menopause
     c. Use of HRT—risks, benefits, and contraindications

Vaginitis

- Definition: A change in the normal vaginal environment which causes mild to severe inflammation with usually significant discomfort to the patient. Each woman will present with own symptomatology but most common are vaginal itching and burning with abnormal discharge.
- Etiology
  1. Lack of exogenous or endogenous estrogen to the vaginal epithelium allowing a more alkaline environment, decreased blood supply, and a thinner, drier epithelium with less cornification. This allows easier infusion of bacteria than would have been suppressed by a healthier mucosa with a more acidic pH.

2. Fungal overgrowth caused mostly by *Candida albicans*.
   a. May be precipitated by use of antibiotics or recent initiation of HRT
   b. Repeated candidal infections can also be secondary to a glucose intolerance, i.e., Diabetes

- Signs and Symptoms
  1. Vaginal burning and itching
  2. Vaginal discharge—may be malodorous or no odor, watery, or thick and white to thin and yellow
  3. Dyspareunia
  4. Post coital bleeding
  5. External dysuria

- Differential Diagnosis
  1. Atrophic vaginitis
  2. Candida vaginitis
  3. Trichomonas vaginitis
  4. Bacterial vaginosis
  5. Foreign body

- Physical Findings
  1. Findings may vary depending on type of infection
     a. Atrophic vaginitis
        (1) Pale mucosa with no rugation
        (2) Some inflamation
        (3) Watery to a thin yellow sticky discharge
        (4) Some excoriation with or without bleeding
        (5) May note petechiae in the vaginal walls
     b. Candida vaginitis
        (1) Erythematous appearance to vagina and/or vulva

(2) Possible excoriations

(3) Clear discharge to white thick placques adhering to vaginal walls

c. Trichomonas vaginitis

(1) Some erythema

(2) May have petechiae on cervix (strawberry patches)

(3) Thin malodorous yellow discharge, may be frothy

d. Bacterial vaginosis

(1) No inflammation

(2) Large amount greyish/whitish/yellow vaginal discharge with fishy odor

- Diagnostic Evaluation/Findings

1. Microscopic evaluation using wet mounts and testing pH of vaginal discharge

a. Atrophic vaginitis

(1) NSS

(a) Increased WBC, bacteria, and RBC

(b) Decreased lactobacilla

(2) KOH: No findings

(3) pH: 5.5–7.0

b. Candida vaginitis

(1) NSS: Some increase in WBCs and lactobacilli

(2) KOH: Pseudohyphae and/or spores

(3) pH: ≤ 4.5

c. Trichomonas vaginitis

(1) NSS: Positive Trichomonads with flagellae and WBCs

(2) KOH: No findings

(3) pH: 5.5–7.0

d. Bacterial vaginosis
   (1) NSS
      (a) Clue cells
      (b) Rare WBCs
   (2) KOH: No findings
   (3) pH: > 4.5
   (4) Positive wiff test—a drop of KOH is placed on a slide with a sample of discharge. An amine or fishy odor is released immediately

- Management/Treatment
  1. Thorough history and pelvic exam
  2. If suspect or known history of STD exposure perform a Gonococcal and Chlamydia screen, serology (RPR or STS) for syphilis, and HIV test (if indicated)
  3. Medical treatment for each is as follows
     a. Atrophic vaginitis
        (1) Use of HRT (p.o. or transdermal) or
        (2) Topical estrogen cream intravaginally
     b. Candida vaginitis
        (1) Effective over the counter medications now available. Miconazole nitrate or Clotrimazole (cream or suppository)
        (2) Terconazole cream or suppositories—applied intravaginally every night for 3 or 7 day regimen
        (3) Butoconazole nitrate cream intravaginally for 3 nights
        (4) With recurrent infections, should be evaluated for glucose intolerance
     c. Trichomonas
        (1) Metronidazole, p.o., one gram initially, then one more gram in 12 hours
        (2) Treatment of sexual partner is essential to avoid reinfection

d. Bacterial vaginosis

(1) Metronidazole, p.o., 500 mg, b.i.d., for one week (most common dosage schedule)

(2) Sexual partner does not need to be treated unless recurrent infections

- Nursing Considerations

1. Patient education regarding

a. Proper use of medications including risks, benefits, and side effects

b. Avoid alcohol with use of metronidazole

c. How to prevent infections

(1) Good personal hygiene

(2) Use of HRT

(3) Use of cotton underwear and loose fitting garments

(4) Avoid intercourse until treatment is complete

d. Approach the issue of sexuality and possible STD to the older person with a great deal of sensitivity in a nonjudgemental manner. Allow privacy with time for questions and discussion. May be most difficult topic for a person who was brought up in an environment where sex was taboo. HIV counseling may also be indicated and must be done if this test is performed.

Vulvar Dystrophies

- Definition: Benign nonneoplastic epithelial disorders of vulva

- Etiology

1. There are 3 major classifications of vulvar dystrophies. These are

a. Lichen sclerosis—etiology is unknown. Major symptom puritis, which worsens with time. Sometimes referred as atrophic dystrophy.

b. Squamous Cell Hyperplasia or Hyperplasitc Dystrophy: Due to chronic irritation or infections. Sometimes associated with forms of atypia.

c. Mixed Dystrophy—Lichen sclerosis with squamous cell hyperplasia.

- Incidence
  1. Thirty percent of these are of an atrophic nature, i.e., lichen sclerosis
  2. About 50% make up the squamous cell hyperplasia
  3. Twenty percent of white lesions are mixed dystrophy
  4. Vulvar intraepithelial neoplasia (VIN) may be present in about 10% of the hyperplastic lesions and in about 15–20% of the mixed dystrophies
- Signs and Syptoms
  1. Mild to severe vulvar itching
  2. Vulvar burning
- Differential Diagnosis
  1. Vulvar Intraepithelial Neoplasia
  2. Paget's Disease
- Physical Findings
  1. White patches on vulva—may be flat, ivory white, diffuse to placque-like lesions
  2. Possible excoriations/fissures due to scratching
  3. Some vulvar edema may occur
- Diagnostic Evaluation/Findings: Vulvar biopsy
- Management/Treatment: Possibility of vulvar cancer—imperative that a biopsy is performed for any vulvar lesion. Referral to a gynecologist is required for a diagnosis and appropriate treatment.
- Nursing Considerations
  1. Patient education regarding importance of evaluation of any vulvar lesion
  2. Stress importance of immediate and continued follow up evaluation for such problem

Genital Prolapse

- Definition: Varying degrees of vaginal relaxation causing displacement of bladder (cystocele), lower rectum (rectocele), uterus (uterine prolapse), and/or peritoneum (enterocele)
  1. First degree—displacement only with straining but not beyond the introitus
  2. Second degree—displacement past introitus with straining
  3. Third degree—displacement past introitus at rest
  4. Procidentia—total eversion of the vagina when cervix and uterus protrude beyond introitus
- Etiology: In addition to parturition, relaxation of pelvis is influenced by the loss of estrogen. Atrophic changes also occur with muscles and ligaments causing loss of strength and tone to these structures.
- Incidence: Gradually decreasing in the U.S. It is assumed this is due to decreased parity in women and earlier surgical intervention.
- Signs and Symptoms
  1. Sensation of fullness or pressure in vaginal pelvic area
  2. Backache
  3. Urinary frequency, retention, and recurrent UTIs
  4. Occasional urinary incontinence
  5. Constipation
- Differential Diagnosis: Pelvic mass
- Management/Treatment
  1. Pending severity of symptoms, refer to gynecologist for evaluation
     a. Surgical correction
     b. Use of pessaries for temporary support or permanent correction to those contraindicated for surgery
  2. Topical estrogen cream or HRT used as adjunctive therapy
- Nursing Considerations
  1. Teach patient about how to reduce intraabdominal pressure
     a. Avoid heavy lifting

b. Weight loss if indicated

c. Avoid constipation

d. Stop smoking

Pelvic Mass

- Definition: Can vary in size, shape, and consistency; may be totally asymptomatic. May be fixed or mobile. Position in relation to other pelvic organs is important, as well as presence or absence of tenderness
- Etiology
    1. Post menopausal pelvic mass, highly suspicious for malignancy, especially ovarian in origin
    2. Tubo-ovarian abscess may occur, especially to those women with earlier history of recurrent pelvic inflammatory disease
    3. Enlargement of the uterus—the principle feature of uterine sarcoma
- Incidence
    1. Risk for ovarian cancer increases throughout life till mid 70's, then declines. Fourth leading cause of death between ages 55–74.
    2. About half of adnexal tumors are malignant in those over 55
    3. Benign tumor of uterus, leiomyoma is not usually found in postmenopausal women because of need for estrogen for growth. However, with increased prescribing of estrogen for HRT, it is possible for preexisting fibroids to reappear.
- Signs and Symptoms
    1. Pelvic pain
    2. Vaginal bleeding
    3. Vague complaints of bloating or "gas"
    4. Pelvic pressure
    5. When no infection/inflamation, may be patient asymptomatic
- Differential Diagnosis
    1. Leiomyoma
    2. Tubo-ovarian abscess

3. Uterine sarcoma
4. Ovarian carcinoma
5. Tubal carcinoma (rare)

- Physical Findings
    1. Palpable ovary in a woman who is in late menopause is an abnormal finding.
    2. Presence or absence of adnexal tenderness
    3. Enlarged uterus
    4. Thrombophlebitis may be secondary to pelvic mass causing partial venous flow obstruction
- Diagnostic Evaluation/Findings
    1. Pelvic examination
    2. Sonography
    3. Computerized axial tomography (CT scan)
    4. Abdominal flat plate
    5. Surgical exploration
- Management/Treatment
    1. Maintain high suspicion for malignancy in postmenopausal women who present with vague complaints
    2. Refer to gynecologic surgeon for further evaluation when a mass is palpated
- Nursing Considerations
    1. Education regarding the importance of follow-up and evaluation of any pelvic mass.
    2. Support and guidance for those diagnosed with a malignancy.

Breast Carcinoma

- Definition: One out of every 10 American women will develop this type of cancer in their lifetime. Slow growing tumor that takes 6–8 years to reach a diameter of one cm, and then almost another year to reach a 2 cm size.

- Etiology
  1. The majority of breast carcinomas are adenocarcinomas
  2. Postmenopausal women are generally at risk for intraductal carcinomas. Frequently infiltrate and become multifocal.
  3. Lobular carcinomas more common in premenopausal age group
  4. Paget's disease presents as a dermatitis or an eczema near the nipple and is a result of intraductal carcinoma invading the skin
- Incidence
  1. Despite its slow growth, it is the 2nd leading cause of death and is also the leading site of cancer in women
  2. Intraductal cancer is responsible for 80–85% where lobular carcinoma makes up about 10–12% of all breast cancers. Paget's disease is rare, making up only 1%.
- Signs and Symptoms
  1. Nontender breast lump found on breast self examination
  2. Nipple discharge or bleeding
  3. Complaint of nipple/areolar itching with open lesion or redness
  4. Unilateral breast tenderness
  5. Associated symptoms may include bone, back, or chest pain; general malaise, weight loss, anorexia; fever, cough, hoarseness, chest pain, or change in bowel movements
- Differential Diagnosis
  1. Fibrocystic breast changes
  2. Fibroadenoma
  3. Papilloma
  4. Breast cyst
  5. Fat necrosis
  6. Mammary duct ectasia
- Physical Findings
  1. Palpable breast lump, usually nontender

2. Early breast cancer, 10% of cases may present with pain
3. Peau d'Orange appearance with late finding or a rapidly growing type of cancer
    a. Induration and dimpling of skin
    b. Ulceration
    c. Inflammation or edema
4. Palpable supraclavicular and/or axillary lymph nodes

- Diagnostic Evaluation/Findings
    1. Mammography
    2. Biopsy (needle or surgical)
- Management/Treatment
    1. Complete history of presenting complaint or symptom including characteristics of pain and nipple discharge, and how lump was discovered
    2. Thorough examination for associated symptoms
    3. Complete breast examination
    4. Refer to gynecologist or surgeon for evaluation of lump
- Nursing Considerations
    1. Patient education for early detection
        a. Teach monthly breast self exam (BSE)
        b. Yearly breast exam by licensed health care practitioner
        c. Yearly mammogram for women 50 years of age and older
    2. Education, support, and guidance with close follow-up of a patient diagnosed with breast cancer
        a. Education regarding symptoms of recurrance or metastasis
        b. Emotional support
            (1) Possible loss of breast
            (2) Threat to life
            (3) Adjustment to the disease with each phase of diagnosis and treatment

c. Anticipatory guidance centering around sexuality and partner's response

d. Referral for social, psychological, or financial assistance

Sexual Dysfunction

- Definition: Morrison-Beedy & Robbins (1989) give four most common types of sexual dysfunction in women:
  1. Inhibited sexual desire
  2. Orgasmic dysfunction
  3. Vaginismus
  4. Dyspareunia
- Etiology
  1. Sexual dysfunction often related to aging process, e.g., estrogen deficiency causes thinning of the vaginal epithelium and the vagina becomes smaller and shorter with decreased elasticity. Also, decreased vaginal blood flow results in decreased vaginal lubrication when stimulated. Repeated episodes of dyspareunia cause vaginismus.
  2. Disease or surgery may alter the self image as well as cause physiologic changes in sexuality of women and their partners:
     a. Coronary artery disease—fears of chest pain or heart damage with sexual activity
     b. Diabetes—can cause alterations in hormonal, psychological, vascular, and neurological functioning
     c. COPD—increased shortness of breath/dyspnea with certain positions
     d. Arthritis—increased pain with decreased mobility
     e. Parkinson's disease—Decreased orgasmic potential, increased fatigue, and increased feelings of worthlessness
     f. Stroke—impaired body image secondary to paralysis and sensory loss
     g. Surgeries—especially
        (1) Hysterectomy

    (2) Vulvectomy
    (3) Breast surgeries
    (4) Ostomy surgeries
3. Depression
4. Drugs—much has been written about side effects of certain drugs that may decrease libido and possibly inhibit sexual response. Examples include certain tranquilizers, antidepressants, antihypertensives, phenothiazines, and alcohol.

- Incidence
  1. Elderly women versus men are more apt to be widowed or living with a husband who is functionally impaired
  2. The actual extent of concern about sexual dysfunction by older women is unknown. Past studies reveal methodologic problems with estimating such prevalence.
  3. It is suggested that the importance and frequency of sexual activity in younger years predicts a couple's sexual motivation in later years
  4. Many studies of couples report cessation of sexual activity is more often related to *men's* inability to perform or their lack of desire rather than their wives
- Signs and Symptoms
  1. History of painful intercourse (dyspareunia) with or without bleeding
  2. Vaginal dryness
  3. Remarks made about "change" in sexual desire
  4. Concern about increased difficulty achieving orgasm
- Differential Diagnosis
  1. Major depression
  2. Loneliness/isolation
  3. Dyspareunia caused by vaginal infections
- Physical Findings
  1. Atrophic vagina

2. Genital prolapse may be found
3. Vaginismus
4. May have negative findings

- Management/Treatment
  1. Thorough history and physical allowing total privacy and reassurance of confidentiality
  2. For vaginal atrophy:
     a. Topical or oral estrogen replacement
     b. Use of artificial, water soluble lubricants
  3. Referral for evaluation for surgical correction of genital prolapse

- Nursing Considerations
  1. Recognize and validate patient's sexuality
  2. Patient Education
     a. Physiologic changes in sexual response
        (1) Longer, slower, and more direct stimulation may be required
        (2) Changes in the male sexual responses
        (3) Vaginismus—practicing contraction and relaxation
  3. Sexual counseling before and after surgery may be helpful for some individuals
  4. Support for other forms of contact and intimacy
  5. Referral for professional counseling for depression
  6. Referral to psychosexual therapist

Questions

1. Mrs. M. comes into the office for an annual gynecological exam. She is 65 years old, has had no hysterectomy and is taking both Premarian and Provera for HRT. She has no significant medical history. Her only complaint is occasional spot bleeding for the last 6 months since starting HRT. All of the following are true except:
   a. If the bleeding occurs during or soon after Provera it is considered withdrawal bleeding and no further work up is needed.
   b. If other than withdrawal bleeding we assure patient this is a side effect of HRT and not to be concerned.
   c. The uterus is most typical site of genital tract bleeding in postmenopausal women.
   d. Postmenopausal vaginal bleeding should always be referred for evaluation.

2. Some of the benign causes of vaginal bleeeding include all but one of the following:
   a. Atrophic vaginitis
   b. Cervical polyp
   c. Endometrial hyperplasia
   d. Trauma

3. Changes in the vagina due to decreased estrogen in postmenopausal women include all of the following except:
   a. Shorter and narrower space within the vaginal vault
   b. Normal rugae
   c. Less cornification of the epithelium
   d. Alkaline pH

4. Mrs. S. who is 60 years old has been diagnosed with atrophic vaginitis. She is very concerned since she thought she always had good personal hygiene habits. Patient teaching for Mrs. S. would include all of the following except:
   a. The vaginal mucosa is expected to become thinner and drier with aging because of estrogen deficiency. Therefore, more susceptible to infection.
   b. Antibiotics is the most effective cure for this problem.
   c. Estrogen replacement, topically or systemic, is usually prescribed for such problem.
   d. HRT can improve the health of the patient as well as ameliorate her vaginal symptoms.

5. An elderly woman presents with severe vulvar itching. On clinical inspection there are excoriations over the vulva which are ivory white in appearance with mild inflamation. The rest of the exam is within normal limits. Management of such a problem would be:

   a. Application of topical steroids since its most likely due to chemical irritants
   b. Refer for biopsy for complete cellular pathology
   c. Application of cool compress
   d. Topical antifungal cream for one week

6. Vulvar dystrophies is the term that is now used for nonneoplastic white lesions of the vulva. When considering management of these disorders the differential diagnosis should include all but:

   a. Mixed dystrophy Malignant melanoma
   b. Lichen sclerosis
   c. Vulvar intraepithelial neoplasia
   d. Paget's disease

7. Besides carcinoma of the vulva, the other most common site of malignancy in the female genital tract is:

   a. The cervix
   b. The endometrium
   c. The vagina
   d. The bladder

8. Genital prolapse includes all of the following except:

   a. Displacement of the cervix beyond the introitus without straining
   b. Shrinking of the vaginal walls
   c. Complaint of vaginal pressure and occasional urinary incontinence
   d. Bulging of the anterior vaginal wall by the bladder

9. Management of uterine prolapse and rectocele on an elderly woman who is high risk for surgical correction may include all but:

   a. Topical estrogen cream vaginally
   b. Placement of a pessary
   c. Teach patient regarding regular bowel elimination and avoidance of heavy lifting
   d. Sitz baths

10. A pelvic mass in a postmenopausal woman:
    a. Is most commonly due to uterine fibroids
    b. Is always symptomatic
    c. Is highly suspicious for ovarian cancer
    d. May be monitored over a period of time

11. Signs and symptoms which raise suspicion of a pelvic mass include:
    a. Vaginal bleeding
    b. Vague complaint of bloating
    c. Pelvic pressure
    d. All of the above

12. The following statement about breast cancer is true.
    a. It is the 2nd leading cause of death in women.
    b. It is usually a fast growing tumor.
    c. The majority of women usually experience breast pain when a malignant lump is found.
    d. Women who have experienced early menopause may be at much higher risk.

13. Prevention of breast cancer includes patient education. Which of the following statements is false?
    a. Yearly mammograms are only recommended for women over age 50.
    b. Women should perform breast self exam on a monthly basis.
    c. Risk of developing breast cancer increases with age.
    d. Breast lumps in postmenopausal women are always malignant.

14. Which of the following does not contribute to sexual dysfunction in the elderly woman?
    a. Lack of male partners
    b. Dyspareunia
    c. Use of estrogen cream vaginally
    d. Depression

15. An elderly woman is found to have significant vaginismus on pelvic examination. Causes of such a problem would include all of the following except:
    a. Atrophic vaginitis
    b. Dyspareunia

c. Vaginal dryness
d. Douching

16. Management of an elderly women with vaginismus includes all of the following except:

    a. Topical estrogen cream
    b. Contraction and relaxation exercises
    c. Vaginal lubricants
    d. Cool compresses

17. Vulvar Intraepithelial Neoplasia is more likely to be associated with which of the following:

    a. Mixed dystrophy of the vulva
    b. Lichen sclerosis
    c. Squamous cell hyperplasia
    d. Vulvar dermatitis

18. The following is true regarding ovarian cancer:

    a. It is the 4th leading cause of death in women between ages 55–74.
    b. Incidence peaks at 60 then declines gradually.
    c. Women are usually symptomatic during the early stages.
    d. Almost all adnexal masses found in women over 55 are malignant.

19. All of the following may cause abnormal vaginal bleeding in a postmenopausal woman except:

    a. Vaginitis
    b. Ovarian cancer
    c. Urinary tract infection
    d. Endometrial polyps

20. Sexual dysfunction in older women may be related to all of the following except:

    a. Certain medical diseases may alter sexual response.
    b. Sexual dysfunction is often related to the physical changes of the aging process.
    c. Vaginismus is not curable in older women.
    d. Depression is a major cause of sexual dysfunction in older women.

21. Which of the following is true about Breast carcinoma?
    a. Because of its slow growth, it is the fifth leading cause of death.
    b. It is the leading site of cancer in women.
    c. Lobular breast carcinoma is the most common type in postmenopausal women.
    d. The incidence of breast cancer has been declining for several years.

22. Standard medical treatment for candida vaginitis includes:
    a. Betadine douche daily for three days
    b. Metronidazole 500 mg b.i.d. for one week
    c. Terconazole cream applied intravaginally at bedtime for three days.
    d. Hydrocortisone topical applications q.i.d. for 5 days

23. Vaginal relaxation can cause displacement of the
    a. Bladder
    b. Lower rectum
    c. Peritoneum
    d. All of the above

Answers

1. b	9. d	17. a
2. c	10. c	18. a
3. b	11. d	19. c
4. b	12. a	20. c
5. b	13. d	21. b
6. a	14. c	22. c
7. b	15. d	23. d
8. b	16. d	

Bibliography

Buxton, B. H., Schinfield, J. S., & Ryan, B. M. (1992). Gynecological problems. In Calkins, Ford, & Katz (Eds.), *Practice of geriatrics* (pp. 474–482). Philadelphia: W. B. Saunders.

Byyny, R. L., & Speroff, L. (1990). *A clinical guide for the care of older women.* Baltimore: Williams & Wilkins.

Dondero, T., & Lichtman, R. (1990). The breasts. In Lichtman & Papera (Eds.), *Gynecology: Well women care* (pp. 141–171). Norwalk: Appleton & Lange.

Eliopoulos, C. (1990). *Health assessment of the older adult* (2nd ed.). Redwood City: Addison Wesley.

Goldstein, M. K., & Teng, N. H. (1991). Gynecologic factors in sexual dysfunction of the older women. *Clinics in Geriatric Medicine, 7*(1), 42–61.

Lichtman, R., & Duran, P. (1990). The vulva and vagina. In Lichtman & Papera (Eds.), Gynecology: Well women care (pp. 173–201). Norwalk: Appleton & Lange.

Morrison-Beedy, D., & Robbins, L. (1989). Sexual assessment and the aging female. *Nurse Practitioner, 14*(12), 35–45.

Stenchever, M. (1991). Vulva and vaginal conditions. In Stenchever & Aargaard (Eds.), *Caring for the older women* (pp. 171–182). New York: Elsevier.

Stenchever, M. (1991). Gynecologic malignancies in the elderly. In Stenchever & Aargaard (Eds.), *Caring for the older women* (pp. 183–203). New York: Elsevier.

Weingold, A. B. (1990). Abnormal bleeding. In Kase, Weingold, & Gershenson (Eds.), *Principles and practice of clinical gynecology* (pp. 511–543) (2nd ed.). New York: Churchill Livingstons.

Hematology Disorders

Molly English

Anemia: A commom phenomenon in the elderly that can mean a decrease in the total number of circulating red blood cells, a decrease in the concentration of hemoglobin in the blood, or a decrease in the volume of packed red blood cells. Anemias can be classified according to the size of the average red blood cell (microcytic, macrocytic, normocytic) and the mean corpuscular hemoglobin concentration (hypochromic, normochromic).

Iron Deficiency Anemia

- Definition: A chronic hypochromic, microcytic (MCV < 80 μ^3) anemia resulting from an inadequate supply of iron needed to synthesize hemoglobin.
- Etiology
  1. Acute or chronic blood loss (esp. from G.I. tract)
  2. Impaired absorption or excessive loss of iron (especially from total gastrectomy or severe generalized malabsorption)
  3. Inadequate dietary intake, high in iron (not as prevalent in the United States)
- Incidence
  1. Iron deficiency is the most common cause of microcytic anemia in the elderly and is high in incidence worldwide.
  2. Anemias in general are more common in the elderly due to the increased prevalence of acute illness, and nutritional deficiency.
- Signs and Symptoms
  1. Vary according to the severity and rate of onset of anemia as well as underlying disease processes:
     a. Specific to elderly (first signs are often confusion or angina)
        (1) Irritablity
        (2) Unusual or bizarre behavior
        (3) Decreased concentration
        (4) Confusion
        (5) Agitation
        (6) Frequent falls

(7) Shortness of breath

(8) Peripheral edema

b. General findings

(1) Fatigue

(2) Headache

(3) Dyspnea

(4) Tinnitus

(5) Dizziness

(6) Lethargy

(7) Weakness

(8) Syncope

(9) Numbness

(10) Tingling

(11) Dysphagia

(12) Angina

- Differential Diagnosis: Rule out other causes of anemia such as anemia of chronic disease, sideroblastic anemia, and anemia caused by certain drugs and toxins.
- Physical Findings
  1. Pallor
  2. Tachycardia
  3. Heart murmurs
  4. Wide pulse pressure
  5. Atrophic glossitis
  6. Dark tarry stools (heme +)
  7. Anorexia
  8. Brittle, spoon shaped nails
  9. Postural hypotension

- Diagnostic Evaluation/Findings
  1. Diagnosis is based on the combination of symptomatology and laboratory findings.
  2. It is important to find the underlying cause of the anemia because anemia is not part of the normal aging process. Anemia is often a sign of illness in the elderly, stemming from ulcers or alcoholism.
  3. Laboratory results reveal
     a. Total iron binding capacity (TIBC) increased
     b. Serum iron decreased
     c. Serum ferritin decreased
     d. Transferrin saturation <10%
     e. Hemoglobin and hematocrit progressively decreased
     f. White blood cell count normal to increased
     g. Platelets increased
     h. Reticulocytes decreased
     i. Mean corpuscular volume (MCV) $<80\ \mu^3$
     j. Mean corpuscular hemoglobin concentration (MCHC) decreased
     k. Red cell volume width (RDW) increased
     l. Bone marrow with absent iron stores
     m. Red blood cells decreased
- Management/Treatment
  1. Identify underlying cause of anemia and correct if possible.
  2. Oral therapy (must be sustained for as long as needed)
     a. Ferrous Sulfate 325 mg;
     b. Ferrous Fumarate 200 mg; or
     c. Ferrous Gluconate t.i.d. between meals for six to twelve months
  3. Indications for parenteral therapy
     a. Noncompliance of patient to other forms of treatment

   b. Intolerance of oral iron therapy
   c. Chronic, continuous, uncorrected bleeding
   d. Patients on parenteral nutrition
   e. Patients with diseases such as ulcerative colitis or malabsorption syndromes
   f. Iron Dextran IM or IV with dose based on patient's weight
4. Evaluate response to oral and parenteral therapy for first two weeks by monitoring reticulocyte count and hemoglobin concentration.

- Nursing Considerations
  1. Educate patient regarding diet, with foods high in iron such as apricots, organ meats, and green vegetables.
  2. Encourage rest periods as needed.
  3. Discuss causes of insufficient iron and provide instructions for medication treatment plan including dosages, side effects, and food/fluid/drug interactions.
  4. Initiate physician referral/consultation for patients with suspected underlying disease, history of undiagnosed bleeding, or positive stool guaic on three separate occasions.
  5. Nurse Practitioners should be involved in the workup and diagnosis of the anemia.

Vitamin B_{12} Deficiency (pernicious anemia)

- Definition: A macrocytic (MCV > 100 μ^3), megaloblastic, normochromic anemia resulting from atrophic gastric mucosa not secreting intrinsic factor.
- Etiology
  1. Development of pernicious anemia
  2. Autoimmune response
  3. Total gastrectomy
  4. Other gastrointestinal disorders
- Incidence: Both men and women are equally affected.

- Signs and Symptoms
  1. The first signs of vitamin B_{12} deficiency in the elderly are often neurological and psychiatric in nature. The most common neuropsychiatric effect of B_{12} deficiency involves the peripheral nervous system.
  2. Other signs and symptoms include sore tongue, indigestion, constipation, diarrhea, tingling in extremities, and chronic numbness.
- Differential Diagnosis
  1. Eliminate other causes of macrocytic anemia
  2. Inquire about neuropathy or family history of pernicious anemia
  3. Rule out anemia of liver disease
- Physical Findings
  1. Elderly often present with well advanced disease.
  2. Physical presentations include pallor, icterus, smooth, beefy red tongue, unstable gait, and difficulty with fine motions of fingers.
- Diagnostic Evaluation/Findings
  1. MCV > 100 μ^3
  2. Schilling test showing inappropriate excretion of B_{12} in urine (intrinsic factor deficit)
  3. Serum bilirubin increased
  4. Hemoglobin/hematocrit decreased
  5. White blood cells decreased
  6. Platelets decreased
  7. Red cell width increased
  8. Reticulocytes decreased
  9. Bone marrow-megaloblastic
  10. B_{12} decreased
  11. Red blood cells decreased
- Management/Treatment
  1. Distinguish between primary and secondary causes.
  2. Recognize that therapy for pernicious anemia is lifelong.

3. Therapeutic
   a. Initial—100ug Vit. B_{12} (Cyanocobalamin) IM daily for three weeks to replenish body stores
   b. Maintenance—1000ug Vit. B_{12} IM every month for life
4. A CBC should be performed on elderly patients monthly for three months to insure appropriate, effective therapy and compliance with drug regimen.
5. When appropriate efficacy of therapy has been established, a CBC should be done once every three to six months.

- Nursing Considerations
  1. Patient Education
     a. Discuss nature and cause of disease
     b. Emphasize need for lifelong treatment with Vit. B_{12} Injections
     c. Teach importance of diet high in Vit. B_{12}
     d. Encourage rest as needed for recovery and safety
     e. Provide instructions to patient or family regarding injection technique or refer to home health service as needed.
  2. Physician referral/consultation for patients who have other hematological disorders or who have been treated with oral B_{12} in the past.

Folic Acid Deficiency Anemia

- Definition: A normochromic, macrocytic anemia resulting from an insufficient amount of folic acid needed for synthesis of deoxyribonucleic acid (DNA).
- Etiology
  1. Alcohol abuse
  2. Inadequate dietary intake
  3. Impaired absorption
  4. Prolonged drug therapy (such as barbiturates and phenytoin) that interferes with nuclear maturation and synthesis of DNA
  5. Overcooking foods
  6. Competition of bacteria for available folic acid

- Incidence: Folic acid deficiency is a common, slowly progressive, megaloblastic anemia that is most prevalent in alcoholics, elderly people, and in people with intestinal or malignant diseases.
- Signs and Symptoms
    1. Progressive and severe fatigue is the cardinal presentation of folic acid deficiency.
    2. Other signs and symptoms include shortness of breath (SOB), palpitations, diarrhea, nausea, anorexia, headaches, irritability, forgetfulness, and depression (most common neuropsychiatric problem in folic acid deficient patients).
- Differential Diagnosis: Rule out Vit. B_{12} deficiency (pernicious anemia) and other causes of macrocytic anemia.
- Physical Findings
    1. Generalized pallor
    2. Generalized wasting
    3. Jaundice
    4. Glossitis
    5. Cheilosis
    6. Absence of neurological signs
- Diagnostic Evaluation/Findings
    1. Hematocrit decreased
    2. Platelets decreased
    3. Reticulocytes decreased
    4. MCV > 100 μ^3
    5. RDW increased
    6. White blood cells decreased
    7. Serum folate decreased (<4mg/ml)
    8. Schilling test within normal limits
- Management/Treatment
    1. Eliminate contributing factor (e.g. alcohol) if possible
    2. Therapeutic

   a. Oral—Folate 2–4mg p.o. daily for most elderly. Can be increased to 5–10mg daily with presence of alcoholism, chronic infection, or hemolytic anemia.
   b. Parenteral—indicated for severely ill patients, patients with malabsorption, and patients who are unable to take oral medications
3. Length of treatment dependent upon underlying cause of deficiency; monitor Hct and reticulocyte count in about four to six weeks; hematocrit begins to rise in seven to ten days.
4. Reticulocyte count rises in two to three days after therapy is started and peaks in five to seven days.

- Nursing Considerations
  1. Advise patient to report any infections, as well as dyspnea, chest pain and dizziness (possible signs of decreased blood flow to vital organs).
  2. Patient Teaching
     a. Reason for folic acid deficiency
     b. Emphasize well balanced diet with foods high in folic acid (oatmeal, broccoli, red beans)
     c. Identify alcohol abusers and other high risk individuals
     d. Reinforce importance of therapeutic supplement
     e. Encourage rest as needed
     f. Establish patient's favorite foods that are high in folic acid
  3. Referral/consultation with physician for patients with suspected concurrent diagnosis of folate and B_{12} deficiency.

Anemia of Chronic Disease

- Definition
  1. A normocytic (MCV 80–100 μ^3), normochromic, chronic anemia due to chronic infections tuberculosis (TB), chronic inflammation (rheumatoid arthritis), and neoplastic diseases, and other chronic illnesses such as liver disease and diabetes mellitus.
  2. Anemia is usually mild, progressive and asymptomatic.

- Etiology
  1. Disruption of iron metabolism
  2. Defect in red cell production within bone marrow
  3. Shortening of erythrocyte life span
- Incidence
  1. Specific incidence not adequately defined.
  2. Possibly second most common to iron deficiency in incidence.
- Signs and Symptoms
  1. Decreased activity level
  2. Easily prone to fatigue
  3. Headache
  4. Dizziness
  5. Tinnitus
  6. Generalized weakness
  7. Dyspnea on exertion
  8. Malaise
- Differential Diagnosis: Rule out other types of anemia
- Physical Findings
  1. Generalized pallor
  2. Lingual surface, buccal surface, conjunctivae, and nail beds pale
  3. Ankle swelling
  4. Visual changes
  5. Dementia
- Diagnostic Evaluation/Findings
  1. Normal to increased iron stores with concurrent low serum iron (hallmark finding of anemia of chronic disease)
  2. Serum iron decreased
  3. Total iron binding capacity decreased
  4. Serum ferritin increased

5. Hemoglobin decreased
6. Hematocrit decreased (seldom below 30)
7. MCV normal (80–100 μ^3)
8. Reticulocytes (hypoproliferative) decreased

- Management/Treatment
  1. Treat primary or underlying cause
  2. Promote rest as needed
  3. Referral and consultation with physician for further evaluation and treatment of underlying problem

- Nursing Considerations
  1. Education
     a. Focus patient teaching on correlation of anemia to underlying chronic disease
     b. Review treatment plan for primary cause of anemia

Questions

1. Iron deficiency anemia is:
   a. Macrocytic
   b. Microcytic
   c. Normochromic
   d. Megaloblastic

2. The primary treatment for iron deficiency anemia is:
   a. Parenteral therapy
   b. Diet of organ meats and green vegetables
   c. Oral iron replacement
   d. Iron dextran

3. Diagnosis of iron deficiency anemia is based on:
   a. History
   b. Physical
   c. Diet
   d. Symptomatology and lab findings

4. The most common neuropsychiatric problem in folic acid deficiency in elderly patients is:
   a. Dementia
   b. Aggressive behavior
   c. Depression
   d. Forgetfulness

5. Betty is a 70 year old widow with persistent indigestion. She complains of a sore tongue and tingling in the hands and feet. These symptoms have been present for two months. She had a partial gastrectomy one year ago. What is the most like diagnosis?
   a. Pernicious anemia
   b. Anemia of chronic disease
   c. Folic acid deficiency

6. Which of Betty's lab tests would likely be abnormal?
   a. Stool guaiac
   b. Schilling test

c. TIBC
d. Folate

7. All of the following physical findings are found in folic acid deficiency except:

   a. Jaundice
   b. Pallor
   c. Wasting
   d. Neurological signs

8. Which of the following is the hallmark finding in anemia of chronic disease?

   a. Decreased hemoglobin
   b. Bilirubin increased
   c. Normal iron stores with low serum iron level
   d. Decreased reticulocytes

9. Mrs. Johnson is 75 years old and a recent widow. She comes to the clinic complaining of fatigue that started six months ago and has become extreme over the last month. She notices that she becomes easily short of breath and has forgotten to feed her cat on three occasions. She also admits that she has not had "any appetite". What is a likely diagnosis for Mrs. Johnson?

   a. Age related changes
   b. Hypochondriasis
   c. Folic acid deficiency
   d. Aplastic anemia

10. After further evaluation, Mrs. Johnson admits that she has about four or five martinis every night to help her sleep since her husband's death six months ago. Which of the following is a likely etiology for Mrs. Johnson's underlying problem?

    a. Anemia of chronic disease
    b. Blood loss
    c. Overcooking foods
    d. Alcohol abuse

11. Which of the following are causes of iron deficiency anemia?

    a. Chronic blood loss
    b. Atrophic glossitis
    c. Both a and b
    d. Impaired absorption of iron

12. All of the following are physical findings of iron deficiency anemia except:
    a. Visual changes
    b. Pallor
    c. Anorexia
    d. Wide pulse pressure

13. The most common neuropsychiatric effect of B_{12} deficiency involves:
    a. Central nervous system
    b. Limbic system
    c. Optic nerve
    d. Peripheral nervous system

14. Which of the following are important aspects of patient education in the client with Vitamin B_{12} deficiency?
    a. Encourage strenuous exercise
    b. Ascertain the client's level of understanding regarding the nature and cause of the deficiency
    c. Emphasize that Vitamin B_{12} injections are only temporary
    d. Encourage rest as needed
    e. Both b and d

15. Anemia of chronic disease can be a result of all of the following except:
    a. Chronic infections
    b. Strenuous exercise
    c. Chronic inflammation
    d. Neoplastic diseases

16. Mr. Cooper is a 69 year old black male who comes to the office complaining of weakness, tinnitus, headache, and syncope. After further evaluation, Mr. Cooper states that he has just recently been in the hospital for treatment of a gastric ulcer. What is the most likely cause of Mr. Cooper's symptoms?
    a. Liver disease
    b. Iron deficiency anemia
    c. Brain tumor
    d. Pernicious anemia

17. Which of Mr. Cooper's laboratory tests would likely be abnormal?
    a. Hemoglobin and hematocrit

b. Electrolytes
c. Serum iron and ferritin
d. Both a and c

18. The etiology of anemia of chronic disease can best be attributed to:

a. Disruption of iron metabolism
b. Both a and d
c. Alcohol abuse
d. Shortening of erythrocyte life span

Answers

1. b
2. c
3. d
4. c
5. a
6. b
7. d
8. c
9. c
10. d
11. c
12. a
13. d
14. e
15. b
16. b
17. d
18. b

Bibliography

Beck, W. S. (Ed.). (1991). *Hematology.* Cambridge: MIT Press.

Bushnell Lopez, F. K. (1992). A guide to primary care of iron deficiency anemia. *The Nurse Practitioner. 17,* (11), 68–74.

Delafuente, J. C., & Stewart, R. B. (Eds.). (1988). *Therapeutics in the elderly.* Baltimore: Williams and Wilkins.

Ebersole, P., & Hess, P. (1990). *Toward healthy aging: Human needs and nursing response.* St. Louis: C.V. Mosby.

Ford, R. D. (Ed.). (1987). *Diagnostic tests handbook.* Springhouse: Springhouse Publishing.

Gambert, S. R. (Ed.). (1987). *Handbook of geriatrics.* New York: Plenum.

Hogstel, M. O. (Ed.). (1992). *Clinical manual of gerontological nursing.* St. Louis: Mosby Year Book.

Kane, R. L., Ouslander, J. G., & Abrass, I. B. (1989). *Essentials of clinical geriatrics.* New York: McGraw-Hill.

Norris, J. (Ed.). (1993). *Diseases.* Springhouse: Springhouse Publishing.

Thompson, J. M., Mcfarland, G. K., Hirsch, J. E., Tucker, S. M., & Bowers, A. C. (1989). *Mosby's manual of clinical nursing.* St. Louis: C. V. Mosby.

ENDOCRINE AND METABOLIC DISORDERS

Pamela Cacchione

Type II Diabetes: Non-Insulin-Dependent Diabetes Mellitus (NIDDM)

- Definition: A clinically and genetically heterogeneous group of disorders that have a common feature of abnormally high glucose levels. NIDDM involves both relative insulin deficiency and resistance to insulin action. NIDDM is distinguished by the absence of ketosis, which signifies the presence of at least some insulin.
- Etiology: Risk factors include age over 40, obesity, familial pattern, sedentary life style, and lower socioeconomic and educational background. There is a strong genetic, familial link. One theory holds that in obesity there is an increased demand on the beta cells, with an impaired insulin production in response to the beta cells. Another theory is that there are post cell receptor defects impairing glucose transport. The last theory is that there is insulin resistance mediated by decreased insulin receptors in the target cells.
- Incidence: The incidence of diabetes in the 65 and over age group is approximately 88.7/1000 persons in the USA. NIDDM accounts for over 80% of all diabetes cases in old age.
- Signs and Symptoms
    1. Symptoms are often subtle therefore a high level of suspicion is required.
    2. Rarely are there ketones in the urine
    3. Polyuria, polyphagia and polydypsia rarely occur
    4. Blurring of vision
    5. Increased susceptibility to infections especially fungal and staphylococcal infections.
    6. Fatigue and weakness
    7. Decreased level of consciousness or acute confusion
    8. Impotence
    9. Arterial disease: involving the cardiovascular, cerebral vascular and peripheral vascular systems.
- Differential Diagnosis
    1. Hyperglycemia due to pancreatitis
    2. Hyperglycemia due to endocrine disorders which interfere with insulin action

3. Hyperglycemia due to drugs that promote hyperglycemia and insulin resistance

- Physical Findings
  1. Dehydrated appearance
  2. Decreased level of consciousness
  3. Fingerstick glucose over 240 mg/dl
  4. Fungal rashes or yeast infections may be present
  5. A wound that will not heal may be present
  6. May present with a fingerstick glucose as high as 1000 mg/dl
- Diagnostic Evaluation/Findings
  1. Fasting glucose levels greater than or equal to 140 mg/dl on two occasions
  2. Glucose tolerance test: Glucose levels greater than or equal to 200 mg/dl two hours after ingesting 75g of glucose
  3. Glycosylated hemoglobin HbA_{1c} levels of > 8 mg/dl
- Management/Treatment
  1. Patient teaching: starts initially in the primary care setting or hospital but must be an ongoing process with follow up at home.
  2. Diet education
     a. Protein 15-20% of intake
     b. Carbohydrates 55-60% of intake
     c. Fat 30% maximum of intake
     d. High fiber diet and low to moderate salt
  3. Exercise: May help patient to require less insulin but should be pursued carefully and glucose levels should be monitored closely before and after exercise.
  4. Life style modification
     a. Decrease or eliminate smoking
     b. Decrease or eliminate alcohol consumption
     c. Integrate glucose monitoring into their routine

Table 1
BASIC PHARMACOKINETICS OF THE ORAL HYPOGLYCEMIC AGENTS

DRUG	*TOLBUTAMIDE (Orinase)*	*ACETOHEXAMIDE (Dymelor)*	*TOLAZAMIDE (Tolinase)*	*CHLORPROPAMIDE (Diabinese)*	*GYBURIDE (Diabeta) (Micronase)*	*GLIPIZIDE (Glucotrol)*
Recommended dose	250-500mg divided doses	250-500mg single or divided	100-500mg single or divided	100-250mg single dose	1.25-5mg single or divided	5-10mg single or divided
Maximum dose	2-3gms/day	1.5gms/day	1.0gms/day	500mg/day	20mg/day	40mg/day
Half Life Hours	6 hours	5 hours	7 hours	35 hours	biphasic 3.2 and 10 hours	3.5-6 hours
Onset	1 hour	1 hour	4-6 hours	1 hour	1.5 hours	1 hour
Duration hours	6-12 hours	10-14 hours	10-14 hours	72 hours	24 hours	12-18 hours
Comments	Least potent, short half-life, useful kidney disease	Essentially no advantage over Orinase. Patients with Orinase intolerence may use Dymelor	Essentially no advantage over Orinase. Equipotent with fewer side effects	Most potent;use with caution in elderly with kidney disease. Hyponatremia may be a problem. Longest half life.	50-200 times more potent than other agents. Use with caution in the elderly	Take on empty stomach. Toxicity low.

5. Long term monitoring of the non-insulin-dependent diabetic includes:
    a. Monitoring for large vessel disease
    b. Monitoring for microvascular disease
    c. Monitoring for peripheral neuropathy
    d. Monitoring for peripheral vascular disease
6. May require insulin to control initial high blood sugars
7. Oral hypoglycemic agents (see Table 1)
    a. First generation sulfonylureas
        (1) Increase secretion of beta cells
        (2) Decrease the resistance at target cells
    b. Second generation sulfonylureas
        (1) Same actions as first generation
        (2) Fewer side effects

- Nursing Considerations
    1. Patient education about disease process and benefits of maintaining good control
    2. Patient education about all the new modifications in their lifestyle: diet, exercise, and medication regimen
    3. Allowing patient to ventilate their feelings about their disease process
    4. Educate the patient regarding the necessity for excellent foot care and podiatry care of their toe nails
    5. Provide direct patient care for exacerbations of disease process
    6. Education of the staff on latest trends in diabetes care and latest technology available
    7. Perform research in area of care of the diabetic patient
    8. Evaluate patient's medications which worsen hyperglycemia
        a. Glucocorticoids
        b. Diuretics (thiazides, chlorthalidone, furosemide)

   c. Estrogens
   d. Nicotinic acid
   e. Phenothiazines
   f. Phenytoins
   g. Sugar-containing medications
   h. Lithium
   i. Sympathomimetic agents

9. Evaluate patient's medications which might potentiate hypoglycemia
   a. Beta-blockers
   b. Monamine oxidase inhibitors
   c. Insulin
   d. Alcohol
   e. Sulfonamides, sulfonylureas
   f. Cimetidine
   g. Bishydroxycoumanin
   h. Phenylbutazone
   i. Salicylates (large doses)
   j. Anabolic steroids

10. Patient education regarding sick day guidelines
    a. Take insulin or oral hypoglycemics as prescribed
    b. Promote fluid intake
    c. Check fingersticks more often

11. Patient education regarding hypoglycemia (Insulin Reaction): Blood glucose < 60 mg/dl, the elderly present with change in mental status due to their decreased beta response. Give 15 gm of carbohydrates (5 Lifesavers)

12. Patient education regarding hyperglycemia: Glucose > 240 mg/dl, the elderly present with lethargy, headache, frequent urination, thirst, nausea, abdominal pain. Urine should be checked for ketones. Insulin is given if indicated.

13. Special problems with diabetes
    a. Diabetic Ketoacidosis (DKA): (Seen primarily in Insulin Dependent Diabetes Mellitus), severe hyperglycemia with ketone bodies in the urine. Fruity or acetone smelling breath. Requires hospitalization. Insulin drips, every hour to two hours, fingersticks, referral, intravenous hydration and evaluation for cause.
    b. Hyperglycemic Hyperosmolar Nonketosis (HHNK): Severe hyperglycemia without ketones, seen in NIDDM. Glucose is usually > 600 mg/dl, can be > 1,000. Serum Osmolality > 340 mOsm/kg. Correct dehydration and hyperglycemia, refer, determine cause.
    c. Somogyi effect—rebound hyperglycemia: Nocturnal hypoglycemia during sleep with rebound hyperglycemia in a.m. Can lead to inappropriate increase in insulin or oral hypoglycemics. Symptoms—unexplained hyperglycemia in a.m., nightmares, ketonuria, headaches. Evaluation—3:00 a.m. fingerstick will show a low blood glucose. Treatment—lower insulin dose.
    d. Dawn phenomenon: Hyperglycemia in morning due to release of counter regulatory hormones. Evaluation: check glucose at 3:00 a.m.; it will be normal. Treatment—increase insulin at the p.m. dose.

Type I Diabetes: Insulin-Dependent Diabetes Mellitus (IDDM)

- Definition: A clinically and genetically heterogeneous group of disorders that have a common feature of abnormally high glucose levels. IDDM patients are ketosis prone.

- Etiology: These individuals have human leukocyte antigens (HLA) which produce autoantibodies which may be responsible for the destruction/inactivation of pancreatic B cells. This type of diabetes usually occurs in people less than 30 years old.

- Incidence: IDDM accounts for only 10% of all diabetes; it affects men as often as women. Some thin adult and elderly patients develop IDDM. Five percent (5%) of the total population have documented diabetes.

- Signs and Symptoms
    1. Rapid onset of flu like symptoms
    2. Polyuria, polydypsia, polyphagia

3. Weight loss
4. Blurred vision
5. Fatigue and weakness
6. Nausea and vomiting
7. Decreased level of consciousness
8. Ketones in urine and ketoacidosis
9. Frequent infections
10. Impotence

- Differential Diagnosis
    1. NIDDM
    2. Hyperglycemia from pancreatitis
    3. Hyperglycemia due to endocrine disorders and other diseases that interfere with insulin action
    4. Hyperglycemia due to drugs that promote hyperglycemia and insulin resistance
- Physical Findings
    1. Dehydrated appearance
    2. Decreased level of consciousness
    3. Fruity smelling breath
    4. Fingerstick glucose over 240 mg/dl
    5. Ketones and glucose in the urine
    6. Fungal rashes or yeast infections may be present
    7. A wound that will not heal may be present
- Diagnostic Evaluation/Findings
    1. Fasting glucose levels equal to or greater than 140 mg/dl on two occasions
    2. Glucose tolerance test: Glucose levels equal to or greater than 200 mg/dl two hours after ingesting 75 g of glucose
    3. Glycosylated hemoglobin HbA_{1C} levels of > 8 mg/dl
    4. Dipstick urine for ketones: Depending on the glucose level present

- Management/Treatment

    1. Patient teaching: Starts initially in the primary care setting or hospital but must be an ongoing process with follow up at home.
    2. Diet education
        a. Protein—15-20% of intake
        b. Carbohydrates—55-60% of intake
        c. Fat—30% maximum of intake
        d. High fiber diet and low to moderate salt
    3. Exercise: may help patient to require less insulin but should be pursued carefully, glucose levels should be monitored closely pre and post exercise.
    4. Life style modification:
        a. Decrease or eliminate smoking
        b. Decrease or eliminate alcohol consumption
        c. Integrate glucose monitoring into routine
    5. Insulin:
        a. Regular (Short acting) 30 minute onset, 2-4 hour peak, 4-6 hours duration
        b. NPH or Lente (Intermediate acting) 2-4 hour onset, peak 6-12 hours, 18-24 hours duration
        c. Ultralente (long acting) unpredictable peak, 30-36 hour duration
        d. 70/30 insulin (short and intermediate acting) 70% NPH, 30% Regular
        e. Starting doses:
            (1) Begin with 10-20 units of intermediate acting insulin
            (2) Adjust dose by 2 units at a time. Change dose no more often than every 2-3 days unless patient is hypoglycemic
        f. Monitoring Insulin Regimen:

(1) Urine testing: Useful for testing for ketones. Not as useful in the elderly due to their high renal threshold for glucose.

(2) Blood glucose monitoring: There are numerous blood glucose monitoring devices available including devices for visually impaired and disabled. Individuals should be monitoring their glucose levels at least four times a day during initial diagnosis and acute management and then twice a day (when fasting and prior to supper once levels have stablized).

- Nursing Considerations
  1. Patient education regarding disease process and benefits of maintaining good control
  2. Patient education regarding all the new modifications in lifestyle: diet, exercise, and insulin regimen
  3. Allowing patient to ventilate feelings about disease process
  4. Educate the patient regarding the necessity for excellent foot care and need for podiatry care
  5. Provide direct patient care for exacerbations of disease process
  6. Education of the staff on latest trends in diabetes care and latest technology available
  7. Perform research in area of care of the diabetic patient

Hypothyroidism

- Definition: Thyroid hormone deficiency
- Etiology: Primary hypothyroidism is thought to be due to an autoimmune process. Primary hypothyroidism often follows Hashimoto's thyroiditis or may be an iatrogenic reaction to hyperthyroidism therapy. Secondary hypothyroidism is due to the inability of the pituitary gland to secrete thyroid-stimulating hormone or the inadequate secretion from the hypothalamus of thyrotropin-releasing hormone.
- Incidence: Is thought to be about 2-5% of all those > 65 years of age and is much higher in women than men at all ages.
- Signs and Symptoms
  1. Atypical presentation

2. Arthralgia
3. Weakness
4. Decreased mental function
5. Depression symptoms
6. Constipation
7. Cold intolerance
8. Weight loss and anorexia
9. Dry coarse skin with yellowish cast
10. Dry sparse hair
11. Masklike, puffy face with periorbital edema

- Differential Diagnosis
  1. Depression
  2. Colon cancer
  3. Normal aging
  4. Dementia
  5. Euthyroid
- Physical Findings
  1. Thinning eye brows
  2. Slowing of relaxation phase of reflexes
  3. Nonpalpable thyroid (this is often a normal finding)
  4. Periorbital edema
- Diagnostic Evaluation/Findings
  1. Thyroid function tests:
     a. Increased TSH greater than or equal to 15 μU/ml
     b. Decreased or normal T_4
     c. Decreased free thyroxine index
- Management/Treatment
  1. Start with Thyroxine 0.025 mg orally daily

2. Monitor TSH level monthly
3. Increase Thyroxine by 0.025 mg in two weeks, then monthly as needed

- Nursing Considerations
  1. Educate patients and their families about the disease process, their medication dosages and side effects
  2. Provide symptom relief whenever possible
  3. Educate staff on the latest treatments and nursing interventions for hypothyroidism
  4. Monitor dietary intake and encourage a high fiber high protein diet

Hyperthyroidism

- Definition: Excessive circulating levels of T_4, T_3, or both.
- Etiology
  1. Multinodular goiter: Makes up 50% of all hyperthyroid cases in those age 60 and over. Multinodular goiters may have been euthyroid for years, then may change to become over productive of thyroid hormones.
  2. Plummer's disease: This nodular form of hyperthyroidism is less common in the elderly. This form is a toxic adenoma found on thyroid scanning to be a solitary hyperfunctioning nodule with suppression of the activity in the remainder of the thyroid gland.
  3. Graves disease: Is an autoimmune disorder that leads to the production of antibodies to the thyroid stimulating hormone (TSH) receptor on the thyroid follicular cells. This antibody is also capable of stimulating the thyroid cell causing excess secretion of hormones.
  4. Thyroiditis: Can either be of the granulomatous or lymphocytic type, characterized by a leakage of thyroglobulin, T_3, and T_4 into the circulation due to damaged follicles.
- Incidence: Hyperthyroidism is seven (7) times more prevalent in people over 60 years of age. The most common type of hyperthyroidism in the elderly is the hyperactive nodules. The incidence of hyperthyroidism is about 0.4% of the population.

- Signs and Symptoms
  1. Atypical: progressive functional decline
  2. Cardiac symptoms: atrial fibrillation, MI and tachycardia
  3. Weakness and easy fatigue
  4. Weight loss and anorexia
  5. Diarrhea
  6. Nervousness: occurs in less than 50% of the elderly
  7. Memory loss
  8. Heat intolerance
  9. Pruritus
  10. Tremor
- Differential Diagnosis
  1. Between the four causes of hyperthyroidism
  2. Thyrotoxicosis: a thyroid storm of hormones which can be fatal
  3. Pituitary disorders causing excess secretion of thyroid hormones
- Physical Findings
  1. Palpable nodules may be present
  2. May have an enlarged thyroid gland
  3. Atrial fibrillation or a pulse >90
  4. A fine regular and rapid tremor may be present
- Diagnostic Evaluation/Findings
  1. Thyroid Function Tests: decreased TSH, increased T_4, and increased T_3
  2. Thyroid radioiodine uptake: An individual is given a dose of radio opaque iodine, then thyroid gland is scanned for active nodules or hot spots.
  3. Referral to an endocrinologist
- Management/Treatment
  1. Radioactive Iodine: To obliterate the thyroid gland followed by thyroid replacement therapy

2. Anti-thyroid drugs:
    a. Propylthiouracil 100-150 mg orally every 8 hours
    b. Methimazole 10-15 mg orally every 6 hours
    c. Saturated solution of potassium iodide (SSKI) 5 drops, orally, three times per day.
    d. Betablockers; Propranolol 10 mg orally every 6 hours
    e. All of these are followed by thyroid hormone replacement
3. Surgical removal of the thyroid gland followed by thyroid replacement

- Nursing Considerations
    1. Evaluate anyone with new onset atrial fibrillation for hyperthyroidism
    2. Patient education on the medications dosages and side effects
    3. Allow patient to ventilate concerns regarding chosen therapy; medication, radioactive iodine, or surgery
    4. Monitor dietary intake and encourage high protein foods
    5. Provide symptomatic relief when possible

Hypokalemia

- Definition: A serum potassium level below 3.8 mEq/L considered severe when potassium level falls below 3.3 mEq/L.
- Etiology
    1. Excessive loss due to:
        a. Medications such as carbenicillin, amphotericin B, diuretics, or steroid therapy.
        b. Treatments such as parenteral fluid therapy without potassium replacement and gastric suctioning
        c. GI disorders, such as diarrhea, vomiting or fistula
    2. Inadequate potassium intake
    3. Alkalosis

- Incidence: Exact incidence is unknown. However, it is thought to be common in the elderly due to frequency with which diuretics and laxatives are used and the frequent occurrence of other predisposing conditions.
- Signs and Symptoms
    1. Confusion and disorientation
    2. Fatigue and weakness
    3. Apathy and anorexia
    4. Muscle cramps and even paralysis
    5. Ventricular arrhythmias (especially in people taking Digitalis)
- Differential Diagnosis
    1. Diabetic Ketoacidosis
    2. Malnutrition
    3. Renal disease
    4. Iatrogenic
- Physical Findings
    1. Physical examination may demonstrate an emaciated and dehydrated individual.
    2. Reflexes may be diminished
    3. Pulse may be irregular
- Diagnostic Evaluation/Findings
    1. Electrolyte panel will demonstrate potassium levels below 3.8 mEq/L
    2. Serum magnesium level may also be low
    3. An electrocardiogram may demonstrate ST depression, U waves, flattened T waves, ectopic beats, and tachyarrhythmias
    4. Blood gas results may demonstrate metabolic alkalosis
- Management/Treatment
    1. A diet rich in potassium
    2. Treatment of cause e.g., diabetic ketoacidosis, diarrhea or vomiting
    3. Potassium replacement therapy:

a. Divided doses of 10% potassium chloride, 20 to 80 mEq/day can be given orally

b. Potassium gluconate, 20 to 80 mEq/day, is more appropriate when metabolic alkalosis is present

c. When potassium can not be taken by mouth, intravenous potassium is available. The dose is not to exceed 40 mEq/L at a rate of 10-20 mEq/hour

d. Removal of potassium depleting diuretics and switching to K-sparing diuretics if possible

- Nursing Considerations
  1. Nurses should keep in mind how susceptible elderly patients are to electrolyte disturbances and monitor test results as available
  2. Patient/client education regarding:
     a. Condition and the treatments being given
     b. Prescribed medications, their dosages, time to be taken and reason for being taken
     c. Foods high in potassium
     d. Necessity of contacting primary care provider if symptoms recur
  3. Monitor their cardiac rhythm
  4. Follow up potassium levels in one month, then every six months for a year, annually thereafter

Hyperkalemia

- Definition: A serum potassium level greater than 5.0 mEq/L.

- Etiology: Age related decreases in renin and aldosterone levels increase the elderly person's risk for hyperkalemia. Medications such as angiotensin-converting enzymes inhibit potassium elimination. Cyclosporin, nonsteroidal anti-inflammatory drugs, and beta-adrenergic blockers may cause hyperkalemia. It is also common in renal failure patients.

- Incidence: Thought to be common due to age-related changes that predispose elderly to this condition. Incidence is unknown.

- Signs and Symptoms
  1. Nausea
  2. Intermittent intestinal colic or diarrhea
  3. Muscle weakness
  4. Flaccid muscle paralysis
  5. Paresthesia of face, tongue, feet, and hands
  6. Ventricular arrhythmias
  7. Cardiac arrest
- Differential Diagnosis
  1. Neuromuscular damage
  2. Dehydration
- Physical Findings
  1. Decreased reflexes
  2. Irregular pulse
  3. Paresthesia of face, tongue, feet and hands
  4. Signs of dehydration
  5. Cardiac arrest
- Diagnostic Evaluation/Findings
  1. Electrolyte panel will demonstrate a potassium level > 5.0 mEq/l
  2. Arterial blood gasses may demonstrate metabolic acidosis
  3. Electrocardiogram will demonstrate: peaked T waves, widened QRS complex, Prolonged P-R interval and ventricular arrhythmias
- Management/Treatment
  1. Restrict the intake of potassium or drugs potentiating hyperkalemia
  2. Elimination of potassium
     a. Sodium Polystyrene Sulfate (Kayexalate): Given orally 15-30 g with sorbitol or rectally 50 g in the form of a retention enema.

b. Potent Diuretic Therapy: This can be helpful to reduce the serum potassium level and reduce fluid overload. IV administration of furosemide (lasix) or ethacrynic acid (Edecrin) should be individually dosed.

c. Dialysis: Is reserved for extreme cases of hyperkalemia. These patients are usually dialysis patients already.

d. Glucose and Insulin: Has been used in emergency situations. Insulin facilitates the movement of potassium into the cells thereby reducing the serum potassium level.

e. Calcium gluconate also is used in emergency situations to protect the heart. It does not reduce the serum potassium level but may provide time to reduce the serum potassium level by providing protection to the myocardium. This should be used when symmetrical peaked T waves and widened QRS complexes are present.

f. Sodium Bicarbonate: Temporarily shifts potasium into the cells lowering the serum potassium level. It is also useful when patient has metabolic acidosis.

- Nursing Considerations

1. Nurses must be aware that this is a common condition that the elderly are predisposed to, and due to its potentially fatal outcome, a high index of suspicion should be maintained and laboratory tests should be monitored.

2. Patient/client education regarding:

   a. Prescribed medications, their dosages, time to be taken and reasons for being taken.

   b. Low potassium foods and which foods to avoid.

   c. Reasons for elimination of potassium sparing medications.

3. Monitor the patient's cardiac rhythm

4. Educate nursing staff about hyperkalemia; signs and symptoms especially EKG changes.

5. Patient follow-up should include serum potassium levels in one month, once stabilized, then every six months for a year, then annually therafter.

Hyponatremia

- Definition: The decrease in serum sodium (Na) concentration to less than 135 mEq/L that occurs when there is an excess of water relative to total sodium. The total extracellular fluid may be increased, normal or decreased.
- Etiology: There are several reasons for hyponatremia in the elderly:
    1. Volume depletion from vomiting, diarrhea, GI suctioning, renal disorders, diuretic therapy
    2. Dilutional hyponatremia from water excess compared with the sodium level caused by heart failure, cirrhosis, and renal disorders.
    3. Syndrome of Inappropriate Antidiuretic Hormone Secretion (SIADH)—total body sodium content is normal but water is retained because of increased ADH secretion. It is defined by these classic findings:
        a. Inappropriate hypertonicity of urine, with osmolality often hypertonic to plasma
        b. Increased excretion of sodium in the urine
        c. Plasma volume dilution: normal or low BUN and creatinine levels
        d. Absence of edema
- Incidence: Elderly are at increased risk for hyponatremia especially if they are hospitalized or institutionalized. Studies have demonstrated a 7% incidence of hyponatremia in hospitalized elderly and a 18-22% incidence of hyponatremia in elderly nursing home residents (Abrams, & Berkow, 1990).
- Signs and Symptoms
    1. Presence of symptoms depends on the magnitude of the hyponatremia.
        a. May be absent if chronic
        b. Lethargy and fatigue
        c. Muscle cramps
        d. GI symptoms: nausea and anorexia
        e. Disorientation to confusion

f. Coma

g. Seizures

- Differential Diagnosis
  1. Types of hyponatremia
  2. Neuromuscular problems
  3. Seizure disorder
- Physical Findings
  1. Signs of hypovolemia, dehydration
  2. Edema (with dilutional hyponatremia)
  3. Depressed sensorium
  4. Decreased deep tendon reflexes
  5. Hypothermia
  6. Seizures
- Diagnostic Evaluation/Findings
  1. An electrolyte panel demonstrates a sodium level below 136 mEq/L
  2. BUN and Creatinine levels are usually normal in dilutional and SIADH hyponatremia
  3. BUN and Creatinine levels are usually high in volume depletion hyponatremia
  4. Urinary sodium levels are low (< 20 mEq/l) in patients with volume depletion or edema and high (> 20 mEq/l) in patients with SIADH.
- Management/Treatment: Depends on the reason for the hyponatremia
  1. Volume depletion hyponatremia
     a. Correct the volume depletion with isotonic saline solution
     b. Sodium levels < 125 mEq/L require a hypertonic saline solution
  2. Dilutional hyponatremia
     a. Fluid restrictions are useful in CHF and Cirrhosis which requires potassium depleting diuretics; 1000 cc to 1500 cc fluid restriction should be sufficient.

b. Decrease fluid volume overload from other sources, e.g., IV therapy or excessive intake of liquids

3. SIADH:

a. Fluid restriction of 1000 cc to 1500 cc daily

b. May require IV infusion of hypertonic saline solution

c. Chronic management includes Demeclocycline, a tetracycline antibiotic which causes increased sodium levels by interfering with the effects of ADH on the kidneys.

- Nursing Considerations

1. Nurses should have a high suspicion for hyponatremia in hospital and nursing home setting.

2. Educate patient and families on fluid restriction and encourage the patient to eat fruit and suck on hard candy rather than drinking fluids

3. Educate the patient on the change in their medications, the dosage, and side effects.

4. Monitor patient's sodium level

5. Monitor patient's intake and output

6. Seizure precautions for patients with sodium levels below 125 mEq/L

7. Educate the nursing staff on the signs and symptoms of hyponatremia and the latest in nursing and medical treatment.

Malnutrition

- Definition: Malnutrition is a negative imbalance between the nutrient supply to tissues and the requirement for that nutrient, whether from an inappropriate dietary intake or defective utilization by the body (Abrams & Berkow, 1990).
- Etiology: There are multiple causes for malnutrition in the elderly: depression, cancer, gastrointestinal disorders, hyperthyroidism, medications, poor intake, cholesterol phobia, and tuberculosis. Social factors causing malnutrition include social isolation and financial difficulties.
- Incidence: malnutrition is frequently encountered in the elderly, especially frail elderly.

- Signs and Symptoms
    1. Loss of appetite
    2. Peripheral edema
    3. Cachexia
    4. Glossitis
    5. Gradual or sudden weight loss
    6. Poor wound healing
- Differential Diagnosis
    1. Depression
    2. Cancer
    3. Anorexia
    4. Tuberculosis
    5. Hyperthyroidism
- Physical Findings
    1. Cachexia
    2. Obesity
    3. Edema
    4. Wounds that will not heal
    5. Signs of illnesses possibly causing malnutrition
- Diagnostic Evaluation/Findings
    1. Weekly weights will document gradual weight loss; dietary history should confirm compromised dietary intake.
    2. Anthropometric measurements are used as general guides; norms have not yet been established for elderly
    3. Laboratory evaluation should include serum hemoglobin, iron, transferrin, total iron binding capacity, folate and B_{12} levels. These levels can all be low for certain types of malnutrition.
    4. Stool for occult blood may be positive in GI disorders or cancer.
    5. Serum cholesterol level, albumin and total protein will be low. Albumin is a late indicator of malnutrition.

6. Geriatric Depression Scale: greater than 15 is indicative of depression in the elderly.

- Management/Treatment
    1. Focuses on treating the underlying cause. Encourage food intake; small frequent meals in congenial setting
        a. Dietary consultation regarding food preferences
        b. Nutritional supplements: milk shakes, ice cream, Ensure or other nutritional supplements.
        c. Monitor weekly weights and monthly laboratory tests
        d. Enteral hyperalimentation, hopefully for short term restorative therapy
        e. Parental hyperalimentation is useful, short term, especially preoperatively and postoperatively.
- Nursing Considerations
    1. Nurses should not be misled by obesity; most obese elderly are malnourished
    2. Monitor weights at least weekly in patients who have demonstrated a gradual weight loss over a year to few months.
    3. Special care is needed in feeding the frail elderly; recruit volunteers to assist with feeding in long term care settings.
    4. Encourage supplements, and encourage family to bring in food from home.
    5. Discourage low cholesterol diets for elderly whose cholesterol levels are below 240.
    6. Educate patient and family regarding proper diet and need for supplements.
    7. Assess patient for depression and make appropriate referrals.
    8. Educate nursing staff regarding signs and symptoms of malnutrition and resulting sequelae.

Questions

1. Changes in mental status can be found in:

    a. Hypoglycemia
    b. Hypothyroidism
    c. Hyperthyroidism
    d. All of the above

2. Insulin-dependent diabetes mellitus:

    a. Is the most common type of diabetes in the elderly
    b. Frequently presents with glucose levels over 1,000 mg/dl
    c. Presents with elevated glucose levels and ketones in the urine
    d. Is due to post receptor deficits that impair glucose transport

3. Non-insulin-dependent diabetes:

    a. Accounts for only 10% of diabetics
    b. May present with glucose levels over 1,000 mg/dl
    c. Always presents with ketones in the urine
    d. None of the above

4. A 78 year old man on micronase 2.5 mg po Q am, is complaining of having a flu. He wants to know what the sick day guidelines are. Which of the following is not a sick day guideline?

    a. He should skip his micronase today
    b. He should push po fluids
    c. He should monitor his glucose level more frequently
    d. He should notify his primary care provider if he can not keep fluids down

5. Patient education for newly diagnosed diabetics should:

    a. Not begin until they are discharged home
    b. Start in the hospital or primary care setting and continue at home
    c. Cover all the complications at once
    d. Should include diet teaching on a low protein and low fiber diet

6. An 80 year old diabetic woman presents with difficulty walking on her right foot. What do you need to assess:

    a. Her blood sugar levels. They may be low causing problems with her balance

b. Her blood pressure. She may be having a stroke
c. Her foot. She may have developed a foot ulcer
d. None of the above

7. An 84 year old female in the nursing home reports complaints of weakness, constipation, and dry skin that started about a month ago. What should be done?
   a. She should have thyroid function tests drawn
   b. One hemoccult should be done to rule out colon cancer
   c. Nothing, this is just normal aging
   d. Depression screening

8. A patient comes into the nursing home from the hospital after having an MI. Now she is weak, tremulous, nervous, confused, and has atrial fibrillation. What is this woman's most likely problem?
   a. She's just making the difficult transition into a nursing home.
   b. She probably had some cerebral anoxia when she had her MI.
   c. She should have thyroid function tests; she may be hyperthyroid.
   d. She has new onset atrial fibrillation and needs to be on digoxin.

9. You notice there are a lot of residents on your unit in the nursing home complaining of yeast infections. So you:
   a. Start treatment and begin monitoring their blood sugars more closely
   b. Evaluate everyone's thyroid function
   c. Tell the staff that they are doing a great job with washing their hands.
   d. None of the above

10. NPH insulin has a (an):
    a. Onset in 2-4 hours and lasts 18-24 hours
    b. Peaks in 6-12 hours and lasts 32-36 hours
    c. Onset in 30 minutes and lasts 4-6 hours
    d. Peaks in 2-4 hours and lasts 16-18 hours

11. When someone is hypoglycemic they need:
    a. Better diabetic teaching
    b. An insulin drip in the hospital
    c. 15 gms of carbohydrates
    d. Fingerstick glucose levels every 15 minutes until they improve

12. On reviewing the am fasting glucose blood levels and am fingerstick glucose levels you find large discrepancies. So you:
    a. Discard the glucose meter you have and buy a new one
    b. Develop a program to standardize the method used for fingersticks and check it for accuracy
    c. Discontinue fasting fingersticks they are obviously a waste of time
    d. Cancel all fasting glucose blood draws. They are obviously inaccurate

13. Treatment for hypokalemia includes all of the following except:
    a. Removing potassium depleting medications as much as possible
    b. A diet rich in potassium
    c. Potassium replacement
    d. Eliminate magnesium rich foods from their diet

14. Hyperkalemia is potentially fatal because:
    a. It is accompanied by flaccid paralysis
    b. Cardiac arrhythmias are common
    c. It results from severe malnutrition
    d. All of the above

15. Treatment for non-emergent hyperkalemia includes:
    a. Insulin and glucose infusions
    b. Calcium gluconate I.V.
    c. Sodium bicarbonate I.V.
    d. Sodium polystyrene sulfate p.o. every 2-4 hours.

16. An 84 year old woman in the hospital is found to have hyponatremia. What tests need to be done to determine what kind of hyponatremia she has?
    a. Serum sodium level, urinary sodium level and Hemoglobin and Hematocrit
    b. Urinary sodium level, BUN and Creatinine and Hemoglobin and Hematocrit
    c. Serum sodium level, BUN and Creatinine and Urinary sodium levels
    d. BUN and Creatinine, Serum sodium levels and Hemoglobin and Hematocrit

17. Common causes of malnutrition include all but the following:
    a. Depression
    b. Cancer
    c. Tuberculosis
    d. Cerebral vascular accidents

18. Your patient is asking why she has to take thyroxine every day when she feels fine. You respond by:
    a. Explaining that since her thyroid gland has been removed she needs to replace the hormone that her gland used to produce in order to stay feeling fine.
    b. Telling her that you will have it discontinued as soon as possible
    c. Explaining to her that this is the way the thyroxine is ordered
    d. Referring her for counselling, she is obviously having trouble dealing with having a chronic disease

19. Nursing considerations for the elderly who have malnutrition include all of the following except:
    a. Assessing the elder for depression
    b. Treating obese elders with high cholesterol diets
    c. Recruiting volunteers to assist with feeding elderly in the long term care setting
    d. Educating elder and their family regarding proper diet

20. Nursing assessment for malnutrition includes:
    a. Drawing cholesterol and albumin levels
    b. Weekly weights and dietary histories
    c. Ppd and chest x-rays
    d. None of the above

21. Signs and symptoms of malnutrition include all of the following except:
    a. Euphoria
    b. Peripheral edema
    c. Poor wound healing
    d. Loss of Appetite

22. Your 83 year old client continues to have high am fasting blood sugars despite the increased dose of pm insulin that has been ordered. What should you do next?

    a. Discontinue their evening snack.
    b. Restrict their diet to 1600 calorie ADA.
    c. Increase the evening dose of insulin until their am fasting blood sugar is within an acceptable range.
    d. Check a 3 am fingerstick.

23. Medications which will increase a client's blood glucose include all but which of the following:

    a. Glucorticoids
    b. Alcohol
    c. Salicylates (large doses)
    d. Sulfa drugs

24. The EKG changes that suggest an elderly client has hyperkalemia include:

    a. Ectopic beats, bradyarrhythmia and ST elevation
    b. Peaked T waves, widened QRS, prolonged P-R interval and ventricular arrhythmias
    c. ST depression, U waves, ectopic beats and tachyarrhythmias
    d. Atrial fibrillation with peaked T waves and tachyarrhythmias

25. The EKG changes that suggest the elderly client is hypokalemic include:

    a. Ectopic beats, bradyarrhythmia and ST elevation
    b. Peaked T waves, widened QRS, prolonged P-R interval and ventricular arrhythmias
    c. ST depression, U waves, ectopic beats and tachyarrhythmias
    d. Atrial fibrillation with peaked T waves and tachyarrhythmias

26. The starting dose of Thyroxine (Synthroid) for an elderly client is:

    a. Thyroxine 0.025 mg, orally, b.i.d. for one month then titrate up by 0.025 mg
    b. Thyroxine 0.25 mg, orally, q.d. for 2 weeks then titrate up by 0.25 mg
    c. Thyroxine 0.025 mg, orally, q.d. for 2 weeks then titrate up by 0.025 mg
    d. Thyroxine 0.25 mg, orally, b.i.d. for one month then titrate up by 0.25 mg

27. Signs and symptoms of hyperthyroidism include all of the following except:

    a. Constipation
    b. Weight loss
    c. Functional decline
    d. Memory loss

28. All of the following are potential causes of hypokalemia except:

    a. Gastric suctioning
    b. Ace inhibitor medications
    c. Poor dietary intake
    d. Metabolic alkalosis

29. Treatments for SIADH include:

    a. A low salt diet
    b. Pushing fluids to 2000 cc a day
    c. Penicillin VK 500 mg orally, q. 6 hours
    d. None of the above

30. Your client presents with symptoms of muscle aches, weakness, constipation, and a puffy face. Your most likely diagnosis would be:

    a. Depression
    b. Hypothyroidism
    c. Colon cancer
    d. Hyperkalemia

31. Which is not a possible cause of hyperkalemia

    a. The use of nonsteroidal anti-inflammatory drugs
    b. Renal disease
    c. Crohn's disease
    d. Use of ACE Inhibitors

32. Nursing considerations for hypokalemia include:

    a. Dietary teaching on which foods are high in potassium
    b. Eliminating all potassium sparing medications
    c. Explaining their condition and why medications are not necessary for its treatment
    d. None of the above

33. Hyponatremia occurs frequently in the elderly due to which of the following reasons:

    a. Dehydration is common in the elderly due to diuretic therapy
    b. Dehydration is common in the elderly due to malnutrition
    c. Volume excess is common in the elderly due to an increased thirst drive
    d. Volume excess due to decreased antidiuretic hormone secretion due to SIADH

34. Treatment options for hyperthyroidism include all of the following except:

    a. Propranolol 10 mg, orally, Q 6 hours
    b. Propylthiouracil 100 mg, orally, Q 8 hours
    c. Furosemide 20 mg, orally, Q 12 hours
    d. Methimazole 10 mg, orally, Q 6 hours

35. What laboratory findings would be diagnostic of hypothyroidism?

    a. Increased TSH, increased T_4 and decreased free thyroxine index
    b. Decreased TSH, increased T_4 and increased T_3
    c. Increased TSH, increased T_4 and increased T_3
    d. Increased TSH, decreased T_4 and decreased free thyroxine index

36. Anthropometric measures are used:

    a. To diagnose malnutrition in the elderly
    b. To suggest and ideal weight for each elderly person
    c. As general guides due to lack of norms for the elderly
    d. Only in those individuals below age 55

37. Which oral hypoglycemic agent is used with caution in the elderly due to its long half life:

    a. Chlorpropamide (Diabinese)
    b. Tolbutamide (Orinase)
    c. Glipizide (Glucotrol)
    d. Acetohexamide (Dymelor)

38. Which of the oral hypoglycemics needs to be taken on an empty stomach:

    a. Chlorpropamide (Diabinese)
    b. Tolbutamide (Orinase)
    c. Glipizide (Glucotrol)
    d. Acetohexamide (Dymelor)

Answers:

1. d
2. c
3. b
4. a
5. b
6. c
7. a
8. c
9. a
10. a
11. c
12. b
13. d
14. b
15. d
16. c
17. d
18. a
19. b
20. b
21. a
22. d
23. a
24. b
25. c
26. c
27. a
28. b
29. d
30. b
31. c
32. a
33. a
34. c
35. d
36. c
37. a
38. c

Bibliography

Abrams, W. and Berkow, R., (1990). *The Merck manual of geriatrics.* New Jersey: Merck Sharp and Dohme Research Laboratories.

American Academy of Family Physicians, The American Dietetic Association, National Council on the Aging, Inc. (1991). *Nutrition screening manual for professionals caring for older americans.* Washington, DC: Greer, Margolis, Mitchell, Grunwald & Associates, Inc.

Bohannon, N. (1988). Diabetes in the elderly. *Post Graduate Medicine, 8*,(5), 283-295.

Brocklehurst, J. C., Jallis, R. C., Fillit, H. M., (Ed) (1992). *Textbook of geriatric medicine and gerontology.* New York: Churchill Livingstone.

Hazzard, W., Andres, R., Bierman, E., & Blass, J., (1990). *Principles of geriatric medicine and gerontology.* New York: McGraw-Hill Information Services Company.

Hogstel, M. (Ed.). (1992). *Clinical manual of gerontological nursing.* St. Louis: Mosby Year Book.

Metheny, N. (1992). *Fluid and electrolyte balance nursing considerations* (2nd ed.). Philadelphia: J. B. Lippincott Company.

Solomon, D. (1987). The elderly patient with thyroid disease. *Geriatric Consultant*, March-April, 20-23.

Tracy, J., & Eufemio, M., (1988). Pitfalls in the diagnosis of hypothyroidism in the elderly. *Geriatric Medicine Today, 17*(8), 47-50.

Tzagournis, M., & Skillman, T., (1989). *Diabetes mellitus an overview.* Kalamazoo: Upjohn.

Psychosocial Problems

Lois S. Walker

Bereavement

- Definition: Bereavement is the process of mourning the death of a loved one. The tasks of bereavement are to accept the reality of the loss, separate emotionally from the deceased, and move on to establish new relationships and lifestyle. The bereavement process takes about two years to complete, but many elders report feelings of loss remain for much longer.
- Etiology: Bereavement occurs in all age groups. Elders report adjusting to the loss of a spouse or child are among the most difficult of life's experiences.
- Incidence
  1. Bereavement is a universal experience in late life. There are more similarities than differences between elderly men and women with this process. Dealing with loneliness and managing the tasks of daily living are considered their greatest problems.
  2. The first year of bereavement is the hardest for widowers. In contrast to widows, they have more health problems (especially CVD) and higher rates of mortality from suicide or natural causes.
  3. Widows are more vulnerable in the second to third years of bereavement. They have more mental health problems (especially depression and anxiety disorders) and more somatic complaints.
  4. An estimated 15% to 25% of elders experience dysfunctional or unresolved grief reactions. Risk factors are: multiple life crises, psychiatric problems, poor health, nonsupportive environment, low socioeconomic status, conflicted or dependent relationship with the deceased, and severe depression in initial phase of bereavement.
- Signs and Symptoms: Common symptoms of uncomplicated bereavement
  1. Initial phase (first several weeks)
     a. Shock and denial
     b. Numbness and emptiness
     c. "Free-floating" anxiety
     d. Somatic symptoms
  2. Second phase (4–6 weeks)
     a. Numbness and anxiety diminish

b. Yearning to be reunited with loved one
c. Anger toward the deceased for leaving
d. Transitory auditory or visual hallucinations and/or a strong ''sense of presence'' of the deceased
e. Crying, depressed mood, loss of energy
f. Chronic sleep disturbance
g. Poor appetite
h. Loss of interest in daily activities
i. Concentration and memory problems
j. Search for explanation of the death
k. Obsessional review of death scene
l. Begin to accept finality of the death

3. Third phase (about one year–24 months.)
   a. Realization its time to get on with life
   b. Renegotiate social identity
   c. Learn to cope with loneliness
   d. New role acquisition and skills

- Differential Diagnosis
  1. Major depressive disorder.
  2. Adjustment disorder with depressed mood
- Physical Findings: In elderly persons, bereavement is usually accompanied by physical symptoms of stomach distress, shortness of breath, frequent sighing, an empty feeling in the abdomen, lack of muscular power, and great ''subjective distress.'' Chronic sleep problems and lack of appetite with subsequent weight loss often motivate the individual to seek medical attention for symptomatic relief.
- Diagnostic Evaluation/Findings: Commonly, the elderly survivor meets the criteria for clinical depression. The bereaved usually regards the feeling of depressed mood as ''normal'' and reports it does not interfere with necessary functioning. Dysfunctional grieving, in contrast, is delayed and/or distorted. Signs are:

a. Acquisition of symptoms belonging to last illness of deceased

b. Significant hostility toward persons connected with the death, especially physicians and nurses

c. Acts in ways detrimental to social or economic existence (giving away belongings or making foolish economic decisions)

d. Agitated depression with feelings of worthlessness, bitter self-accusation and obvious need for punishment

e. False euphoria

f. Self-destructive impulses

g. Overidentification with decreased

h. Failure to progress through the usual phases

- Management/Treatment

1. Uncomplicated bereavement

a. Provide information about the grieving process

b. Facilitate process of grieving

c. Assist to manage somatic symptoms

d. Refer to self-help and support groups

e. Assess need for help with financial matters, living arrangements and personal care. Involve family members in decision-making and refer to appropriate legal and social services.

f. Caution not to make major life decisions until main period of grieving has passed.

g. Provide information about anniversary reactions

2. Dysfunctional grieving

a. Refer for psychiatric evaluation

b. Assess suicide risk

- Nursing Considerations

1. Uncomplicated bereavement

a. Facilitate healthy resolution

(1) Encourage to verbalize feelings
(2) Empathetic listening
(3) Validate feelings and experiences
(4) Work with family members and close friends to provide support
(5) Assist to work through any unfinished business with deceased (journal writing, visits to grave, prayer)
(6) Provide in-home or telephone contacts for homebound elder
(7) Prevent isolation and loneliness
    (a) Promote peer involvement
    (b) Refer to support groups
(8) Reinforce strengths and self-esteem

b. Assist to meet physical needs
    (1) Monitor eating patterns
    (2) Monitor sleep patterns
    (3) Reinforce medical care regimens

2. Dysfunctional grieving
    a. Identify elders at risk
    b. Assess response to grief process
    c. Provide grief counseling
    d. Refer for psychiatric consult and/or psychotherapy
3. Primary prevention
    a. Participate in community education programs
    b. Assess community resources
    c. Advocate for needed resources and services

Depression

- Definition: Clinical depression is a syndrome consisting of a constellation of physical, affective and cognitive symptoms that range in severity from mild to severe. Depression in late life is underdiagnosed because clinicians and elders incorrectly attribute the symptoms to the aging process or medical problems. Because depression is underdiagnosed, many elders do not receive adequate treatment.

- Etiology: Depression in late life is multifactorial in origin involving a combination of psychosocial, biological and genetic factors.
  1. Genetic
     a. More common in women than men (2:1)
     b. Family history of depression is statistically greater than chance but less than in younger depressives
  2. Biochemical
     a. Levels of norepinephrine and serotonin decrease with age
     b. The enzyme monoamine oxidase and the metabolite 5-hydroxyindoleacetic acid increase with age
  3. Dysregulation of the hypothalamic-pituitary-adrenal (HPA) axis.
     a. Cortisol levels are increased in depression
     b. Nondepressed elders have a higher incidence of false positive responses to the dexamethasone suppression test (DST) than younger persons
  4. Dysregulation of the thyroid axis and in growth hormone release
     a. Blunted responses of thyroid stimulating hormone (TSH) to the administration of thyroid releasing hormone (TRH) are found in many normal elders and in depressed patients
     b. Growth hormone is secreted only during sleep in the elderly and may cease altogether.
  5. Desynchronization of circadian rhythms
     a. Depressive illnesses are cyclic and cause insomnia and diurnal variation of mood
     b. Sleep cycle disrupted in old age
  6. Learned helplessness hypothesis
  7. Sociodemographic risk factors
     a. Female

b. Unmarried, particularly the widowed

c. Lack of supportive social network

d. Co-occurrence of physical conditions such as stroke, cancer and dementia

8. Negative cognitive-behavioral reinforcements
9. Reactivation of unresolved early losses

- Incidence

1. Approximately 15% of community resident elders have depressive illness. The prevalence of major depression among these elderly is about 3%. The rates of depressive illness among nursing home residents is estimated as 15% to 25%. In addition, 13% of nursing home residents are reported to develop a new episode of major depression during any given year and another 18% develop new depressive symptoms. (NIH Consensus Development Panel on Depression in Late Life, 1992)
2. The elderly age group is least likely to receive treatment for depression. It is estimated that only 10% of the elderly who are in need of psychiatric treatment ever receive it.
3. Mortality rates for depressed elders are much higher than for their nondepressed peers.
4. The course of depression in elderly adults is similar to that in younger age groups. An estimated 70% of patients treated for depression recover, but future episodes of depression do recur in about 40% of these people.

- Signs and Symptoms

1. Physical symptoms

   a. Decrease or increase in appetite/weight (– or +5 lb)

   b. Insomnia or hypersomnia

   c. Psychomotor agitation or retardation

   d. Fatigue or lack of energy

2. Emotional symptoms

   a. Depressed or dysphoric mood

TABLE 1

Diagnostic Criteria for Depressive Disorders

	Major Depression	*Dysthymia*	*Depressive Disorder NOS*	*Adjustment Disorder Depressed*
Episode	Daily for at least 2 weeks	Continuous symptoms for 2 years	Variable	Occurs within 3 months of identified stressor
Intensity	Depressed mood or anhedonia and at least 4 symptoms	Depressed mood and at least 2 symptoms	Depressed mood and 2 or 4 symptoms	Depressed mood and impaired function or symptoms in excess of those expected for the degree of stress
Course	Variable onset and duration. Can be superimposed upon dysthymia	No clear onset, has chronic course.	Variable	Symptoms ease as stress decreases. Can lead to major depression.

Note. From *Diagnostic and Statistical Manual of Mental Disorders* (3rd ed. rev.) by American Psychiatric Association, 1987, Washington, D. C.: Author. Adapted by permission.

b. Anhedonia (inability to experience pleasure)

c. Low self-esteem

d. Feelings of hopelessness, worthlessness, or guilt

3. Cognitive symptoms

   a. Difficulty thinking, concentrating or making decisions

   b. Thoughts of death or suicide

   c. Cognitive deficits (''pseudodementia'')

   d. Delusions, often of persecution, incurable illness, or nihilism

4. Diagnostic criteria for depressive disorders (see Table 1)

   a. Major depression

      (1) Symptoms are severe and disabling

      (2) ''Pseudodementia'' may be present

      (3) Seasonal affective disorder (SAD)

   b. Dysthymia (depressive neurosis)

      (1) Loss of self-esteem prominent

      (2) Introjection and guilt usually absent

      (3) Poor coping skills

c. Depressive disorder not otherwise specified (NOS)
   (1) Symptoms moderate to severe
   (2) Does not meet criteria for dysthymia or major depression
d. Adjustment disorder with depressed mood (reactive depression)
   (1) Precipitating stressor present
   (2) Depressed mood with hopelessness
e. Organic mood syndrome
   (1) Major depressive episode due to a specific medical or pathophysiological condition
   (2) Medications most common cause
   (3) Fearfulness, anxiety, or irritability often present

- Differential Diagnosis
  1. Medical conditions

TABLE 2

Medical Conditions and Medications that Cause Depression

Neurological	**Medications**
Dementias	Antipsychotics
Parkinson's disease	Barbiturates
Stroke	Benzodiazepines
ALS	Meprobamate
Multiple sclerosis	Corticosteroids
Seizure disorders	Methyldopa
Brain tumors	Digitalis
Metabolic	Beta-blockers
Hypothyroidism	Reserpine
Hyperthyroidism	Antidepressants
Addison's disease	Estrogens
Hypokalemia	Hydralazine
Severe anemia	Anti-Parkinsonians
Diabetes Type II	**Others**
Vitamin B_{12} deficiency	Alcohol abuse
Hepatitis	Chronic pain
Cushing's disease	Cancer
Cardiovascular disease	Rheumatoid arthritis
Hypertension	Chronic infection
Myocardial infarction	COPD
Coronary artery bypass surgery	Sleep disorders
Congestive heart failure	Impaired renal function

TABLE 3

Clinical Characteristics of Depression and Dementia

Depression	*Dementia*
Clear onset of cognitive problems	Insidious onset
Symptoms of relatively short duration	Symptoms present for longer time period
Consistent depressed mood	Mood usually labile or blunted. May be depressed
Patient complains of cognitive loss	May complain of cognitive loss but tends to conceal problems
Makes little effort to perform tasks	Struggles to perform tasks and reply appropriately
Attention and concentration often good	Attention and concentration often poor
Responds with many ''Don't know'' answers	Attempts to answer questions

The clinical evaluation of depression is complex and challenging. Many medical conditions and medications have depressive symptoms as part of their clinical syndrome. Others mask depressive symptoms or lead to a secondary depression. (see Table 2)

2. Dementia

   Depression can be superimposed upon dementia or cognitive deficits can be symptoms of depression and not dementia (''pseudodementia''). Correct diagnosis and treatment for depression will often lead to a return of cognitive function. (see Table 3)

- Physical Findings

  1. Appearance: Depressed elders may resemble the depressed person of any age. It is more likely, however, that the elderly mask their symptoms by

     a. Expressing depressive symptoms through somatic complaints, most commonly, gastrointestinal problems.

     b. Conveying feelings of helplessness, despair and worthlessness in an indirect manner during an interaction

     c. Agitated and anxious behaviors (handwringing, pacing, twisting a handkerchief, etc.)

     d. Appearing apathetic and expressionless with poor attention and difficulty in establishing rapport

  2. Comprehensive physical examination including neurological status, to rule out medical causes

3. Specific diagnostic tests for depression

   a: The dexamethasone suppression test (DST) and other laboratory tests for depression are not deemed reliable for clinical practice at this time.

- Diagnostic Evaluation/Findings

  1. The assessment interview: Provides data for making a diagnosis and prescribing treatment. It is also the first therapeutic interaction between the nurse and the depressed elder. The clinician, therefore, needs to be sensitive to the relationship-building aspects of the interaction by:

     a. Introducing self by name and title

     b. Explaining the purpose of the interview in clear terms and stating briefly what the client can expect as a result of the assessment.

     c. Conducting the interaction in a comfortable setting that assures privacy.

     d. Discussing issues of confidentiality and answering any questions the client may have about who will have access to information that was discussed.

     e. Addressing the client formally as Mr., Mrs., etc.

     f. Maintaining eye contact and sitting close enough so a hearing or visually impaired person can understand what is said.

     g. Pacing the interaction so the client has sufficient time to respond without feeling rushed.

     h. Using a conversational style to gather information. This does not rule out the use of standardized instruments to evaluate depressive symptoms or mental status.

     i. Summarizing what was discussed at the end of the interaction and making some brief comments about your preliminary impressions. Be careful to comment on strengths as well as problems that were discussed.

     j. Inviting the elder to ask you any concluding questions.

     k. Bringing closure to the interaction by informing the elder what you will do with the information and what outcomes can be expected.

2. Psychosocial Assessment for Depression
   a. Patient and family history
      (1) Length of current depressive episode
      (2) History of previous depressive episodes
      (3) History of drug and alcohol use
      (4) Response to previous therapeutic interventions
      (5) Family history of depression, suicide, and/or alcohol abuse
   b. Presenting problem
      (1) Description in client's words
      (2) Onset, duration, symptoms noted and progression
      (3) Solutions attempted
      (4) Significant changes in client's life
      (5) How responsibility for problem is viewed
   c. General observations
      (1) Appearance and response to interview
      (2) Consistency of behavior
      (3) Nonverbal behavior, i. e., posture, mannerisms, facial expression, etc
      (4) Clinician's response to client
   d. Mood
      (1) Description of mood
      (2) Suicidal/homicidal ideas or plan
   e. Thought content and processes
      (1) Preoccupations
      (2) Do thoughts flow logically
      (3) Delusions

f. Perceptions
   (1) Illusions
   (2) Hallucinations

g. Problems with self esteem and feelings of guilt

h. Coping mechanisms and strengths

i. Mental Status
   (1) Concentration
   (2) Memory retention and immediate recall
   (3) Comprehension
   (4) Counting and calculation
   (5) Judgment

3. Specific Mental Status Tests
   a. Folstein's Mini-Mental State
   b. Pfeiffer's Short Portable Mental Status Questionnaire

4. Specific Depression Schedules
   a. Yesavage's Geriatric Depression Scale
   b. Beck Depression Inventory
   c. Zung Self-Rating Depression Scale

- Management/Treatment
  1. Goals of treatment
     a. Partial or complete remission of depressive symptoms
     b. Reduce risk of relapse and recurrence
     c. Improvement of the pain and suffering associated with physical illnesses.
     d. Enhancement of general mental, physical and social functioning and personal well-being
     e. Minimization of cognitive disability
     f. Reduction of health care costs and mortality

TABLE 4

Common or Troublesome Side Effects of Antidepressants

Anticholinergic -Dry mouth and nasal passages -Constipation -Urinary hesitancy -Blurred vision -Tachycardia -Poor concentration -Memory dysfunction -Temperature dysregulation **Autonomic** -Orthostatic hypotension -Palpitations -Increased sweating -Tremor -Cardiac conduction delays	**Central Nervous System** -Stimulation -Sedation -Delirium -Myoclonic twitches -Nausea -Seizures (esp. high doses of maprotiline & buproprion) -Extrapyramidal reactions (amoxapine) **Others** -Allergic skin rashes (esp. maprotiline) -Impotence -Priapism (trazadone) -Agitation -Psychosis -Weight gain (except fluoxetine, bupropion, sertraline) -Tricyclics highly lethal with overdoses

2. Antidepressant medications

   a. Indicated for a major depressive episode or recurrent depressive illness. Consider medication when symptoms are moderate to severe. Approximately 60% of patients clinically improve with medication, but many elders do retain significant residual symptoms.

   b. Choice of specific drug is based on side effects profiles and potential adverse drug interactions (see Table 4).

   c. Avoid drugs with high anticholinergic, cardiovascular, and sedative side effects as elderly persons are especially sensitive to them. Also, avoid drugs that cause orthostatic hypotension which can lead to falls and fractures (see Table 5).

   d. Monoamine oxidase inhibitors, especially Nardil, are generally safe and effective, but have not been widely used with elderly patients.

   e. Many clinicians favor the newer drugs trazodone, fluoxetine, bupropion and sertraline because they have fewer anticholinergic and cardiovascular effects, and do not cause weight gain. They are not as well studied as the tricyclics and little is known of their effectiveness with the most severe depressions.

TABLE 5

Antidepressants: Degree of Major Side Effects

Generic (Trade name)	*AntiCholinergic Side Effects*	*Sedation*	*Ortho-Static Hypotension*	*Seizures*	*Conduction Abnormalities*
Tricyclics					
Amitriptyline (Elavil)	+4	+4	+3	+3	+4
Imipramine (Tofranil)	+3	+3	+4	+3	+4
Nortriptyline (Aventyl)	+3	+3	+1	+2	+3
Desipramine (Norpramin)	+2	+2	+3	+2	+3
Doxepin (Sinequan)	+3	+4	+2	+3	+2
Protriptyline (Vivactil)	+3	+1	+2	+2	+4
Trimipramine (Surmontil)	+4	+4	+3	+3	+4
MAO Inhibitors					
Phenelzine (Nardil)	0	+1	+3	+2	+1
Tranylcypromine (Parnate)	0	0	+3	+2	+1
Isocarboxazid (Marplan)	0	0	+2	+2	+1
Newer Agents					
Maprotiline (Ludiomil)	+3	+3	+2	+4	+3
Amoxapine (Asendin)	+3	+2	+1	+3	+2
Fluoxetine (Prozac)	0	0	0	+1	+1
Trazodone (Desyrel)	0	+4	+4	+1	+1
Bupropion (Wellbutrin)	0	0	0	+4	+1
Sertraline (Zoloft)	+1	0	0	?	0

Note. +4 = high, +3 = moderate, +2 = low, +1 = very low, 0 = none, ? = unknown, but probably minimal if at all. From "Practical Psychopharmacologic Considerations in Depression" by K. H. Brasfield, 1991, *Nursing Clinics of North America, 26*, p. 654. Copyright 1991 by Nursing Clinics of North America. Adapted by permission.

f. Significant antidepressant response takes 6 to 12 weeks in elderly patients.

g. Blood levels of tricyclic antidepressants should be closely monitored to avoid adverse reactions.

h. The dosage of antidepressants in late life should be case specific but generally is less that for younger adults. Increases are done slowly while closely monitoring the elder's response.

i. Lithium is indicated for bipolar depression and seasonal affective disorder (SAD). Serum levels in elderly patients should range from 0.5–0.8 mEq/L (versus 0.8–1.2 mEq/L in younger persons).

3. Electroconvulsive therapy (ECT)

   a. The 1991 NIH Consensus Development Panel on Depression in Late Life concluded that ECT has an important role in the treatment of serious depression in the elderly.

   b. ECT is usually considered when antidepressant medication has been ineffective or the patient's medical condition contraindicates their use.

   c. ECT is more effective than antidepressants in all age groups. Its efficacy rate is 80%, but it also has a high relapse rate.

   d. There is some evidence that advancing age heightens the probability of transient post-ECT confusion, especially in the very old.

   e. Prior to receiving ECT, all medication should be discontinued, if possible. MAO inhibitor antidepressants should be stopped 10 days to two weeks before and lithium should be stopped 48 to 72 hours before. Both these drugs cause problems with the anesthetic used during ECT.

   f. Treatments are usually given three times a week for a total of 6 to 12 treatments.

   g. Contraindications for ECT are presence of intracranial mass, fragile cardiovascular status, or aneurysm.

4. Psychotherapy: The combination of antidepressant medication and psychotherapy has consistently yielded better results for depressed elders than medication alone. Common themes that are addressed in psychotherapy with elders are maintenance of self-esteem, fear of pain and suffering, helplessness and hopelessness, isolation and loneliness, loss and competency and a need to rely on those who may abandon them (Turner 1992). Frail elders are treated with supportive psychotherapy that focuses on reassurance, education, ventilation, reminiscence and validation of the elder's self worth.

   a. Cognitive behavioral therapy
   b. Interpersonal therapy
   c. Life Review therapy
5. Group psychotherapy
6. Family psychotherapy

- Nursing Considerations
  1. Monitor responses to antidepressants
     a. Monitor client's standing and sitting blood pressures and pulse rate and rhythm
     b. Assist client to manage common side effects
     c. Report adverse effects promptly
     d. Teach clients and families about medication uses, side effects and adverse effects. Advise side effects may be noticed before therapeutic effect reached. Encourage not to discontinue medication and assist to manage side effects.
     e. Instruct to rise slowly from sitting position; dangle at side of bed before standing.
  2. Promote adequate nutrition, hydration and elimination
     a. Monitor intake and output
     b. If client has little appetite, suggest six small meals a day in place of three larger ones, encourage family to supply favorite foods, use of liquid supplements
     c. Increase fluid intake to counter anticholinergic side effects of antidepressants
     d. Encourage foods high in fiber to prevent constipation
  3. Promote an adequate balance of rest, sleep and activity.
     a. Assess sleep patterns
     b. Teach relaxation techniques, etc.
     c. Encourage physical exercise
     d. Explore activities client might pursue

   e. Encourage interaction with other people
   f. Help client structure time in meaningful way
4. Assess suicide risk, especially when client begins to respond to antidepressant medication
   a. Make safety contract
   b. Provide telephone backup
5. Assist client to recognize, accept, understand and verbalize feelings, especially anger
   a. Use empathetic approach to help client identify feelings
   b. Observe and comment on the verbal and nonverbal expression of feelings
   c. Assist client to link feelings to specific thoughts, events, issues, etc.
6. Promote client's feelings of self-worth
   a. Reinforce client's strengths
   b. Assist with activities of daily living
   c. Give honest praise for accomplishment of small activities or tasks
7. Build a trust relationship
   a. Demonstrate ongoing interest in client
   b. Use simple, direct sentences
   c. Avoid asking too many questions
   d. Focus interactions on pertinent topics
   e. Be consistent
   f. Schedule frequent, brief appointments until client can tolerate longer sessions
8. Collaborate closely with others involved with client's care
   a. Family members
   b. Other professional providers

9. Develop training programs for care providers, nursing staff and others working with the elderly in various community and institutional settings about the recognition of behavioral manifestations of depression and how to obtain help for the depressed elder.
10. Participate in the development of outreach and case-finding services to locate and identify depressed older people who need treatment.

Suicidal Behavior

- Definition
  1. Completed suicides are more frequent among older persons than any other age group. Unlike younger persons, elders rarely attempt suicide as a "cry for help." Instead, they make serious attempts to kill themselves using means that are highly lethal.
  2. Institutionalized elders may attempt indirect suicide by stopping eating, refusing medications, or refusing various tests and examinations.
- Etiology: Clinical depression is a significant factor among elderly suicides. Other risk factors are:
  1. Unemployed
  2. Socially isolated and often widowed or divorced
  3. Serious physical illness with considerable pain
  4. Chronic sleep problems
  5. Alcohol abuse
  6. Low self-esteem and feeling inadequate and useless
  7. Feeling rejected
  8. History of mental illness and previous suicide attempts
  9. Expressed fears about nursing home placement or hospitalization

  Several studies report that most elderly suicides had been seen by a physician within the month prior to their death and many were seen within one week prior to their suicide.
- Incidence: Suicide and suicidal behavior are currently the 10th leading cause of death in the over 65 age group (Blazer, et al., 1986). The rate is highest in those over the age of 80, although there is a marked sex and race differential. Suicides among men outnumber those among women,

and suicides among whites outnumber those among nonwhites. Elderly white men are at highest risk. The NIH Consensus Panel (1992) reported the suicide rate in 80–84 year olds was 26.5 per 100,000 in contrast to the suicide rate in the general population of 12.4 per 100,000.

- Signs and Symptoms
  1. Clinical depression often present. Risk of suicide is greatest when the person is recovering from a serious depression.
  2. Direct verbal clues may be given.
  3. More often, elderly express indirect verbal clues such as stating that their family would be better off without them.
  4. Behavioral changes:
     a. Purchasing a gun
     b. Changing a will
     c. Showing sudden uncharacteristic actions or agitation
     d. Complaining of peculiar somatic complaints
- Differential Diagnosis:

  Evaluate for depression and feelings of hopelessness
- Physical Findings:

  (See section on depression)
- Diagnostic Evaluation/Findings
  1. Evaluate for depression
  2. Evaluate suicide potential
     a. Ask directly about suicide intent
     b. Determine if the person has a specific plan
     c. Determine if the person has the means to carry out the plan
- Management/Treatment
  1. Do not leave the suicidal person alone
  2. Arrange to hospitalize the suicidal elder in a psychiatric treatment setting, by legal commitment if necessary
  3. Treat the underlying depression
  4. ECT is often first choice of treatment for seriously suicidal elders

5. Arrange for long-term follow-up care and treatment prior to hospital discharge.

- Nursing Considerations
  1. Suicide prevention in late life
     a. Develop training programs for long-term care, mental health and community nurses, physicians and others working with the elderly. Include the assessment of suicidal risk in the elderly as well as the use of the Geriatric Depression Rating Scale and other depression screening instruments.
     b. Provide educational programs for elderly persons and their families and caregivers. Include information on the aging process, signs of depression and suicidal characteristics. Emphasize suicide is preventable and depression is treatable.
     c. Advocate for community outreach treatment teams composed of mental health professionals to travel to the elderly in need of help. Few elderly persons seek treatment in community mental health centers.
  3. Nurses working with old people should focus on helping to strengthen kinship ties and the closer involvement of family members with isolated elders.
  4. Strengthen social support networks of older persons by encouraging use of senior citizen centers, peer helper programs, volunteer activities.
  5. Encourage use of grief support groups to bereaved widows and widowers.
  6. Nurses working in settings where they come in contact with older persons can readily recognize an elder who may be at risk for suicide, do an assessment and actively intervene to see that treatment is received.

Delirium (Acute Confusion)

- Definition: Transient confusional state characterized by a global disturbance of attention and cognition, a reduced level of consciousness, abnormally increased or reduced psychomotor activity, and a disturbed sleep-wake cycle. Its onset is rapid, often occurring at night, and its duration is brief. Acute confusion is a common disorder in the elderly, especially the very old.

TABLE 6

Medical Conditions and Medications that Cause Delirium (Acute Confusion)

Medications	Systemic Illness
Anticholinergics	Congestive heart failure
Antipsychotics	Pulmonary insufficiency
Tricyclics	Uremia
Antispasmotics	Hepatic insufficiency
Antiparkinsonians	Lupus erythematosus
Corticosteriods	Infections
Cimetidine	Burns and multiple trauma
Benzodiazepines	AIDS
Levodopa	Cancer
Narcotic analgesics	Malnutrition
NSAIs	Dehydration and Na depletion
Diuretics	Hypoglycemia
Digoxin	Hypokalemia
Antihypertensives	**Others**
Antiarrhythmics	Stroke
	Epilepsy
	Postoperative state
	Withdrawal from alcohol, sedative/hypnotics

- Etiology
    1. Delirium results from a widespread reduction in cerebral metabolism and an upset in the neurotransmission processes which are brought on by a wide range of medical conditions (see Table 6).
    2. The most common cause of delirium in the elderly is intoxication due to medications, particularly anticholinergics.
    3. Several factors, often acting concurrently, are responsible for delirium in the elderly:
        a. Aging processes in the brain
        b. Reduced resistance to stress and acute illnesses
        c. Visual and hearing impairments
        d. High prevalence of chronic diseases
        e. Sleep loss
        f. Sensory overload
        g. Relocation to unfamiliar environment

- Incidence
    1. An estimated 40% (Lipowski, 1989) to 80% (Foreman, 1992), of elderly patients hospitalized for acute physical illness are admitted with delirium or develop it shortly after admission. General surgery in later life is followed by delirium in 10% to 15% of patients. About 50% of patients treated for femoral neck fractures develop delirium.
    2. Acute confusion, or delirium, is associated with increased morbidity, increased intensity of nursing care, longer hospitalization, increased rates of nursing home admission, and increased mortality.
    3. Delirium can be followed by dementia or some other organic mental syndrome, especially if cause not identified and treated.
- Signs and Symptoms
    1. The most prominent feature is disorder of attention manifested by impaired ability to sustain attention to environmental stimuli, carry on a conversation, engage in goal-directed thinking or perform goal directed behavior.
    2. In contrast to dementia, disorders of memory and orientation are secondary rather than primary. Because of attention deficits, the patient is unable to register and retain new information and has little memory of the period of delirium once it has been resolved.
    3. Level of consciousness can vary from drowsiness or stupor to excessive alertness and severe insomnia.
    4. Perceptual disturbances occur.
        a. Vivid dreams and nightmares are common and may merge with hallucinations occurring in periods of wakefulness.
        b. Misinterpretations and illusions.
        c. Hallucinations are commonly visual, but can be auditory.
    5. Acute paranoid delusions accompanied by fear, anxiety, attempts to escape or destructive rage episodes.
    6. Cognitive impairment often fluctuates, and lucid intervals may occur, especially during the daytime hours.
    7. Disturbance of sleep-wake cycle with insomnia or daytime sleepiness

- Differential Diagnosis
  1. Dementia
     a. Prior history
     b. Insidious onset
     c. Attention normal except in severe cases
     d. Hallucinations and delusions usually absent
     e. Orientation impaired
     f. Psychomotor activity often normal
     g. Patient has difficulty finding words, perseveration
     h. Absence of physical illness or drug toxicity
  2. Functional psychosis
     a. History of psychiatric illness
     b. Tends to have markedly depressive or manic behavior
     c. Symptoms do not fluctuate or get worse at night
     d. Cognition may be selectively impaired
     e. Predominantly auditory hallucinations
     f. Delusions sustained and systematized
     g. Orientation may be impaired
     h. Speech normal, slow or rapid
     i. Involuntary movements usually absent
     j. EEG usually normal
- Physical Findings
  1. Temperature may be elevated
  2. Focal neurologic findings may be present
  3. Restlessness, aggressiveness, dazed expression
  4. Anxiety and lack of cooperativeness
  5. Behavior fluctuates unpredictably
  6. Tachycardia, sweating, dilated pupils, elevated BP

- Diagnostic Evaluation/Findings
  1. Physical examination including neurological examination
  2. Routine laboratory tests
  3. Special tests as needed
     a. EEG to rule out seizure disorder. In delirium, EEG often reveals a generalized slowing of background activity.
     b. CT scanning
     c. MRI
  4. Identify all medications, toxicology screen
- Managment/Treatment
  1. Diagnosis of underlying cause or causes
  2. Discontinue or reduce dosage of all medications
  3. Treatment should be related to both the cause and the symptoms of the delirium
     a. Remove underlying cause whenever possible or treat
     b. Adequate fluid and electrolyte balance, nutrition and vitamin supply should be ensured
     c. Provision of reassuring, supportive nursing care that assists the patient in reestablishing orientation is critical
     d. Environmental controls to avoid overstimulation or understimulation
     e. Attention to patient's concerns and fears which may be expressed in content of delusions or hallucinations
     f. Sensitivity to patient's degree of stress
     g. Family members should be reassured that delirium is a transitory disorder
     h. Sedation may be needed if patient is agitated and restless
        (1) Use short-acting antianxiety agent with no active metabolites (Serax 10–50 mg/day; Ativan 0.5–2 mg/day; Xanax 0.5–4 mg/day)
        (2) Antipsychotics (Haldol 0.25 mg up to three times a day)

4. Preventive measures
   a. Avoid polypharmacy
   b. Monitor drug intake and patient's responses closely
   c. Early recognition of onset of delirium so assessment and interventions can be started sooner rather than later.

- Nursing Considerations
  1. Anticipate or predict who is likely to suffer delirium.
     a. Persons over the age of 80 are most vulnerable
     b. Men are more vulnerable then women
     c. Persons who live alone and lack social supports. Family members and familiar people help maintain contact with reality and provide reminders of one's identity and life history.
     d. Relocation, especially if the move is rapid, sudden and unplanned.
     e. Confinement to a restricted space where there is a lack of familiar objects.
     f. Disruption of the sleep cycle and distortion of light and darkness.
     g. Disruptions of patterns of daily living.
     h. Pain or discomfort from unmet physical needs.
     i. Drugs
     j. Lack of prostheses, including eyeglasses, hearing aids, dentures or artificial limbs that enhance and complete the body image.
     k. Bed confinement, particularly in the horizontal position.
     l. Loss of control over body functions, including bowel and bladder incontinence, impactions and diarrhea, and in particular, the presence of tubes such as catheters, IV therapy lines and nasogastric tubes.
     m. Restraints
     n. Lack of contact with caring people
     o. Amnesia, as a result of drugs, surgery, or trauma.

- Nursing Actions
  1. Provide orientation measures
     a. Uncovered windows or artificial illumination to correspond to day and night
     b. Clock within patient's line of vision with a face large enough for client to read.
     c. Calendars
     d. Personal objects belonging to the client, especially photos of loved ones.
     e. Adequate light to illuminate the area
     f. Eye contact maintained with caregivers. Many problems with confusion clear when the client is placed in a chair rather than the horizontal position in bed.
     g. Describe the setting and the equipment in it to cut down on misperceptions and illusions.
     h. Explain daily procedures, rules, who to ask for help etc so client knows what to expect and how to summon help.
     i. Explain any IV lines, catheters, etc. in use and their purpose.
  2. Help client maintain a sense of body integrity
     a. Help in using body in its normal or expected manner.
     b. Verbally reinforce things client is able to do.
     c. Nursing care should complement and supplement what client is unable to do for self.
     d. Active range of motion, bathing, and back rubs restore a sense of body integrity.
  3. Provide sense of personal continuity and identity
     a. Reduce the total number of persons the client comes in contact with. Consistent staff members caring for client will reduce confusion.
     b. Determine by what name the client prefers to be addressed.
     c. Encourage family members to visit often and stay to provide links between past and present. Use telephone to call if unable to come in person.

   d. Speak to client about photos and other personal objects in room.
   e. Encourage life review/reminiscence.

4. Managing agitation
   a. Agitation is related to fear or lack of control. Important for caregiver to remain calm and in control.
   b. Speak always in firm, gentle voice.
   c. When client is sitting, maintain eye contact so patient does not feel threatened.
   d. Offer drink of water or towel so patient has something to hold in her hands instead of grabbing for tubing, etc.
   e. Use touch in a soothing way.

5. Safety measures
   a. If patient attempts to pull out tubing, remain calm, speak gently, and maintain steady pressure on his arm to prevent the tube from coming out. Stay with patient, talking gently until he/she eventually releases the tube.
   b. Have someone sit with client to remind him not to pull out tubes and distract attention. Family members and friends can be encouraged to visit to help with this. Some families are willing to hire ''sitters'' to provide this service if it becomes a serious problem.
   c. Avoid use of restraints as they tend to increase confusion. If some restraining is necessary, use mitten and soft elbow restraints. They should be removed every hour so the hands and elbows can be exercised.
   d. Try using creative measures before resorting to restraints. Try telephoning a close friend and letting the client hear a familiar reassuring voice to calm agitation.

6. Helping the client deal with illusions/hallucinations
   a. Listen to the patient's statements and try to determine what is being misperceived.

   b. Do not support the illusion.
   c. Validate reality. Clear up any mistakes and arrange the environment to preclude more errors.
7. Confusion at night
   a. Assess events occurring at end of day to determine what may be precipitating factors. Fatigue, unmet toileting needs, increased noise, decreased light, the effect of medication, pain after a day of activity, etc.
   b. Try to meet identified needs.
   c. "Sundown syndrome" often occurs when there are fewer personnel such as at change of shifts. Encourage family members to come in at these times if possible.
   d. Keep night light on.
8. Client who screams out at night
   a. Assess what the client fears. Is it pain? Being alone?
   b. The presence of a calm person and adequate light in the room can reduce the problem. Helping client express concerns and feelings may often resolve screaming.
   c. Set up program of behavior modification.

Dementia

- Definition
  1. Dementia is an organic mental syndrome that is characterized by impairment in short- and long-term memory with impairment in at least one other aspect of intellectual function such as abstract thinking, judgment, aphasia, or personality.
  2. It has a chronic, insidious, progressive course.
  3. Although, long lasting, some types of dementia may be arrested or reversed.
  4. Dementia occurs in all age groups, but its highest incidence is in persons over the age of 75 years.

- Etiology: Dementia, a clinical syndrome, can be produced by numerous pathological states that affect the brain. Some of these states are progressive or fixed, such as Alzheimer's disease, and others are arrestable or reversible, such as malnutrition. Frequently, more than one pathological cause is present.

1. Arrestable or reversible causes of dementia
   a. Intoxications
      (1) Medications (See Table 6)
      (2) Heroin, volatile chemicals and other substances of abuse
      (3) Carbon monoxide, carbon disulfide
      (4) Lead, mercury, and manganese
   b. Infections (see causes of delirium)
   c. Metabolic disorders (see causes of delirium)
      (1) Dehydration (most common metabolic cause)
      (2) Wilson's disease
      (3) Hypothyroid
      (4) Hypoglycemia
   d. Nutritional disorders
      (1) Thiamine deficiency
      (2) Pernicious anemia
      (3) B_{12} deficiency
      (3) Folate deficiency
      (4) Niacin deficiency (pellagra)
   e. Vascular problems
      (1) Severe hypertension
      (3) Arteriosclerosis
      (4) Vasculitis
      (5) Emboli
      (6) Episodes of cerebral ischemia and hypoxia

f. Space-occupying lesions

   (1) Chronic subdural hematoma

   (2) Brain tumors, benign and malignant

   (3) Obstructive hydrocephalus

g. Normal-pressure hydrocephalus

h. Depression

   (1) Occurring alone

   (2) Occurring with Alzheimer's disease and other types of progressive dementia

i. Mnemonic for reversible causes of dementia: DEMENTIA

   Drugs or delirium

   Ethanol or eyes and ears (visual or hearing deficits)

   Metabolic changes

   Endocrine

   Nutritional causes and normal pressure hydrocephalus

   Trauma, tumor, toxins

   Infections

   Affective disorder, arteriosclerosis

2. Irreversible causes of dementia

   a. Alzheimer's disease (most common cause)

   b. Multi-infarct dementia

   c. Jakob-Creutzfelt

   d. Pick's disease

   e. Parkinson's disease

   f. Huntington's disease

   g. Cerebellar degenerations

   h. Amyotrophic lateral sclerosis

   i. AIDS

   j. Down's syndrome

k. Korsakoff's syndrome

- Incidence: Dementia affects about 4% of the population over the age of 65. About two-thirds of the elderly with dementia have Alzheimer's disease. It is predicted that 20% of the general population will develop severe dementia by the age of 80. A consistent 10% of AIDS cases have been in people over 50 years of age. The neurological syndrome, known as AIDS dementia complex (ADC) is increasingly seen in persons with no other manifestations of AIDS (Scharnhorst, 1992)
- Signs and Symptoms
    1. Memory impairment is usually the first and most prominent symptom in dementing disorders. Early in the disorder, this memory loss tends to be most marked for recent events. As the dementia progresses, remote and highly learned memory traces are also lost and the patient may not even recognize close family members.
    2. Impairment in abstract thinking
    3. Impaired judgment
    4. Other disturbances of higher cortical functions:
        a. Aphasia (disorder of language)
        b. Apraxia (inability to carry out motor activities despite intact comprehension and motor function)
        c. Agnosia (failure to recognize or identify objects despite intact sensory function)
        d. Constructional difficulty (inability to copy three-dimensional figures or arrange blocks or sticks in specific designs)
    5. Personality change, most often apathy displayed as self-centeredness with no interest or empathy for the needs of others.
    6. Symptoms are severe enough to interfere with work or usual social activities or relationships with others.

- Differential Diagnosis: The clinical diagnosis of dementia with identification of the pathological state that causes it should not be considered a onetime process. Repeated evaluations over time are required to establish the diagnosis and to identify and treat complicating or superimposed conditions.

1. Delirium, either alone or occurring concurrently with dementia.
2. Depression, though depression superimposed upon dementia is more common than a depressive illness with a cognitive disturbance severe enough to mimic the dementia syndrome.
3. Arrestable or reversible causes
4. Progressive degenerative causes

- Physical Findings
  1. The history, obtained from both the patient and the family, is the most important component of the initial evaluation.
     a. Chronological account of current problems
     b. Onset and progression
     c. Specific cognitive, memory, and behavioral changes
     d. Medical history
        (1) Relevant systemic diseases
        (2) Trauma and surgery
        (3) Psychiatric disorders
        (4) Nutrition
        (5) Alcohol and substance abuse
        (6) Exposure to environmental toxins
        (7) Medications, prescribed and OTC
        (8) Hachinski scale—organizes data relevant to cerebral vascular disease and MI
     e. Family history
        (1) Dementia
        (2) Down's syndrome
        (3) Psychiatric disorders
  2. Physical examination
     a. Neurological exam and localizing signs
     b. Vision and hearing screening

c. Mental status (use published mental status test to provide baseline for subsequent evaluations)
   (1) Memory
   (2) Orientation
   (3) Ability to calculate
   (4) Aphasia, apraxia
   (5) Visual spatial skills
   (6) Mood
   (7) Hallucinations and delusions
   (8) Impulse control
   (9) Level of consciousness and cooperation

d. Other screening tests
   (1) Ask to write his/her name
   (2) Write a dictated sentence
   (3) Write numbers in a circle to correspond to a clock's face
   (4) Functional assessment (ADL, IADL)

3. Laboratory testing
   a. CBC with differential and platelets—anemia, infection, hematologic disorders
   b. Iron studies—if anemia found on CBC
   c. Serum electrolytes—metabolic abnormalities
   d. Thyroid function tests
   e. Vitamin B_{12} and folate panels
   f. BUN, creatinine, bilirubin, albumin/globulin—liver disease
   g. Blood glucose (fasting)
   h. VDRL/HIV, depending on history
   i. Urinalysis
   j. EKG

k. Chest X-ray

l. Drug levels—may reveal improper dosing

4. Additional tests as needed

   a. CT scan, head (without contrast)—intracranial mass lesions, subdural hematoma, normal-pressure hydrocephalus, multi-infarct dementia (MID)

   b. Blessed Dementia Scale (high correlation with neuritic plaque counts in Alzheimer's disease (AD)

   c. Mattis Dementia Rating Scale (correlates well with the functional capacity of AD patients)

   d. EEG—with altered consciousness or suspected seizures

   e. Formal psychiatric evaluation when depression is suspected

5. Hospitalize when

   a. History is unclear

   b. Patient is suicidal

   c. Acute deterioration without apparent cause

   d. Social situation precludes adequate observation

6. Order neuropsychological evaluation

   a. Obtain baseline information when diagnosis is in doubt

   b. Before and after treatment evaluations

   c. Cases of exceptionally bright persons suspected of early dementia

   d. Ambiguous imaging findings that require further elucidation

   e. Distinguish dementia from depression and delirium

   f. Extent and nature of impairment following focal or multifocal brain injury

7. Speech and language evaluation

   a. Rule out complex language disorders

   b. Enhance communication between patient and family

8. MRI—if suspect small infarcts, mass lesions, atrophy of brain stem and other small subcortical structures
9. Lumbar puncture—if suspect active infection or vasculitis

- Diagnostic Evaluation/Findings
  1. The diagnosis of dementia is based on the history and evaluation of clinical, functional and laboratory data. Test results, however, cannot substitute for clinical judgment.
  2. Look for progressive decline in memory, other areas of judgment and daily functioning in both the instrumental activities of daily living (IADL) and the activities of daily living (ADL).
  3. Memory loss is prominent, but the first sign may actually be visual-spatial abnormalities, such as problems managing a checkbook or following a recipe.
- Management/Treatment
  1. Specific treatment of underlying disease or disorder
  2. Maximize client's functional abilities.
  3. Modify client's environment to compensate for deficits and ensure safety.
  4. Promote optimal orientation and communication.
  5. Manage behavioral problems with psychosocial and behavioral strategies.
  6. Discontinue nonessential medications, particularly antipsychotics, benzodiazepines, and sedatives/hypnotics.
  7. Provide for client's comfort and safety.
  8. Limit use of restraining devices.
  9. Maintain in home setting as long as possible.
  10. Provide adequate nutrition and hydration.
  11. Promote mobility and weight-bearing exercise.
  12. Manage incontinence problems.
  13. Help family cope with client's illness and caretaking responsibilities.

14. Anticipate legal and ethical decisions and assist client and family to make decisions about guardianship, life support measures and other matters before the need arises.
15. Facilitate a smooth transition to hospital or long-term care facility.

- Nursing Considerations
  1. Reducing caregiver burden: Most patients with Alzheimer's disease or other dementing disorder will be cared for at home by spouses and other family members for the greater part of their illness. Supporting the morale and caregiver skills is critical if the patient is to receive optimal care. The burden experienced by family caregivers is enormous.
     a. Provide information about the dementing illness and the progression of symptoms the family can expect.
     b. Assist family to assess their capabilities for providing needed care. Provide information about in home services that are available in their community and make appropriate referrals.
     c. Assist family to understand the effects of the illness on the patient's behavior and personality. Knowing such changes as apathy, emotional lability and wandering result from brain damage and are not under the patient's control will help dispel any anger they may have and foster appropriate expectations.
     d. Supportive relationship should be established with family members and professional providers. Families need to know whom they can call when they have questions or concerns.
     e. Regular visits should be scheduled to assess cognitive function, activities of daily living and other problems that develop. Brief, supportive interactions and counseling with family caregivers during these visits is important.
     f. Family caregivers should be linked with support groups in their community such as those provided by the Alzheimer's Disease and Related Disorders Foundation.
     g. Respite services are available in most communities and families should be encouraged to use them. Emphasize that family caregivers need time away from the patient to maintain their own health and well being.

h. Families experiencing conflicts and tension should be referred for appropriate counseling services for individual, family or group psychotherapy.

i. Help families realistically assess the care they are able to provide. Many patients reach the time when they do require institutional care. The decision to enter a long-term care facility is very difficult for many families to make. They benefit from support and counsel

2. Verbally or physically abusive behaviors

   a. Assess instances of aggressive behavior directed toward others to identify precipitating factors. These could be:

      (1) Reaction to new environment by person with cognitive impairment

      (2) Lack of choice about daily care regimes, seating at mealtime, timing of procedures, etc.

      (3) Social isolation with no opportunity to express opinions, interact with others, release tension in acceptable ways

      (4) Reactions to disabilities in self and others around them

      (5) Inability to deal with an environment that provides too much stimulation (too many people, too much noise, being rushed or hurried)

   b. Determine unmet need being expressed through abusive behavior. Listen to patient's words for clues.

   c. Develop a plan for managing the patient's behavior in future situations. Set a time frame for implementing the plan realizing that change may not occur immediately. Evaluate and revise approaches as need be.

   d. Strategies that have worked:

      (1) Approach patient in full view, addressing by name, and refrain from touching the patient.

      (2) Requests should be simple and nondemanding, use one-step commands (avoid multiple requests at same time).

      (3) Avoid hurrying or rushing patient. If patient appears agitated, consider withdrawing request and returning a short time later when patient may be more agreeable.

(4) Remember that patient's behavior is a result of brain damage, not deliberate action.

(5) Modify environment as feasible to avoid over- and under-stimulation.

(6) Decrease patient's isolation. Encourage staff members to interact with patient while giving care. Too often, the only conversation an aggressive patient hears is directions and orders. Involve patient in diversional and recreational activities. If patient refuses, try again at another time.

(7) Assign same staff members to work consistently with the aggressive patients. Patient and staff will become familiar with one another and staff will be better able to understand the patient's needs and wants.

(8) Nursing staff confronted with an abusive patient need to remain calm. Two agitated persons will escalate the situation. Staff can always withdraw for a few minutes, if need be.

(9) Set up a program of behavior modification. Reinforce positive behaviors with staff attention. Reduce undesirable behavior by leaving patient at first sign of abuse. Increase contacts with patient during calm periods.

3. Wandering behavior

   a. Assess when, where and under what circumstances a resident wanders to determine precipitating factors (Evans, 1991). These may be:

      (1) Lifelong patterns of walking to relieve stress

      (2) Feelings of insecurity

      (3) Boredom and restlessness

      (4) Need for physical exercise

      (5) Escape from noisy or overstimulating environment

      (6) Personal space has been violated

      (7) Side effect of antipsychotic or antidepressant medication

b. Strategies to manage wandering behavior

(1) Accompany resident during wanderings, speaking in conversational tone, and gently direct back to "home" area.

(2) Participation in a regular program of physical exercise or walking activity (out of doors in good weather) will meet needs for physical exercise and eliminate need to wander.

(3) Providing a secure area in the facility where residents can wander at will without harm coming to them. Some facilities provide a wander garden or patio.

(4) Restrict access to unsafe or undesireable areas.

(5) Provide environmental cues to help wanderer who is merely "lost."

(6) Develop alternatives to restraints using comfort support pillows (Kallmann, et al., 1992).

4. Alteration of sleep-wake pattern

a. Develop a routine for physical exercise and daytime activities.

b. Anticipate needs to use toilet during the night by providing bedside commode or urinal, lighted route to bathroom and low bed with partial side rails. Check with persons during rounds and, if found awake, offer to assist to bathroom.

c. Keep night light on in resident's room.

d. Avoid intake of caffeine after 12 noon.

e. Establish bedtime routines such as established bedtime, warm bath and back massage. Some residents enjoy soft music playing on the radio.

f. Discourage naps during the day.

g. If resident awakens, permit to get out of bed and offer small snack or warm milk. Allow to sit up for awhile until becomes drowsy and can return to bed.

5. Restless or agitated behavior

a. Assess to determine what need is not met.

(1) Need to use toilet and/or constipation

(2) Physical pain or discomfort from medical problem

(3) Side effect of antidepressant or antipsychotic medication

(4) Social isolation

b. Strategies to manage

(1) Staff approach with warm, supportive manner. Holding a resident's hand while talking can be soothing and comforting.

(2) Some patients are helped by regular program of physical exercise. Other patients respond to exercise by becoming more restless.

(3) Validation therapy (Feil, 1992).

6. Suspiciousness and paranoid accusations

a. Lack of trust and fear behind most suspicious behavior

b. Hearing impaired individuals are more likely to develop paranoid thoughts and delusions. Use hearing aid if problem is correctable.

c. Do not argue about delusional material, simply state you have a different understanding.

d. Refocus conversation on reality based topics.

e. Do not make promises you cannot keep.

7. Social Isolation

a. Demonstrate interest and concern.

b. Help maintain communication with family.

c. Socialization experiences

(1) Remotivation group

(2) Activity groups

(3) Movement therapy

Late-Life Delusional (Paranoid) Disorder

- Definition: The onset of persistent, persecutory delusions or delusional jealousy, with or without auditory hallucinations, in a person over the age of 65 that is not due to other medical or psychiatric disorders.
- Etiology
  1. Hearing loss and impaired vision correlate highly with delusional thinking and auditory hallucinations.
  2. Social isolation resulting from loss of family members and friends combined with a relatively isolated life-style.
  3. Difficulty coping with loss, especially in persons who tend to use the defense mechanism of projection.
- Incidence: Geriatric clinicians report a greater frequency of persons with extreme suspiciousness and persistent delusions than is reflected in the literature. Several community surveys report the incidence of delusional disorder as two to four percent of the total elderly population. Women are at increased risk with an estimated ratio of 11:1 females to males.
- Signs and Symptoms
  1. Presence of persistent, nonbizarre delusions that concern everyday experiences, such as neighbors are scheming to burglarize their home, or a spouse is having extramarital sexual relations.
  2. The individual's affect and behavior is appropriate to the content of the delusional system. May display resentment and anger. On rare occasion, the anger is so intense it leads to violence.
  3. Auditory hallucinations may be present but are not prominent as in schizophrenia.
  4. Apart from their delusional thinking and general suspiciousness, the person's behavior is not odd or eccentric.
  5. There is no impairment in cognitive or daily functioning.
  6. Estranged family and social relationships
  7. The individual rarely seeks treatment for the symptoms. Often family members are distressed and seek help from health care providers.

- Differential Diagnosis
  1. Schizophrenic disorders, either late-onset or chronic. Gross disturbances of affect, volition or functioning are present.
  2. Dementia
     a. Paranoid thinking occurs in 20% of individuals with dementia.
     b. Suspiciousness is associated with loss of memory or inability to organize or comprehend environmental stimuli (complain of objects being stolen, or indiscretions on the part of staff members).
     c. Personality and self-care abilities deteriorate over time.
  3. Delirium (acute confusional state)
     a. Paranoia is only one feature with disorder of attention as most prominent symptom.
     b. Fluctuating course with lucid intervals.
     c. Unconnected and transient episodes of paranoid thinking and/or delusions of persecution occur in as many as 40–55% of elders with delirium.
  4. Major depression
     a. Other physical, emotional and/or cognitive symptoms present.
     b. Delusional thinking centers around incurable illness or nihilism, but could be persecutory.
  5. Paranoid symptoms secondary to medical illness
     a. Rule out circulatory, metabolic, infectious, and neurological disorders.
     b. Transient paranoid delusions and aggressiveness can occur after drinking alcohol.
- Physical Findings
  1. Cranky, touchy, or angry demeanor
  2. Usually reports good physical health, but often has hearing or visual impairments.
  3. Lack of warmth or empathy. Appears unlikely to experience intimacy in close relationships.

4. May be belligerent, hostile, or agitated.
5. At high risk for victimization by others and self-neglect or abuse (refusal to eat, take prescribed medications, or attend to hygiene needs).

- Diagnostic Evaluation/Findings
  1. Paranoid delusions and hallucinations are often extensions of the physical and psychological losses the elder has undergone. For example, persons who believe that talk is being directed at them from next door often have significant hearing loss. Feelings of being unwanted or of being subjected to annoyances may also become more intense in the elderly.
  2. Assess physical health and functioning, especially if suspect delusional thinking is affecting judgment and self-care.
  3. Although rare, some pose risk to others. Assess potential for violence towards self or others. Hospitalize under court order, if necessary.
- Management/Treatment
  1. Refer for psychiatric evaluation.
  2. Antipsychotic medication

Outcome studies report treatment success greatest with antipsychotic medications. However, persons with delusional disorder rarely seek treatment and are often suspicious of psychotropic medication and other forms of therapy. Some authorities believe the elderly person may be more comfortable with treatment provided by a general practitioner rather than a psychiatrist.

  3. Psychotherapy
  4. Family therapy
  5. Correct visual and hearing impairments.

- Nursing Considerations
  1. Administer and monitor responses to antipsychotic medications (see Table 7).
     a. Assist to manage common side effects.

Table 7

Side Effects and Adverse Effects of Antipsychotics

Anticholineric Dry mouth Nasal stuffiness Delirium Blurred vision Urinary hesitancy Constipation Tachycardia Agitation Aggravation of narrow-angle glaucoma	**Extrapyramidal** Acute dystonia (rare) Pseudoparkinsonism Acute akathisia (restlessness) **Allergic Reactions** Agranulocytosis Jaundice (rare) Skin rashes Photosensitive skin reactions
Others Sedation Seizure threshold lowered Ejaculatory incompetence	**Cardiac** Orthostatic hypotension EKG abnormalities
Short-term Life Threatening Neuroleptic malignant syndrome	**Long-term Adverse Reactions** Tardive Dyskinesia Tardive Akathisia Retinopathy

   b. Monitor sitting and standing blood pressure and pulse rate and rhythm.

   c. Advise to avoid direct sunlight, wear sunglasses and use lotions with sun-blocking agent.

   d. Help to overcome any resistance to taking medication by exploring person's feelings, explaining its use to relieve symptoms of distressing thoughts and sleep problems, and managing possible side effects.

2. Observe for signs of tardive dyskinesia (TD).

   a. Involuntary movements of mouth, tongue, jaw.

   b. Assess with Abnormal Involuntary Movement Scale: AIMS (Laraia, 1991).

   c. Discontinue medication at first signs of TD.

3. Observe for symptoms of neuroleptic malignant syndrome.

   a. Fever, severe extrapyramidal signs, hypertension, tachycardia, prominent diaphoresis, incontinence

   b. Obtain emergency medical treatment.

4. Establish trusting relationship.
   a. Be consistent, honest, and dependable.
   b. Discuss confidentiality issues.
   c. Avoid promises to keep secrets.
5. Dealing with delusions (See section on Dementia, Nursing Considerations)
6. Assist to establish more satisfactory family and social relationships.

Alcohol Abuse in Late Life

- Definition
  1. Alcohol abuse is drinking behavior that interferes with a person's ability to carry out usual daily activities and/or adversely affects his or her health and interpersonal relationships.
  2. Studies at the National Institute on Aging report that alcohol causes serious problems in late life on a number of important behavioral measures, including reaction time and delayed recognition (memory). Aging does not impair alcohol metabolism but does impair physiological tolerance to alcohol. Elders are not only more severely impaired immediately after drinking but also take longer to recover from its effects.
  3. Alcohol use leads to increased mortality in both middle age and late life. The causes of death among chronic alcohol users include suicide, accidents, cardiovascular disease, cancer, and cirrhosis of the liver.
- Etiology
  1. Alcohol is often used as a means of stress reduction. A lifelong habit of controlled drinking can become more pronounced and uncontrolled as life stresses increase in old age.
  2. Alcohol is used to "self-medicate" the pain of depression, grief, and loneliness experienced by some in old age.
  3. Personality factors and genetic predisposition appear less related to late-onset alcoholism.
  4. Studies of treatment outcome indicate that social isolation is strongly correlated with continued alcohol abuse in late life.

- Incidence
  1. An estimated 10-15% of elders abuse alcohol with evidence that the rates are increasing. Over one-third of these elderly alcoholics developed the illness in old age. Males have a higher prevalence of alcohol abuse than females.
  2. Alcohol use is a "hidden condition" in late life, and therefore is unreported. Clinicians often fail to identify the alcohol-related problems presented by elderly clients.
  3. The interaction of alcohol with the relatively great number of prescription and nonprescription drugs taken by the elderly leads to serious consequences. Alcohol:
     a. Potentiates the depressant effects of antipsychotics, antidepressants, antianxiety agents, analgesics (especially opiates), and anticonvulsants.
     b. Causes unpredictable plasma glucose concentrations when taken concurrently with the oral hypoglycemic agents used to treat Type II diabetes.
     c. Blocks the effectiveness of some drugs, such as anticoagulants.
- Signs and Symptoms
  1. Diagnostic criteria and alcholism screening tools are not valid or reliable with elders because they fail to incorporate age-related adjustments. For example, tolerance for alcohol decreases in old age so that intoxication occurs with lower quantities of alcohol.
  2. Alcohol abuse is suggested by any symptoms that represent evidence of physiological dependence (withdrawal symptoms, blackouts, high blood levels without seeming intoxicated) or psychological dependence (continues to drink despite medical advise to stop or family/social problems clearly caused by drinking).
  3. Other clinical signs that could indicate alcohol abuse suggested by Butler, Lewis, and Sunderland (1991) are:
     a. Insomnia
     b. Impotence
     c. Problems with control of gout
     d. Rapid onset of confusional state

e. Uncontrolled hypertension
f. Unexplained falls/bruises
g. Excessive sleepiness
h. Flushed face
i. Bloated appearance

- Differential Diagnosis: Assess alcohol intake and evaluate extent of the problem. Perform blood alcohol level if individual appears intoxicated.
- Physical Findings: Chronic use of high concentrations of alcohol leads to addiction, or a preoccupation with the use of the drug, the securing of its supply, and a high tendency to relapse after withdrawal. Older adults manifest their addiction when placed in a situation where alcohol is not available, such as a hospital or nursing home.
  1. Symptoms of alcohol withdrawal are:
     a. Initially, anxiety, tremors, nausea, vomiting, perspiration, elevated blood pressure and pulse rate
     b. If withdrawal syndrome is not medically managed, symptoms progress in one to two days to hallucinations, confusion, agitation, disorientation, and withdrawal seizures.
     c. Alcohol withdrawal syndrome can be life-threatening, especially in an older adult with compromised health.
- Diagnostic Evaluation/Findings: The effects of alcohol intake on the body are cumulative. Evaluate the interaction between alcohol use and chronic or episodic illness in the elderly, especially liver function, cardiomyopathies, gastrointestinal function, nutritional deficiencies, and neuropsychological and cognitive (especially memory) problems.
  1. A comprehensive history to obtain detailed information on what the individual drinks and how often, to estimate alcohol consumption. Does the individual drink constantly? Are there episodes of binge drinking?
  2. Whenever possible, information about drinking patterns should also be obtained from family members.
  3. Assess physical health, family health problems, interpersonal difficulties and work-related problems.
  4. Evaluate

a. Neurologic problems such as episodes of amnesia, headaches, and peripheral neuropathy.

b. Evidence of falls such as bruises, cuts, sprains, and cigarette burns, or skin diseases that can result from neglect secondary to alcohol.

c. Gastrointestinal symptoms such as nausea, vomiting, diarrhea, abdominal pain, and unexplained gastrointestinal hemorrhages.

d. Psychiatric symptoms including a detailed evaluation of cognitive status, history of major depression, generalized anxiety, and psychotic symptoms (delusions and hallucinations). Assessment of suicidal ideation is critical because the risk for suicide is significantly high due to both old age and alcohol use.

e. Relationship problems with spouses, children or close friends are often indicators of emerging alcohol problems.

5. Physical examination to:

   a. Screen for medical problems that may exacerbate problems with alcohol. Also, assess medical problems and medications that contraindicate the use of alcohol.

   b. Identify signs of overt alcohol abuse, such as signs of personal neglect.

6. Mental status testing and follow-up testing if cognitive problems are apparent, ideally after two or three weeks of abstinence.

7. A standard laboratory evaluation with special attention to liver-function and electrolytes, especially serum magnesium and levels of serum and urinary amylase

8. EKG to rule out alcoholic cardiomyopathy

- Management/Treatment

  1. Assess degree of alcohol abuse. If the person suffers from acute intoxication that leads to a stuporous or comatose state, hospitalization must be instituted for alcohol withdrawal. In milder cases of alcohol dependence, outpatient treatment is possible for persons who accept they have a problem with alcohol and are motivated to overcome it. The initial treatment step is always to stop drinking.

  2. Treatment of chronic alcohol abuse consists of detoxification with

medical supervision, vitamin supplements, restoring fluid and electrolyte balance, nutritious meals, and rest.

3. Antianxiety agents, commonly diazepam/Valium or chlordiazepoxide/Librium, are used to manage the withdrawal process. Because these drugs potentiate the effects of alcohol as well as lead to their own state of dependency, they are usually used only on an inpatient basis.
4. Following detoxification, the long-term goals of treatment and rehabilitation are emphasized. Education, social support, group and family therapies are used.
5. Disulfiram (Antabuse), a drug used to avert drinking, is used cautiously in elders. Both the patient and family have to be warned of the potential adverse effects that will result if alcohol in any form is ingested (or used in skin care products, such as after-shave lotion).
6. Family therapy and support
7. Participation in Alcoholics Anonymous for long-term support and help in maintaining sobriety. Unfortunately, few of today's elders are in tune with the recovery movement and self-help groups. The recovering elder can be helped to mobilize his or her social network to provide the support and encouragement needed to cope with an alcohol-free lifestyle.

- Nursing Considerations
  1. Assess drinking behavior and confront client's denial
  2. Describe treatment options
  3. Consult with physician regarding detoxification
  4. Provide options for treatment and appropriate referral and follow-up
     a. Reinforce need to abstain from alcohol
     b. Involve family members in treatment process
     c. Maintain contact to reinforce treatment objectives and monitor health status
     d. Maintain accepting, nonjudgmental attitude
  5. Emphasize sobriety is a continuing process. Encourage participation in Alcoholics Anonymous and Alanon for family members.

6. Coordinate treatment goals of the various health care providers involved with the client.
7. Develop educational programs about signs and symptoms of alcohol abuse in late life for consumers, health care providers and staff in long-term care facilities.
8. Advocate for self-help programs specifically designed for older adults.

Questions

1. The process of bereavement:

   a. Occurs only in humans.
   b. Functions to free the individual from too close an attachment to the lost object.
   c. Lasts about one year.
   d. Is significantly different for elderly women as opposed to elderly men.

Mrs. Rowe, an 82 year old resident in a life care community, spent the weekend at her married daughter's home. On Sunday morning her son-in-law tearfully told her that her daughter had died unexpectedly during the night. When Mrs. Rowe heard the news, she grabbed onto her dead daughter, weeping uncontrollably. She refused to let go and, said "It's alright, she's only asleep. She'll wake up soon."

2. Mrs. Rowe is:

   a. Probably demented and likely to decompensate in a similar fashion when under any stress.
   b. Demonstrating massive denial.
   c. Likely to be angry with her son-in-law.
   d. Experiencing a dysfunctional grief reaction.

3. Several months after her daughter's death, Mrs. Rowe is still preoccupied with thoughts of her daughter. All of the following are normal ways in which this is manifested except:

   a. Intrusive, unwanted memories, especially when seeing photos or other reminders of the deceased.
   b. Dreams of the deceased.
   c. Hearing the deceased's voice speaking to her.
   d. Asking her friends to address her by her daughter's name.

4. Mrs. Rowe joins a bereavement group that meets in the senior center. The primary object of the group is to:

   a. Help members develop new relationships.
   b. Assist members to resolve any conflicts they still have with the deceased.
   c. Support members as they deal with the grieving process.
   d. Facilitate working through feelings associated with survivor guilt.

5. Depression in the elderly:
    a. Rarely responds to treatment.
    b. Is usually characterized by guilt and self-accusations.
    c. Occurs primarily in persons who have had depressive episodes earlier in life.
    d. May be precipitated by losses of friends, prestige and a sense of mastery.

6. The elderly are particularly vulnerable to depressive illness because:
    a. Of the physical changes associated with the aging process.
    b. They are too rigid and set in their ways to benefit from psychotherapy.
    c. Of increased longevity with more years spent in retirement.
    d. The enzyme, monoamine oxidase, decreases in normal aging.

7. A 63 year old woman visits the health clinic with complaints of fatigue, difficulty sleeping and a variety of vague muscular aches and pains. While the nurse practitioner talks with her, she mentions that a year ago she retired from her job as executive director of a large nonprofit association. Her daughter is getting divorced and just moved back home with her two school age children. Her husband is pressuring her to move to Florida to golf and relax. She:
    a. Needs a careful physical examination because she is vulnerable for physical or psychiatric illness.
    b. Is probably a hypochondriac who worries needlessly about every ache and pain.
    c. Should be counseled to relax more and enjoy her retirement years.
    d. Should be grateful that she can be of use to her daughter who needs all the help she can get.

8. Her exam is essentially normal. The nurse comments that she is about 25 lb. overweight. As she states this, the patient bursts into tears and sobs that none of her clothes any longer fit and she feels "so old." What additional information would most help you to make a diagnosis?
    a. How long has she had these symptoms?
    b. Has she ever had psychiatric treatment in the past?
    c. What is the quality of her relationship with her husband?
    d. How has she coped with similar events in the past?

9. You consider prescribing an antidepressant for this patient. Of the following drugs, which would be the best choice for her?
    a. Imipramine
    b. Doxepin
    c. Lithium
    d. Sertraline

A 72 year old widower, who was a marathon runner and had been in excellent health had a TUR for enlarged prostate. Four weeks after surgery he still complained of bladder burning despite his urologist's repeated exams which revealed no abnormality. He also complained of insomnia, weakness, and worry about his health. He called his physician's office almost daily to complain about his discomfort. He comes to the office because he thinks he is getting weaker. While there, he mentions that he had been arrested the night before for firing a gun in an alley because he "wondered how it worked." He denied any thoughts of suicide.

10. He is:
    a. Responding normally to the stress of his illness.
    b. Moderately depressed.
    c. Anxious with antisocial tendencies.
    d. At risk for suicide.

11. He should:
    a. Be committed immediately because of his potential for dangerous behavior.
    b. Be told that worrying is what is making him worse.
    c. Be reminded that he is in much better condition than most of his peers.
    d. Have a psychiatric evaluation.

12. If the patient is treated with antidepressant medication, it should be remembered that:
    a. Psychotherapy and drugs together are usually more effective than either alone in the treatment of depression in late life.
    b. He will probably need a higher dose than normal because of the severity of his symptoms.
    c. Antidepressants are expensive and the potential results may not be worth the cost.
    d. Antidepressants will not help his sleep disturbance.

13. ECT:

    a. Usually requires 10 days to two weeks before symptoms of depression improve.
    b. Is the treatment of choice for severely depressed people who have not responded to antidepressants.
    c. Results in a high incidence of chronic memory problems.
    d. Is effective in 40%–50% of patients.

14. Which of the following responses is not true? Dementia in the elderly:

    a. May often be confused with depression.
    b. May often coexist with depression.
    c. Is not usually effected by medications.
    d. May be concealed by denial.

A 72 year old widow is brought by ambulance to the psychiatric hospital from a nursing home where she has been a resident for 3 months. Transfer data indicate that she has become increasingly confused and disoriented and has become a management problem. Her illness is diagnosed as undifferentiated dementia.

15. In which of the following ways should the hospital admission routine be modified for an older confused person like this patient?

    a. The patient should be put to bed and left alone to recover her faculties and composure.
    b. The patient should be medicated to ensure her calm cooperation during the admission procedure.
    c. The patient should be allowed sufficient extra time in which to gain an understanding of what is happening to her.
    d. The patient should be given a tour of the unit to acquaint her with the new environment in which she will live.

16. The patient is to undergo a series of tests to determine whether or not her organic mental syndrome is treatable. Treatable forms of dementia that can be arrested or reversed include all of the following except:

    a. Dehydration.
    b. Normal-pressure hydrocephalus
    c. Cerebral abscess
    d. Multiple sclerosis.

17. Which of the following statements by the nurse would be best to make to this patient, Mrs. Mills, when she awakens in the morning?

    a. "Good morning, Mrs. Mills. This is your second day at Virginia Dare Hospital and I am your nurse today. My name is Cathy."
    b. "Do you remember who I am, Mrs. Mills, or where you are?"
    c. "Hello Mrs. Mills. Did you sleep well? Which dress would you like to wear today, the blue one or the flowered one?"
    d. "Hi, Mrs. Mills. How are we feeling today?"

18. Mrs. Mills's daughter and son-in-law come to visit. The visit goes well until they get ready to leave when Mrs. Mills grasps her daughter's hand and begins to cry, saying "Don't leave me here. I'll die in this place." The daughter is visibly upset when she leaves Mrs. Mill's room. She asks the nurse if she should visit again since her mother is so upset by her leaving. The best reply for the nurse to make is:

    a. "Perhaps it would be best for you not to return for several days until she gets accustomed to the hospital."
    b. "Let me give you the name and telephone number of her social worker. She can schedule a family meeting."
    c. "This has been an upsetting experience for you both, but it is important for you to continue to visit as often as you can. I will go sit with her for a few minutes until she feels better."
    d. ' Why don't you try telephoning her next time instead of visiting. That way she will know you are thinking of her.'

19. The night nurse finds Mrs. Mills at 3:00 am trying to open the janitor's closet down the hall from her room. The nurse notices that the front of her night gown is wet. Which comment by the nurse shows the best understanding of Mrs. Mills' condition?

    a. "Mrs. Mills, it's three o'clock in the morning. What are you doing out of bed?"
    b. "Look at yourself. You are barefoot in the hall and your nightgown in wet. Come back to your room with me, now."
    c. "Goodness, look at you. Next time please use your call light so I can help you."
    d. "Mrs. Mills, are you looking for the bathroom. Let me show you where it is."

20. The next afternoon, Mrs. Mills says to the nurse, "I have to meet with my church choir in an hour." Which response would be best by the nurse?

    a. "The choir's secretary called and said they had canceled today's meeting."
    b. "I understand that you enjoy singing in the choir, Mrs. Mills. I'd like to hear more about it."
    c. "You can't meet with your choir, Mrs. Mills. You are in the hospital now."
    d. "No, Mrs. Mills. You have not belonged to the choir for quite some time."

21. All of the following are common side effects of tricyclic antidepressants, except:

    a. Orthostatic hypotension.
    b. Confusion.
    c. Blurred vision.
    d. Pseudoparkinsonism.

22. A 73 year old man with a diagnosis of dementia is taking haloperiodol (Haldol) 2 mg hs and hydrochlorothiazide 50 mg each morning. The nurse observes him in the lounge. He repeatedly stands, paces, then sits. When she asks him how he feels, he replies, "I don't know what is wrong with me. I feel so jittery." He most likely is exhibiting:

    a. Akathisia.
    b. Dyskinesia.
    c. Ataxia.
    d. Dystonia.

23. The preferred antidepressant for an elderly patient is:

    a. Maprotiline (Ludiomil).
    b. Amitryptyline (Elavil).
    c. Trazodone (Desyrel)
    d. Fluoxetine (Prozac).

24. Mr. W , a 78 year old nursing home resident, is ambulatory with a cane even though he has very poor vision secondary to diabetes mellitus. He had been a successful businessman who ran his own business for many years. The staff describe him as "cantankerous." His wife lives in the same community with

their only child, a son, and visits often. Mr. W frequently demands to be discharged to his son's home; however, the family has unequivocally stated they cannot manage him at home. A licensed practical nurse reports to Ms. N, the nursing supervisor, that Mr. W. has begun to strike out at staff with his cane. She is vague about the exact nature of his behavior. Which assessment approach should Ms. N. use initially?

a. Keep a log of striking-out episodes.
b. Discuss the behavior at a nursing staff meeting.
c. Discuss the behavior with Mr. W.
d. Ask the physician to examine Mr. W.

25. Ms. N discovers that Mr. W's striking-out behavior always occurs immediately following a visit from his family. Based on the available data, a nursing diagnosis for Mr. W would be:

a. Hostile behavior related to the physical changes of aging.
b. Potential for violence directed at others related to unmet needs for closeness to significant others.
c. Ineffective individual coping related to identity crisis.
d. Organic mood disorder related to diabetes mellitus.

26. Mr. W continues to strike-out with his cane. The staff becomes concerned that he will hurt someone. The best intervention related to this behavior is:

a. Take away his cane.
b. Allow him his cane only when he needs to walk.
c. Give him a walker instead of a cane.
d. Engage him in an activity after visiting hours.

27. Mr. C, age 76, makes an appointment with the nurse practitioner at his HMO. He is appears worried but is able to describe his concerns clearly and lucidly. He explains that his wife of 40 years has been accusing him of marital infidelity for quite some time which he denies is true. He lowers his head and says, "I might as well tell you everything. I have been impotent for at least 10 years." Recently, his wife has been going through his pockets and wallet looking for "evidence" of his infidelity. If she finds any sales receipts or credit card charges, she goes into a rage of verbal abuse. Last night she threw a heavy glass ashtray at him that grazed the side of his head. He reports his wife is in good health and is able to function well at home. Since she retired as a nurse, she has become somewhat reclusive leaving the house only to shop or

go to church on Sunday. He asks the NP what he should do. Her best recommendation would be:

a. Reassure his wife of his continued faithfulness to her.
b. Schedule an appointment as soon as possible for his wife to come in for her annual physical exam and a comprehensive assessment.
c. Schedule an appointment for his wife with a psychiatrist.
d. Refer him to the social worker for a couples session.

28. Of the following actions, which one has priority for the NP to carry out before Mr. C leaves the office?

a. Recommend he see the urologist to have his impotence evaluated.
b. Discuss the possibility of hospitalizing his wife if her condition becomes worse.
c. Give him the telephone number of the psychiatric crisis team and the police to call if his wife's behavior escalates.
d. Obtain the names and telephone numbers of their adult children.

29. Mrs. Duke, age 72, comes to the clinic with a temperature of 102 degrees, blood pressure of 150/110, and tachycardia. She has been taking haloperidol (Haldol), 1 mg three times a day for the past three months. These symptoms indicate a diagnosis of:

a. Aranulocytosis.
b. Hpertensive crisis.
c. Trdive dyskinesia.
d. Nuroleptic malignant syndrome.

30. In taking an alcohol history, which one of the following inquiries has least significance for diagnosing alcohol abuse in older adults?

a. The person's definition of "one drink".
b. Concurrent use of other prescription and nonprescription drugs.
c. Circumstances of the alcohol use.
d. Drinking a fifth of whiskey a day, or its equivalent in wine or beer, for a 180 pound person.

Answers

1. b	11. d	21. d
2. b	12. a	22. a
3. d	13. b	23. d
4. c	14. c	24. c
5. d	15. c	25. b
6. a	16. d	26. d
7. a	17. a	27. b
8. a	18. c	28. c
9. d	19. d	29. d
10. d	20. b	30. d

BIBLIOGRAPHY

American Psychiatric Association. (1987). *Diagnostic and statistical manual of mental disorders* (3rd ed. rev.). Washington, DC: Author.

Blazer, D. G. (1989). Affective disorders in late life. In E. W. Busse & D. G. Blazer (Eds.), *Geriatric Psychiatry* (pp. 369–401). Washington, DC: American Psychiatric Press.

Blazer, D. G., Bachar, J. R., & Manton, K. G. (1986). Suicide in late life: Review and commentary. *Journal of the American Geriatrics Society, 34,* 519–525.

Brasfield, K. H. (1991). Practical psychopharmacologic considerations in depression. *Nursing Clinics of North America, 26*(3), 651–663.

Butler, R. N., Lewis, M. I., & Sunderland, T. (1991). *Aging and mental health: Positive psychosocial and biomedical approaches* (4th ed.). New York: Macmillan Publishing Co.

Christison, C., Christison, G., & Blazer, D. G. (1989). Late-life schizophrenia and paranoid disorders. In E. W. Busse & D. G. Blazer (Eds.), *Geriatric psychiatry* (pp. 403-414). Washington, DC: American Psychiatric Press.

Cohen-Mansfield, J. (1991). The agitated nursing home resident. In M. S. Harper (Ed.), *Management and care of the elderly: Psychosocial perspectives* (pp. 89–103). Newbury Park, CA: SAGE Publications.

Dementia Consensus Conference. (1987). Differential diagnosis of dementing diseases. *Journal of the American Medical Association, 258*(23), 3411–3416.

Evans, L. K. (1991). Nursing care and management of behavioral problems in the elderly. In M. S. Harper (Ed.), *Management and care of the elderly: Psychosocial perspectives* (pp. 191–206). Newbury Park, CA: SAGE Publications.

Farberow, N. L., Gallagher-Thompson, D., Gilewski, M., & Thompson, L. (1992). Changes in grief and mental health of bereaved spouses of older suicides. *Journal of Gerontology, 47*(6), 357–366.

Feil, N. (1992). *V/F validation: The Feil method: How to help disoriented old-old* (rev. ed.). (Available from Edward Feil Productions 4614 Prospect Ave. Cleveland, OH 44103).

Foreman, M. D., & Grabowski, R. (1992). Diagnostic dilemma: Cognitive impairment in the elderly. *Journal of Gerontological Nursing, 18*(9), 5–12.

Gallagher, D., & Thompson, L. W. (1989). Bereavement and adjustment disorders. In E. W. Busse & D. G. Blazer (Eds.), *Geriatric psychiatry* (pp. 458–473). Washington, DC: American Psychiatric Press.

Kallmann, S. L., Denine-Flynn, M., & Blackburn, D. M. (1992). Comfort, safety, and independence: Restraint release and its challenges. *Geriatric Nursing, 13*(3), 143–148.

Laraia, M. T. (1991). Psychopharmacology. In G. W. Stuart & S. J. Sundeen (Eds.), *Principles and practice of psychiatric nursing* (4th ed.) (pp. 697-737). St. Louis: Mosby Year Book.

Lipowski, Z. J. (1989). Delirium in the elderly patient. *New England Journal of Medicine, 320*(9), 578–582.

McDougall, G. J. (1990). A review of screening instruments for assessing cognition and mental status in older adults. *Nurse Practitioner, 15*(11), 18–28.

Mellick, E., Buckwalter, K. C., & Stolley, J. M. (1992). Suicide among elderly white men: Development of a profile. *Journal of Psychosocial Nursing, 30*(2), 29–34.

NIH Consensus Development Panel on Depression in Late Life. Diagnosis and treatment of depression in late life. (1992). *Journal of the American Medical Association, 268*(8), 1018–1024.

Raskind, M. A. (1989). Organic mental disorders. In E. W. Busses & D. G. Blazer (Eds.), *Geriatric psychiatry* (pp. 313–368). Washington, DC: American Psychiatric Press.

Reynolds, C. F. (1992). Treatment of depression in special populations. *Journal of Clinical Psychiatry, 53*(9, Suppl.), 45–53.

Scharnhorst, S. (1992). AIDS dementia complex in the elderly: Diagnosis and management. *Nurse Practitioner, 17*(8), 37; 41–43.

Schor, J. D., Levkoff, S. E., Lipsitz, L. A., Reilly, C. H., Cleary, P. D., Rowe, J. W., & Evans, D. A. (1992). Risk factors of delirium in hospitalized elderly. *Journal of the American Medical Association, 267*(6), 827–831.

Turner, M. S. (1992). Individual psychodynamic psychotherapy with older adults: Perspectives from a nurse psychotherapist. *Archives of Psychiatric Nursing, 6*(5), 266–274.

Wolanin, M. O., & Phillips, L. R. (1981). *Confusion: Prevention and care.* St. Louis: C. V. Mosby Co.

Drug Therapy

M. Eletta Morse

Drug Use

- Incidence
    1. Twelve and a half percent (12.5%) of the population are over 65 years of age
    2. The elderly utilize 40–50% of acute hospital days
    3. Elderly clients consume over 30% of prescription drugs and 40% of over the counter (OTC) preparations
    4. Medications averaging 7.5–17.9 prescriptions per year are received by persons over sixty five
    5. The elderly spend more than $3 billion per year on medications
    6. Adverse drug reactions are responsible for 27% of hospital admissions of patients 65 or over
- Factors Responsible for Inappropriate Drug Therapy in the Elderly
    1. Multiple pathologies
    2. Inaccurate diagnosis
    3. Non-specific presentation of illness
    4. Atypical presentation of illness
    5. Multiple providers
    6. Use of OTCs (40% of people >65 use daily)
- Characteristics of Appropriate Drug Therapy in the Elderly
    1. High ratio of efficacy to toxicity
    2. Simple mechanism of action targeted to specific site
    3. Minimal effect on other sites
    4. Reliably absorbed
    5. Minimally bound to protein
- Adverse Drug Reactions (ADRs)
    1. Incidence
        a. Twenty percent (20%) of readmissions to hospital of elderly patients are related to ADRs
        b. Occur in 25% of hospital patients >80 yrs. old

   c. Contribute significantly to mortality, morbidity and institutionalization

2. Categories of ADRs
   a. Allergic
   b. Non-allergic
   c. Idiosyncratic

3. Risk factors for ADRs
   a. Age
   b. Gender
   c. Race
   d. Number of drugs used
   e. Dosage
   f. Duration of prescription
   g. Compliance
   f. Co-mordibities

4. Most common drugs causing ADRs
   a. Psychotropics
   b. Cardiovascular
   c. Noncompliance-intentional or non-intentional of the above drugs leads to increased incidence of ADRs.
      (1) Narrow therapeutic-toxic range of these drugs
      (2) Altered renal excretion
      (3) May necessitate yet another drug to relieve symptoms contributing to polypharmacy

5. Adverse drug INTERactions
   a. Drug displacement from protein binding sites by other protein binding drugs
   b. Induction or suppression of metabolism of other drugs
   c. Additive effects on blood pressure and cognitive function
   d. Adversely effect other medical conditions

e. Drugs with similar actions can cause a cumulative effect or toxicity.

   (1) Orthostatic hypotension

      (a) Antihypertensives

      (b) Diuretics

      (c) Antidepressants

      (d) Antipsychotics

   (2) Anticholinergic effects

      (a) Antidepressants

      (b) Antihistamines

      (c) Phenothiazines

      (d) Disopyramide

   (3) Sedation

      (a) Beta blockers

      (b) Benzodiazepines

      (c) Antihistamines

      (d) Phenothiazines

      (e) Antidepressants

      (f) Alcohol

      (g) Narcotics

      (h) Muscle relaxants

   (4) Gastrotoxic effects

      (a) Nonsteroid anti-inflammatory drugs (NSAIDs)

      (b) Salicylates

      (c) Corticosteroids

      (d) Potassium

      (e) Alcohol

      (f) Estrogens

6. Identifying potential ADRs
    a. Never assume a change in behavior is the result of aging.
    b. In the elderly, toxic reactions can occur even at low drug dosages.
    c. The likelihood of an adverse reaction increases the longer the person is on the drug.
    d. Do consider OTC preparations when evaluating for ADR.
    e. Adverse drug reaction symptoms can occur singly or in symptom clusters (confusion,unsteady gait).
    f. Be watchful for any signs of involuntary movements. Drug-induced Parkinsonism is a frequent side effect of anti-psychotic medication use in the elderly.
    g. Assess patient for signs of tardive dyskinesia (abnormal movements of the lips, tongue and jaw) and akathisia (restlessness, continuous agitation).
    h. Evaluate every complaint of dizziness to rule out othostasis secondary to drug side effect. Drugs are a major cause of dizziness in persons over age 60.
    i. Inappropriate timing of diuretic administration is a common and easily reversible cause of urinary incontinence.
    j. Fatigue and weakness can be caused by many drugs commonly prescribed for the elderly (beta-blockers, diuretics, tricyclic antidepressants, benzodiazepines, and some antihypertensives).
    k. Ataxia or unsteady gait can be a side effect of drugs such as anticonvulsants, hypnotic-sedatives, tranquilizers, and anti-Parkinson's drugs.
7. Drug review
    a. Reduces ADRs
    b. Conducted at least annually, including all prescription drugs, OTC drugs and alcohol use.
    c. Assess patient compliance, response to therapy, possible side effects, drug interactions. Rate of noncompliance high in elderly.

d. Encourage patient to use ONE pharmacy with computer profile capability to assist in detecting potential drug interactions.

e. Advise patient to ask for samples or two prescriptions when a new drug is being prescribed. This can be less expensive for the patient in the event of an adverse reaction or side effect.

f. Enlist help of all health care team members to reinforce proper drug use.

Other Factors Influencing Drug Therapy

- Pharmacokinetics—(What the body does to drugs).

  1. Physiological changes of aging

     a. Decrease in normal renal function

     b. Decrease in lean body mass and total body water

     c. Increase in total body fat per unit of body weight

     d. Decrease in hepatic blood flow

     e. Other changes are common but variable, i.e., cardiac function, cognitive function, sensory changes

  2. Absorption

     a. Mildly decreased gastrointestinal function

     b. Decreased gastric emptying time

     c. May be affected by nutritional deficiencies of Vitamin B_{12} or intrinsic factor

     d. Drug interactions—laxatives, antacids

     e. Most drugs absorbed in small intestine. Notable exceptions are aspirin and alcohol.

     f. Increased gastric pH

     g. Alterations in absorption common in patients with congestive heart failure, bowel resections.

  3. Distribution

     a. Decreased serum albumin production (a major drug binding protein)

(1) Common protein-bound drugs are: warfarin, diazepam, phenytoin, tolbutamide, meperidine.

(2) Clinical effect—large amount of free unbound drug available for action

b. Normal aging changes in body composition

(1) Decrease in total body water and lean body mass results in lower volume distribution and higher concentration of drug

(2) Increase in body fat results in increase of volume distribution of fat distributed or stored drugs.

4. Metabolism

a. Effects of normal aging on metabolism include decreased liver mass, and liver blood flow which may affect metabolism of some drugs such as propranolol

b. Common diseases of the elderly that affect liver function are hepatitis and congestive heart failure.

5. Excretion

a. Renal function declines by 50% between age 20–90. Wide variations in individuals.

b. Decreased renal function affects pharmacokinetics if drug is more than 60% excreted by kidney

c. Drugs that are eliminated by the kidney:

(1) Clear body more slowly

(2) Half-lives (and duration of action) are prolonged

(3) Tend to accumulate to higher drug concentrations.

(4) Some common drugs that are renally excreted: digoxin, atenolol, lithium, diuretics, NSAIDs, captopril.

d. Serum creatinine does not reflect renal function in elderly as accurately as in younger persons.

(1) Decreased muscle mass equals decrease in endogenous creatinine production

(2) Decline in production may give "false normal" serum creatinine

(3) Creatinine clearance is most accurate measure of renal functions in the elderly. Formula for estimating creatinine clearance:

$$\frac{(140-\text{age}) \times \text{body wt.(kg)}}{72 \times \text{serum creatinine (mg/dL)}} = \text{(mL/min)}$$

(For women multiply result by 0.85)

e. Other factors affecting renal clearance

(1) State of hydration

(2) Cardiac output

(3) Intrinsic renal disease

(4) Number of drugs patient is taking that are renally excreted.

(5) Chronic diseases such as hypertension, diabetes, congestive heart failure

6. Baro-receptor activity

a. Decreased sensitivity and responsiveness result in postural hypotension

b. Exacerbates orthostatic side effects with: short acting nitrates, phenothiazines, diuretics, antihypertensives.

7. Fluid and electrolyte balance affected by

a. Diuretic use

b. Obstructive uropathy secondary to benign prostatic hypertrophy

c. Diminished fluid intake secondary to functional or cognitive impairments, urinary incontinence, blunted "thirst" response.

8. Patient evaluation should include

a. State of hydration

b. State of nutrition

(1) Of institutionalized elderly 40% are clinically malnourished

(2) Obtain/monitor serum protein and serum albumin levels routinely

c. State of cardiac output

(1) Decrease in ventricular function without overt heart disease

(2) Diuretic therapy leads to decreased blood volume which can lead to decreased organ perfusion.

- Pharmacodynamics—(What drug does to your body)

1. Tissue sensitivity or responsiveness to drug effects
2. Variable in the elderly
3. Greater tissue sensitivity to central nervous system (CNS)-active drugs
4. Lesser sensitivity to beta-blockers
5. State of nutrition affects drug effectiveness

- Compliance (The extent to which the patient's behavior conforms with medical advice.)

1. Factors associated with noncompliance

a. Diagnosis e.g., Alzheimer's disease

b. Severity of illness

c. Degree of disability

d. Duration of illness (longer duration decreases likelihood of compliance)

e. Clinical response (Good and fast response decreases compliance)

f. Duration and number of treatments

g. Frequency of dosing

h. Side effects

i. Cost

j. Satisfaction with provider

k. Education

l. Income

m. Socioeconomic status

n. Failure to understand instructions

o. Concurrent self-administration of OTC or alcohol

p. Social isolation

2. Factors that affect compliance
   a. Failure to obtain prescription
      (1) 7–10% never filled
      (2) Cost
      (3) Delay in treatment. "Wait until I really need it."
   b. Improper administration of medication
      (1) Incorrect dose
      (2) Improper frequency of administration
      (3) Improper timing or sequence of administration
         (a) With meals ASSUMES three meals a day
         (b) Empty stomach is two hours after or one hour before eating.
      (4) Wrong route or technique (crushing for tube feeding)
      (5) Medication taken for wrong purpose by self medicating patient
   c. Premature discontinuation of medication

3. Compliance tips
   a. Assess for risk factors for noncompliance
   b. Simplify drug regimen by arranging drug schedule to coincide with regular activities
   c. Don't switch brands frequently
   d. WRITE specific directions for use in LARGE type
   e. Don't say "Take as directed" with only verbal directions.
   f. Know the therapeutic goal
   g. Use blister packs, other medication dispensers and compliance aids

h. Be knowledgeable about side effects. Inform patient of side effects.

i. Verify patient's understanding of instructions

j. Encourage regular visits with same provider

k. Encourage self-monitoring and self-reporting

l. Use of support groups

m. Make sure patient can open medication container

n. Instruct patient to discard old or unneeded drugs

4. Clinical consequences of noncompliance

   a. Insufficient treatment

   b. Need for additional medication

   c. Cost

   d. Accumulation of "leftover" medications which are likely to be used inappropriately.

General Principles of Prescribing

- Factors That Complicate Prescribing for the Elderly

  1. Multiple interacting factors which influence age related changes (genetic and environmental)

  2. Each individual must be considered and evaluated each time a drug is considered for use

  3. Limited research available at this time on drug effects on the elderly

- General Recommendations for Prescribing for the Elderly

  1. Evaluate elderly persons thoroughly in order to identify all conditions that could benefit from drug treatment, be adversely affected by drug treatment or influence the efficacy of drug treatment.

  2. Manage medical conditions without drugs as often as possible.

  3. Know the pharmacology of drugs being prescribed. A few drugs should be used well, rather than many poorly.

  4. START LOW, GO SLOW

5. When evaluating patient compliance pay special attention to impaired cognition, diminished hearing and vision, and functional deficits.
6. Evaluate the entire drug regimen any time you add or discontinue a medication.

- Questions to Consider When Prescribing an Additional Drug.
    1. Is the drug necessary? Can a non-pharmacological method be tried first?
    2. What is the therapeutic purpose of the drug—and are we achieving it?
    3. Is the dosage correct? Is the dosage form correct?
    4. What drug interactions may occur?
    5. Is the drug correctly labeled and packaged for this patient's level of function?
    6. Who is responsible for drug administration for this patient?
    7. Can any medication be discontinued?

Medication History

- Demographic Information
    1. All medical conditions
    2. Allergy history for each allergic medication
        a. When did reaction occur—how long ago?
        b. Description of the reaction.
        c. How was the reaction treated?
- Social/Medical/Developmental History
    1. Habits
        a. Caffeine use
        b. Smoking
        c. Alcohol
        d. Herbal tea use
    2. Home remedies

3. Nutrition
    a. Total parenteral nutrition (TPN)
    b. Tube feedings—continuous or intermittent
4. Ostomy—where is it? May affect absorption, excretion.
5. Difficulty swallowing
6. Financial resources
7. Pharmacy
    a. Use of same pharmacy consistently
    b. Where do you store medications?
    c. What do you do with leftover medications?
    d. Current practice different than instructions on label?
    e. Do you share medications?

- Prescription Drugs—Review Each Drug for
    1. Dose and frequency
    2. Route of administration
    3. Start date and discontinue date. Reason for discontinuing?
    4. Prescribing physician(s).
- Nonprescription Medications. Review Each Class of Drug.
    1. Antacids
    2. Antidiarrheals/laxatives
    3. Hemorrhoidal products
    4. Emetic/antiemetic
    5. Cough/cold products
    6. Analgesics
    7. Vitamins/minerals/iron
    8. Sleep aids/sedatives (include alcohol)
    9. Ophthalmic/otic products
    10. Topical preparations

Cardiovascular Drug Therapy

- Digoxin—most commonly prescribed cardiovascular drug
  1. Action/Pharmacokinetics
     a. Increases force and velocity of myocardial contraction (positive inotropic action). Increases contractility of heart muscle.
     b. Slows heart rate (negative chronotropic effect) by vagal and extravagal mechanism.
     c. Rate of absorption slower in the elderly, prolonging attainment of peak plasma digoxin concentrations.
     d. Hyperthyroidism increases renal clearance and reduces volume of distribution of digoxin. Hypothyroidism diminishes renal clearance and expands volume of distribution of digoxin. Important to monitor serum digoxin concentrations for these patients.
     e. Renal and liver dysfunction may increase the drug's half-life from 30–40 hours to as much as 70 hours. Normal age-related decline in renal and hepatic function also affect the drugs half-life.
  2. Indications
     a. Treatment of congestive heart failure, especially low-output failure associated with depressed left ventricular function.
     b. Treatment of certain cardiac arrhythmias, including atrial fibrillation, atrial flutter, and paroxysmal atrial tachycardia, especially where the ventricular rate is elevated.
     c. Treatment of cardiogenic shock, especially if accompanied by pulmonary edema.
  3. Dosage—for all cardiac therapy drugs dosage is individualized based on patient condition, weight etc.
  4. Side effects/ADRs
     a. Cardiac—Atrioventricular nodal and sinus nodal conduction or rhythm disturbances are the predominant cardiac side effects.
     b. Noncardiac side effects include mental status changes (most

common in elderly), anorexia, nausea, vomiting, diarrhea, visual disturbances

5. Contraindications
   a. Ventricular tachycardia or fibrillation
   b. Severe myocarditis
   c. Hypersensitive carotid sinus syndrome
   d. Hypersensitivity
6. Drug Interactions
   a. Antiarrhythmic agents
      (1) Decreased total body clearance of digoxin with quinidine, amiodarone and propafenone which INCREASES the effect of digoxin.
      (2) Recommended to decrease the dose by 25–50% and moniter serum digoxin.
   b. Calcium channel blocking drugs
      (1) Verapamil, diltiazem and nifedipine may DECREASE the elimination of digoxin.
      (2) It is recommended to lower maintenance dose by 25% and monitor serum digoxin.
   c. Miscellaneous agents
      (1) Antacids, colestipol, and cholestyramine, neomycin, cancer chemotherapy, sulfasalazine, and aminosalicylic acid DECREASE the absorption of digoxin.
      (2) Indomethacin, ibuprofen, and diclofenac may decrease elimination of digoxin. Moniter the serum digoxin concentration.
      (3) Rifampin may increase elimination of digoxin. Monitor the serum digoxin concentration; the digoxin dose may need to be increased.
7. Nursing interventions
   a. Monitor serum electrolytes, especially serum potassium, renal and liver function tests and EKG periodically.

b. Monitor intake and output (I & O); note weight changes and signs of edema.

c. Teach patient and/or family

(1) To inform health care provider when protracted diarrhea or vomiting occur: these conditions can alter the electrolyte balance and lead to digitalis toxicity.

(2) Importance of strict observance of the prescribed regimen and avoidance of extra doses to make up for missed doses

- Nitrites and Nitrates

1. Action

a. Nitrates dilate smooth muscle of the venous system which inhibits venous return leading to decrease in ventricular volume. The decrease in left ventricular work and wall tension results in improved subendocardial perfusion.

b. Nitrates have the direct capability to dilate the coronary arteries.

2. Indications

a. Relief of pain of acute anginal attacks (rapid acting drugs only).

b. Prevention of anginal episodes; reduction in frequency and severity of acute attacks (long-acting nitrates, transdermal nitroglycerin, sustained-release forms).

c. Reduction of the cardiac work load in patients with myocardial infarction or congestive heart failure (CHF).

3. Side effects

a. Common—headache, flushing, dizziness, palpitations, burning sensation in sublingual area, skin rash, weakness, tachycardia

b. Life-threatening—orthostatic hypotension, hypersensitivity reaction characterized by syncope, hypotension and collapse.

4. Contraindications

a. Severe anemia

b. Marked hypotension

c. Increased intracranial pressure, cerebral hemorrhage

d. Acute stages of myocardial infarction

5. Interactions

a. The hypotensive effects of nitrites and nitrates may be INCREASED by alcohol, beta-blockers, antihypertensives, narcotics, and tricyclic antidepressants.

b. Nitrates can INCREASE the effects of antihistamines, tricyclic antidepressants and other anticholinergic drugs.

c. Cross-tolerance can occur between nitrites and nitrates.

6. Nursing interventions

a. Use nitrites and nitrates cautiously in patients with glaucoma because increased intraocular pressure can result from generalized vasodilation.

b. Assess for blurring of vision, dry mouth, or severe headache. The dose may need to be adjusted.

c. Teach the patient or family

(1) That dizziness, weakness, syncope and other signs of orthostasis can occur following administration, especially sublingually. Advise the patient to sit or lie down when taking medication and to rest for ten to fifteen minutes after taking medication.

(2) To take one sublingual tablet at five minute intervals during an anginal attack. The health care provider should be contacted or the patient should report to a hospital if the pain persists after fifteen minutes or three tablets.

(3) To avoid alcohol consumption in conjunction with nitroglycerin.

(4) To be alert for the development of a tolerance to the rapid-acting drugs, marked by a lack of relief of pain following several tablets. Temporary discontinuation of the drug (several days) is usually sufficient to restore sensitivity.

- Thiazide Diuretics

  1. Action

     a. Diuretic effect—Impairs active sodium and chloride reabsorption in the early portion of the distal segment of the renal tubule resulting in excretion of these ions with an osmotically equivalent volume of water.

     b. Antihypertensive effect—The mechanism of action of thiazide diuretics as antihypertensive agents is not known. A higher percentage of blacks and older patients appear to respond to thiazide diuretics better than beta-blockers.

  2. Indications

     a. Treatment of edema associated with CHF, hepatic cirrhosis, renal dysfunction, and steroid or estrogen therapy.

     b. Management of all forms of hypertension, either alone (mild) or in combination with other antihypertensive drugs (moderate to severe).

  3. Side effects

     a. Hyponatremia, hypokalemia, hypercalcemia, hyperuricemia.

     b. Hyperlipidemia, hyperglycemia

     c. Phototoxicity

     d. Sexual dysfunction

  4. Contraindications

     a. Anuria or renal decompensation

     b. Hypersensitivity to sulfonamide-derived drugs

     c. Impaired hepatic function; may precipitate renal and hepatic failure

     d. Use with caution in patients with bronchial asthma, diabetes, gout, lupus, advanced heart disease, and debilitated frail elderly

     e. Use with caution in patients receiving digitalis drugs or in patients with a history of cardiac arrhythmias; hypokalemia can precipitate development of arrhythmias

5. Interactions

   a. Thiazide diuretics INCREASE the effects of other antihypertensive agents, amphetamines, quinidine, lithium.

   b. Diuretic effect is DECREASED by use with indomethacin and the pyrazolones.

   c. DECREASES the effects of oral anticoagulants, vasopressors, hypouricemic drugs, and sulfonlyureas.

   d. INCREASES the risk of orthostatic hypotension due to alcohol, narcotics, barbiturates, and other CNS depressants.

   e. Hypokalemia my be intensified if thiazide diuretics are combined with corticosteroids

   f. Hypercalcemia can occur if thiazide diuretics are given with calcium carbonate or other calcium containing products.

6. Nursing interventions

   a. Monitor I&O and be alert for the development of excessive diuresis which can lead to severe electrolyte imbalance.

   b. Teach patient and/or family

      (1) Signs of possible electrolyte imbalance (thirst, dry mouth, anorexia, weakness, muscle pain, oliguria, tachycardia, paresthesias, confusion, irritability).

      (2) To include foods high in potassium in daily diet

      (3) To make positional changes slowly to minimize the danger of orthostatic hypotension.

      (4) That elderly have decreased total body water, and diminished thirst response and are at high risk for dehydration.

- Loop Diuretics

  1. Action—Inhibits active tubular reabsorption of sodium and chloride in the thick ascending loop of Henle, as well as other segments of the proximal and distal tubules resulting in excretion of large quantities of urine high in sodium.

2. Indications
   a. Treatment of refractory edema associated with CHF, hepatic cirrhosis, and renal disease.
   b. Management of hypertension complicated by renal failure (serum creatinine above 2–2.5mg/dl) or CHF which cannot be controlled with a thiazide diuretic.
   c. Ascites due to malignancy, idiopathic edema, and lymphedema.
3. Side effects
   a. Orthostatic hypotension, dysrhythmias
   b. Ototoxicity
   c. Gastric upset
4. Contraindications
   a. Anuria, severe dehydration or electrolyte depletion.
   b. Hepatic coma
   c. Use cautiously in patients with: diabetes, gout, cardiogenic shock, hearing impairment, lupus, postural hypotension.
5. Interactions
   a. INCREASES the effects of antihypertensive agents, theophylline.
   b. Diuretic effect may be DECREASED by phenytoin, indomethacin and other NSAIDs, and probenecid.
   c. Ethacrynic acid may displace oral anticoagulants from their protein binding sites
   d. May INCREASE the toxicity of aminoglycoside antibiotics (ototoxicity), cephalosporins (nephrotoxicity), salicylates, lithium, and cardiac glycosides.
   e. Increased potassium loss may occur when corticosteroids are given with loop diuretics.
   f. Increased orthostasis may occur with narcotics or barbiturates.
   g. May elevate blood glucose levels.

6. Nursing interventions
   a. Monitor serum electrolytes during prolonged drug therapy.
   b. Discontinue the medication if profound hypotension, hypovolemia, hematuria, or profuse diarrhea occur.
   c. Teach patient or family
      (1) Signs of electrolyte imbalance (see thiazide diuretics).
      (2) To change position slowly as orthostasis can result in dizziness or falling.

- Calcium Channel Blockers
  1. Action—Inhibits influx of extracellular calcium ions into cardiac muscle and smooth muscle cells through specific "slow calcium channels." Antianginal effects include dilation of coronary arteries and arterioles and prevention of coronary artery spasm. Dilation of peripheral arterioles also occurs, reducing total resistance.
  2. Indications
     a. Coronary artery vasospasm
     b. Angina pectoris
     c. Supraventricular arrhythmias
     d. Hypertension
  3. Side effects
     a. Flushing, headaches
     b. Ankle edema
     c. Reflex tachycardia, bradycardia, conduction abnormalities
     d. Constipation is most common
  4. Contraindications
     a. CHF
     b. Sick sinus syndrome, A-V conduction disturbance
     c. Cardiogenic shock
  5. Interactions
     a. Drug effect INCREASED by propranolol, cimetidine.

b. Drug effect DECREASED by phenytoin, rifampin.

c. Calcium channel blockers INCREASE effect of digoxin, prazosin, cyclosporin, quinidine.

d. Verapamil and diltiazem reduce clearance of theophylline

6. Nursing interventions

a. Moniter blood pressure during initial stages of therapy and when doses are changed.

b. Assess for development of bradycardia.

c. Assess for mild peripheral edema, usually of the lower extremities.

d. Assess for constipation. Provide preventive bowel regimen when appropriate.

- Beta-adrenergic Blocking Agents

1. Action—Reversible competitive blocking action at beta-adrenergic receptor sites resulting in decrease in heart rate, force of contraction, and plasma renin, slowed A-V conduction, and lowered blood pressure.

2. Indications

a. Hypertension

b. Angina

c. Arrhythmias

d. Reduction in risk of reinfarction after myocardial infarction (M.I.)

3. Side effects

a. Fatigue, insomnia, nightmares

b. Asthma, CHF

c. Depression, confusion

d. Hyperlipidemia

e. Masks symptoms of hypoglycemia

f. Impotence

4. Contraindications
   a. Sinus bradycardia
   b. Right ventricular failure
   c. CHF, bronchial asthma
   d. Cardiogenic shock
   e. Peripheral vascular disease
   f. Diabetes mellitus
5. Interactions
   a. INCREASED effect of beta-blockers by chlorpromazine, cimetidine, furosemide, hydralazine, other antihypertensives.
   b. NSAIDs, barbiturates, phenytoin may DECREASE antihypertensive effect of beta-blockers
   c. Combination therapy with verapamil and beta-blockers may cause CHF.
   d. Cumulative cardiac depressant effects with digitalis, phenytoin, verapamil, and quinidine.
   e. Beta-blockers may prolong insulin-induced hypoglycemia and mask symptoms of hypoglycemia.
6. Nursing interventions
   a. Assess for conditions that might be worsened by beta-blocker therapy (diabetes, asthma).
   b. Moniter the diabetic patient carefully.
   c. Teach patient or family
      (1) Not to stop drug abruptly. This can lead to arrhythmias or myocardial infarction.

- Angiotensin-Converting Enzyme (ACE) Inhibitors
  1. Action—Inhibits ACE which reduces the formation of pressor substance angiotension II and decreases the angiotensin-mediated secretion of aldosterone from the adrenal cortex. Peripheral vascular resistance is lowered, and salt and water is reduced. Degrades bradykinin, resulting in a blood pressure lowering effect.

2. Indications
    a. Treatment of all degrees of hypertension, alone or combined with other drugs, especially diuretics.
    b. Adjunctive treatment of refractive CHF, usually with digoxin and a diuretic.
3. Side effects
    a. CNS—insomnia, paresthesias, headache, dizziness
    b. GI—nausea, vomiting, diarrhea, altered taste, constipation, peptic ulcer.
    c. CV—chest pain, hypotension, palpitations
    d. GU—polyuria, oliguria, renal insuffiency
    e. HEMA—neutropenia,
4. Contraindications
    a. Use with extreme caution in patients with severe renal dysfunction, lupus, valvular stenosis, and diabetes.
5. Interactions
    a. Effects of ACE inhibitors may be INCREASED by diuretics, adrenergic-blocking agents, other antihypertensive drugs, nifedipine, and by severe salt or fluid restriction.
    b. Antihypertensive efficacy can be DECREASED by indomethacin and aspirin and other salicylates.
    c. Concurrent use of ACE-inhibitors and potassium-sparing diuretics or potassium supplements can elevate serum potassium levels.
    d. ACE inhibitors INCREASE the effects of vasodilators such as the nitrites.
6. Nursing interventions
    a. Moniter urinary proteins and CBC periodically.
    b. Teach patient or family
        (1) To continue with moderate salt intake as excessive hypotension may occur with salt restriction.

(2) That any condition causing dehydration may also cause a further reduction in blood pressure.

(3) That captopril must be taken on an empty stomach for best absorption.

- Oral Anticoagulants

1. Action/pharmacokinetics

   a. Interferes with blood clotting by indirect means; depresses hepatic synthesis of vitamin K

   b. Metabolized by liver, excreted in urine, 99% bound to plasma protein.

2. Indications

   a. Atrial fibrillation

   b. Cardiac valvular problems

   c. Pulmonary embolus, deep vein thrombosis

3. Dosage considerations

   a. Individualize dosage to maintain therapeutic range

      (1) 1.3–1.5 times prothrombin time control values for above indications (see #2)

      (2) 1.5–2.0 times prothrombin time control values for mechanical valve prophylaxis and recurrent systemic emboli

4. Side effects/Adverse reactions

   a. Common—diarrhea, rash, fever

   b. Life-threatening—bleeding, hepatitis

5. Contraindications

   a. Hypersensitivity

   b. Bleeding disorders, leukemia, blood dyscrasias

   c. Acute nephritis, hepatic disease, peptic ulcer

6. Interactions
   a. INCREASED action of anticoagulant when taken with: allopurinol, heparin, steroids, cimetidine, disulfiram, quinidine, sulindac, sulfonamides, salicylates, ethacrynic acid, indomethicin.
   b. DECREASED action of anticoagulant when taken with: barbiturates, haloperidol, rifampin, phenytoin, vitamin K, oral sulfonylureas

7. Nursing interventions
   a. Evaluate therapeutic response via prothrombin time, decrease in symptoms
   b. Assess for signs and symptoms of bleeding
   c. Teach the patient and/or family
      (1) To use same brand, same dose tablet rather than mixing different tablets for correct amount
      (2) That medication can be taken at any time of day; choosing same time increases compliance
      (3) About the importance of follow-up for prothrombin time test
      (4) About potential drug interactions
         (a) Review all drugs including OTCs
         (b) No aspirin
      (5) To avoid foods high in vitamin K, e.g., broccoli, licorice, cauliflower, liver.
      (6) Caution about regular and/or excessive use of alcohol; Affects metabolism of warfarin
      (7) To watch for signs and symptoms of bleeding, e.g., "smoky urine," black stools, bruising, bleeding gums.
      (8) To use emergency ID, e.g., Medic-Alert

Hypoglycemics

- Goals of Therapy for Insulin and Oral Agents
  1. Normalize blood glucose levels

2. Normalize serum lipid levels
3. Achieve and maintain ideal body weight
4. Prevent acute and chronic complications
5. Promote physical and psychological well-being

- Insulin Therapy
  1. Action/Pharmacokinetics
     a. Decreases blood sugar, phosphate and K+
     b. Increases blood pyruvate and lactate
  2. Indications
     a. Insulin dependent diabetes mellitus (IDDM)
     b. Ketoacidosis
  3. Dosage—individualized
  4. Side effects/ADRs
     a. Hypoglycemia
     b. Hypersensitivity
  5. Contraindications—hypersensitivity
  6. Interactions
     a. Insulin effect is INCREASED by: Salicytates, alcohol, oral hypoglycemics, beta-blockers, MAO inhibiters.
     b. Insulin effect is DECREASED by: Thiazides, thyroid hormones, corticosteroids, estrogens, dobutamine, smoking
  7. Nursing interventions
     a. Assess patient's visual, cognitive status and fine motor skills.
     b. Teach patient and/or family
        (1) How to draw up and inject insulin
        (2) To rotate injection sites
        (3) To store insulin at room temperature up to one month
        (4) How and when to check blood glucose

(5) How to manage hypoglycemia and hyperglycemia

(6) About symptoms of ketoacidosis

(7) About nutrition/meal planning tips

(8) When and who to call for help

(a) Follow-up with health care provider

(b) Medic-Alert ID

(9) To avoid OTC drugs unless approved by health care provider

- Oral Antidiabetics

1. Action/pharmacokinetics

a. Stimulate functioning beta cells in the pancreas to produce insulin

b. Increase number of insulin receptors or improve insulin binding

c. Absorbed by GI route, metabolized in liver, excreted in urine, 90% plasma protein bound

(1) Avoid first generation sulfonyureas which have prolonged half-life of 60–90 hrs. Second generation drugs have shorter half-life.

2. Indications—stable Non-insulin dependent diabetes mellitus (NIDDM)

3. Dosage—individualized

4. Side effects/ADRs

a. Common-headache, rash, weakness, disulfiram reaction (Flushing, nausea, vomiting)

b. Life-threatening—hepatotoxicity, leukopenia, aplastic anemia, hypoglycemia

c. Primary failure (no response after one month) and secondary failure (decreasing effect after initial good response)

5. Contraindications

a. Hypersensitivity

b. Brittle diabetes

6. Interactions

a. Drug effect INCREASED by: Insulin, MAO inhibiters, cimetidine, oral anticoagulants, methyldopa, NSAIDs, salicylates

b. Drug effect DECREASED by: Calcium channel blockers, corticosteroids, thiazide diuretics, thyroid preparations, estrogens, phenothiazines, phenytoin, and sympathomimetics

(1) May precipitate hyperosmolar nonketotic syndrome (HNKS)

c. Decreases digoxin levels

d. Beta-blockers mask symptoms of hypoglycemia

7. Nursing interventions

a. Assess vision, cognition and fine motor skills for blood glucose monitoring

b. Refer to CDNE and diabetic support groups

c. Teach the patient or family

(1) To moniter blood glucose levels

(2) Symptoms of hypo/hyperglycemia

(3) To take drug in AM to avoid night time hypoglycemia

(4) To avoid OTCs unless approved by health care provider

(5) To carry Medic-Alert ID

Drug Therapy for Arthritis and Anti-inflammatories

- NSAIDs

1. Action/pharmacokinetics

a. Inhibition of prostaglandin synthesis. Analgesic, anti-inflammatory and antipyretic properties.

b. Highly bound to plasma protein, metabolized in the liver with metabolites excreted in the urine.

2. Indication

a. Pain control of mild to moderate pain

b. Inflammation secondary to acute and chronic arthritis

3. Dosage—varies dependent on product

4. Side effects
   a. Common—nausea, vomiting, anorexia, dyspepsia
   b. Life-threatening—nephrotoxicity, blood dyscrasias, GI bleeding
      (1) Significant increased incidence of gastric ulcer secondary to decrease in gastric prostaglandin production. GI bleeding in patients on NSAIDs occurs without preliminary symptoms of gastric distress.
         (a) To decrease incidence or prevent GI bleeding replace lost mucosal prostaglandins with oral prostaglandin MISOPROSTIL which is more efficacious than H_2 blockers in preventing and healing NSAID induced gastric ulceration.
      (2) Increased risk with chronic, full dose therapy
      (3) Increased risk with concomitant NSAID and steroid therapy
   c. ADRs—many NSAID products are OTC medications not supervised by medical care provider
      (1) Increased risk with alcohol use
      (2) Increased risk with smoking

5. Contraindications
   a. Hypersensitivity
   b. History of gastric or duodenal ulcer or bleeding, impaired renal function, CHF
      (1) Cautious use in patient on diuretics
      (2) Increases serum creatinine and fluid retention.
      (3) Increases risk of hyperkalemia

6. Interactions
   a. INCREASED effect of medication when used with phenytoin, sulfonamides or sulfonylureas.

b. DECREASED effect when used with aspirin

c. INCREASES the effect of oral anticoagulants

7. Nursing interventions

a. Administer with food or milk

b. Monitor for GI symptoms, tarry stools

c. Monitor BUN, CBC, Hgb & Hct and prothrombin time

d. Teach the patient or family

(1) Not to exceed recommended dose

(2) That therapeutic response can take up to two weeks for arthritis

(3) To avoid use of alcohol

(4) To avoid aspirin use.

- Salicylates

1. Action/pharmacokinetics

a. Anti-inflammatory and analgesic effect via inhibition of prostaglandin synthesis

b. Antipyretic action from inhibition of hypothalamic heat regulating center.

c. Onset is slow; metabolized by liver, excreted by kidney.

2. Indications

a. Mild to moderate pain or fever

b. Inflammatory conditions

3. Dosage—variable depending on indication and patient

4. Side effects/ADRs

a. Common—nausea, vomiting, rash

b. Life-threatening—thrombocytopenia, GI bleed, hemolytic anemia

c. ADR—tinnitus or impaired hearing

5. Contraindications
   a. Hypersensitivity
   b. Persons with bleeding disorders, GI bleeding, vitamin K deficiency, on heparin or warfarin
6. Interactions
   a. INCREASES effects of anticoagulants, insulin, heparin, valproic acid, sulfonylureas.
   b. DECREASES the serum levels of NSAIDs
7. Nursing interventions
   a. Administer with food or milk
   b. Evaluate for GI distress, tarry stools
   c. Assess for ototoxicity, tinnitus
   d. Provide for audiometric testing before and after long term therapy
   e. Teach the patient or family
      (1) Not to exceed recommended dosage
      (2) To avoid alcohol
      (3) Therapeutic response for arthritis may be up to two weeks

- Corticosteroids (glucocorticoids)

1. Action
   a. Decreases inflammation by suppression of migration of polymorphonuclear leukocytes and fibroblasts
   b. Modifies body's immune response to different stimuli
2. Indications
   a. Inflammation
   b. To produce immunosuppression
   c. Allergy, cerebral edema
3. Dosage—depends on product, indication

4. Side effects
   a. Behavioral
      (1) Insomnia
      (2) Euphoria, depression
   b. GI irritation, peptic ulcer disease
   c. Hypokalemia
   d. Hyperglycemia
   e. Sodium and fluid retention, hypertension
5. Contraindications
   a. Hypersensitivity
   b. Psychosis
6. Interactions
   a. DECREASED action of corticosteroid with cholestyramine, barbiturates, rifampin, phenytoin, theophylline.
   b. DECREASES effects of anticoagulants, antidiabetics, toxoids, vaccines.
   c. INCREASED side effects with alcohol, salicylate, and digitalis use.
7. Nursing interventions
   a. Monitor blood sugar, serum K+
   b. Monitor weight
   c. Assess for signs of infection
   d. Assess for signs of adrenal insufficiency i.e. nausea, anorexia, fatigue, joint pains.
   e. Assess mental status
   f. Teach the patient and/or family
      (1) Not to discontinue the drug abruptly
      (2) Single daily doses should be taken in morning before 9:00 a.m.
      (3) To take with meals or snack
      (4) Medic-Alert ID should be used with chronic therapy.

Drug Therapy of Gastrointestinal Disease

- Goal of Therapy
  1. Neutralize or diminish secretion of gastric acid
- Antacids—Magnesium or Aluminum Based
  1. Action
     a. Reduces gastric acidity by neutralizing secreted gastric acid and inhibiting formation of acid-pepsin complex
     b. Provides adequate buffering for 30 minutes in fasting state
  2. Indications—treatment of gastric or duodenal ulcer; gastric ulcers more prevalent in elderly
  3. Dosage
     a. Efficacy requires doses of 30 ml. seven times daily (1 and 3 hrs. p.c. and h.s.)
     b. Alternating preparations may decrease ''taste fatigue'' and improve compliance
  4. Side effects
     a. Products with aluminum cause constipation
     b. Products with magnesium cause diarrhea
     c. Belching, flatulence
  5. Contraindications
     a. Patients with chronic renal disease may have increased serum levels of aluminum and magnesium.
     b. Hypersensitivity to aluminum or magnesium
  6. Interactions
     a. INCREASES the effects of quinidine, amphetamines, pseudoephedrine, levodopa, valproic acid
     b. DECREASES the effects of cimetidine, corticosteroids, ranitidine, phenothiazines, phenytoin, digitalis, salicylates
  7. Nursing interventions
     a. Administer with 8 ounce glass of water to ensure absorption in stomach.

b. Incidence of epigastric pain can be used as effectiveness indicator

c. Teach patient not to take other drugs within two hours of antacid to avoid impairment of absorption.

- Histamine H_2 Receptor Antagonists

1. Action

   a. Inhibits histamine at H_2 receptor site of parietal cells, thus decreasing gastric acid secretion; possible cytoprotective effect

   b. Metabolized by liver, excreted in urine

2. Indications—current preferred treatment for peptic ulcer disease.

3. Dosage—treat gastric ulcer for 12 weeks, duodenal ulcer for eight weeks to maximize healing rates

4. Side effects—delirium, confusion with cimetidine. Rare with other agents

5. Contraindications

   a. Renal insufficiency

   b. Hypersensitivity

6. Interactions

   a. INCREASES effects of warfarin, metoprolol, benzodiazepines, phenytoins, quinidine, theophylline, tricyclic antidepressants, lidocaine.

   b. DECREASES effect of ketoconazole

   c. Drugs with narrow therapeutic indices need to be avoided e.g., warfarin, diazepam, phenytoin, theophylline, propranolol and lidocaine.

7. Nursing interventions

   a. Administer with meals for prolonged effect

   b. Teach patient and/or family

      (1) To avoid black pepper, caffeine, alcohol, harsh spices.

      (2) To complete recommended course of therapy for effectiveness.

- Sucralfate
  1. Action—enhances mucosal defense by forming a viscous adhesive substance which protects mucosa from acid, pepsin; duration of action up to five hours
  2. Indication—alternative to H_2 blockers
  3. Dosage
     a. Twice daily dosing (2 Gm.b.i.d.) as effective as 1 Gm. q.i.d.
     b. Combination therapy with H_2 antagonists can be used
  4. Side effects—constipation, dry mouth
  5. Contraindications
     a. Poor renal function
     b. Hypersensitivity
  6. Interactions
     a. DECREASES effects of tetracycline, phenytoin, fat-soluble vitamins
  7. Nursing interventions
     a. Teach patient or family
        (1) To take on an empty stomach
        (2) To avoid black pepper, alcohol, caffeine, and strong spices
        (3) To avoid using antacids within one-half hour of drug ingestion.

Central Nervous System (CNS) Altering Drugs

- General Considerations to Prevent Misuse.
  1. Complete medical evaluation to rule out medical cause of psychiatric symptoms. Anxiety symptoms are prominent in cardiovascular disease, pulmonary disease, metabolic and endocrine disorders.
  2. Thorough evaluation of "agitation," "disruptive behavior" for remedial causes. Appropriate evaluation and diagnosis of psychiatric disorders by psychiatric health care provider.

3. Consider non-pharmacological treatments as adjuvant therapies.
   a. Relaxation therapy
   b. Psychotherapy
   c. Support group to increase coping skills
4. Thorough knowledge of drug side effects. Great variety among psychotropics.
5. Start low, go slow.
6. Careful, regular assessment of response of target symptoms to psychotropic drugs.
7. Be aware of tendency for elderly patients to focus on physical symptoms of anxiety, not psychological ones.

- Antianxiolytics
  1. Alcohol—most widely used as self medication
  2. Benzodiazipines—most commonly prescribed drug
  3. Tricyclics
  4. MAO inhibiters
  5. Beta blockers
  6. Buspirone
- Benzodiazepines
  1. Action—divided into two groups based on half-life (short or long acting)
     a. Short acting
        (1) Must be administered 2–4 times daily for continuous effect.
        (2) More problems with withdrawal
        (3) Moderately lipid soluble
     b. Long acting
        (1) Active metabolites of drug present up to 200 hours after dosing

(2) Dose should be increased very gradually

(3) Less problems with withdrawal

2. Indications
   a. Anxiety disorders
   b. Anxiety related to medical illness
   c. Agitation
   d. Adjustment disorder with anxiety response related to significant life change
3. Dosage—smallest effective dose of short-acting, low-potency benzodiazepine for limited period of time. Taper gradually after long term therapy.
4. Side effects
   a. Sedation, impaired concentration, amnesia
   b. Weakness, dizziness
   c. Blurred vision
   d. Orthostatic hypotension leading to falls; injury potential more severe with long-acting benzodiazepines
5. Contraindications
   a. Hypersensitivity
   b. Narrow angle glaucoma
   c. Alcohol abusers, drug addicts, polydrug abusers
6. Interactions
   a. INCREASED effect of benzodiazepines with other CNS depressants, alcohol, cimetidine, disulfiram.
   b. DECREASED effect of benzodiazepines with rifampin, valproic acid.
7. Nursing interventions
   a. Assess for fall risk secondary to orthostasis
   b. Assist with ambulation if gait unsteady
   c. Offer ice chips, hard candy for dry mouth

d. Evaluate mood, sensorium

e. Teach patient and/or family

(1) To follow prescription directions carefully

(2) To avoid driving

(3) To avoid alcohol use

(4) To rise slowly to standing position

- Hypnotics

1. Action/pharmacokinetics

   a. Produces CNS depression causing sleep

   b. Metabolized by liver, excreted by kidney, and highly protein bound

2. Indications

   a. Short term use for situational insomnia related to illness, grief, etc.

   b. Should never be used on a long term basis

   c. Complete evaluation of insomnia should be conducted before medication therapy initiated.

3. Dosage—Prescribe short acting hypnotics which have minimal effect on sleep stages; start at one-third to one-half usual dose.

4. Side effects

   a. CNS "hangover" effects, sedation, confusion

   b. Hypertension, ataxia, falls

   c. Drug dependency with prolonged use.

5. Contraindications

   a. Hypersensitivity

   b. Severe renal and hepatic disease

6. Interactions—INCREASES the action of warfarin, furosemide, cimetidine, disulfiram, alcohol, other CNS depressants

7. Nursing interventions
    a. Evaluate for safety considerations e.g., environmental hazards, poor vision, need for assistive device for ambulation
    b. Assist with ambulation if gait unsteady
    c. Assess for prolonged CNS effect e.g., confusion, short term memory deficits, dependency
    d. Teach patient and/or family
        (1) To avoid driving
        (2) To avoid alcohol and other CNS depressants
        (3) Alternate measures to improve sleep (good sleep hygiene)

- Antipsychotics
    1. Action/pharmacokinetics
        a. All block postsynaptic dopamine receptors in various pathways within the brain.
        b. Subgroups: phenothiazines, thiothixenes, thioridazine HCl, butyrophenones, di-benzodiazipines and others
        c. Products are metabolized by liver, excreted in urine, are highly bound to plasma protein; half-life can be greater than three days
    2. Indications
        a. Schizophrenia
        b. Acute mania
        c. Agitation associated with delirium, dementia
    3. Dosage—lowest appropriate doses, increased slowly with periodic re-evaluations
    4. Side effects/ADRs
        a. Extrapyramidal symptoms
            (1) Pseudo Parkinsonism
            (2) Akathisia

(3) Dystonia
(4) Tardive dyskinesia

b. ADRs
(1) Hypotension
(2) Agranulocytosis
(3) Laryngospasm

5. Contraindications
   a. Patients with pre-existing liver damage, severe hypertension or cardiovascular disease, bone marrow depression
   b. Alcohol or barbiturate dependency or withdrawal
6. Interactions
   a. INCREASES the effect of other CNS depressants, beta adrenergic blockers
   b. DECREASES effects of anticholinergics, levodopa, lithium
   c. Decreases absorption of antacids
7. Nursing interventions
   a. Monitor for urinary retention
   b. Assess CNS for level of consciousness (LOC), gait, affect, sleep pattern.
   c. Ambulation supervision until stabilized on medication
   d. Increase fluids to prevent constipation
   e. Assess for extrapyramidal symptoms
   f. Provide quiet, low stimulation environment for agitated patients
   g. Teach patient and/or family
      (1) To rise slowly to standing position
      (2) To avoid hot showers or baths
      (3) To wear sunscreens or protective clothing
      (4) To avoid overheating during hot weather.

- Antidepressants—Cyclic and MAO Inhibiters. Depression is the most common psychiatric disorder in the elderly. Characterized as early or late onset (after age 60). Late onset is often correlated with medical illness.

  1. Cyclic drugs
     a. Action—selectively inhibits serotonin uptake by the brain.
     b. Metabolized by liver, excreted by kidneys. Half-life 18–28 hours.
  2. Indications—depression
  3. Dosage
     a. One-third to one-half usual adult dose
     b. Therapeutic response in 2–3 weeks
     c. Reaches steady state in 4–19 days
  4. Side effects
     a. EKG changes, tachycardia, cardiac toxicity
     b. Memory loss, sedation, orthostasis
     c. Urinary retention, anticholinergic toxicity
     d. Agitation, headache, insomnia
     e. Convulsions with fluoxetine; use with caution in the elderly
  5. Contraindications
     a. Hypersensitivity
     b. Myocardial infarction
     c. Convulsive disorders
  6. Interactions
     a. INCREASES the effects of epinephrine, alcohol, benzodiazipine, CNS depressants
     b. DECREASES the effects of guanethidine, clonidine, ephedrine
     c. Incompatible with hyperpyretic crisis, convulsions, severe hypertension, MAO inhibitors
  7. Nursing interventions
     a. Monitor blood pressure for orthostasis

b. Monitor weight
c. Monitor EKG for changes, dysrhythmias
d. Increase dietary fluids and fiber to offset constipation, urinary retention.
e. Assess for extrapyramidal symptoms e.g., dystonia, tardive dyskinesia
f. Assess mental status for mood, suicidal tendency, confusion
g. Teach patient and/or family
    (1) Therapeutic effects may take 2–3 weeks
    (2) To use caution in driving
    (3) Not to discontinue drug abruptly
    (4) To avoid sun exposure

Pain Control—Chronic Pain.

- General Concepts
    1. Patients on opioids for a period of time can develop physical dependence
    2. Physical dependence is NOT addiction
    3. Intra-muscular opioid administration on a prn basis leads to inadequate pain control
    4. "Prn" dosing is associated with an increase in toxicity symptoms such as hypoventilation, confusion and sedation.
    5. Meperidine should be avoided in the elderly
    6. Patient controlled analgesia (PCA) is effective even in the frail elderly.
    7. Pain remains one of the most undertreated conditions of the elderly.
- Recommended Drugs for Elderly
    1. Morphine sulfate
    2. Hydromorphone
    3. Fentanyl

- Adjuvant Analgesics
  1. NSAIDs
  2. Corticosteroids
  3. Heterocyclic antidepressants, especially with neuropathic pain

- Chronic Pain—General Concepts
  1. Oral route always approach of first choice
     a. Other routes for pain control are rectal, parenteral, intravenous and sub-cutaneous
     b. Transdermal—no good studies yet as to effectiveness in the elderly
  2. Increase to stronger drug when smaller doses of a more potent agent will be more effective and less toxic
  3. Neuropathic pain usually requires an opioid AND an adjuvant
  4. Analgesics are administered on around-the-clock schedules, NEVER prn
  5. Always check equianalgesic dose when changing route
  6. Assess pain using visual analog scale (VAS)
  7. Start low, go slow
  8. Side effects common to most pain medications
     a. Sedation—especially early in use
        (1) No problem if easily arousable
        (2) Respiratory depression—not a problem with chronic oral morphine use; no changes measured in pCO_2 and pO_2.
     b. Constipation
        (1) Treat early with stool softener and stimulant cathartic

- Narcotics
  1. Action—Depress pain impulse transmission by interacting with opioid receptors. Onset is immediate by IV route, and rapid by oral route.

2. Indications
    a. Moderate to severe pain post-op
    b. Chronic cancer pain
3. Dosage—titrated according to need and drug
4. Side effects
    a. Constipation, occasionally nausea and vomiting
    b. Respiratory depression, although not common with chronic use even in COPD patients
5. Contraindications—hypersensitivity
6. Interactions—INCREASES effects of other CNS depressants
7. Nursing interventions—(see general concepts)

Questions

1. Factors negatively affecting drug use in the elderly include all of the following except:
   a. Multiple pathologies
   b. Multiple providers
   c. Method of administration
   d. Non-specific presentation of illness

2. ADRs most commonly occur with these classes of drugs:
   a. Inhalers and sprays
   b. Cardiovascular and psychotropic
   c. NSAIDs and salicylates
   d. Insulin, oral diabetic agents

3. Adverse drug interactions include all of the following possibilities except:
   a. Hypersensitivity
   b. Suppression of metabolism of other drugs
   c. Cumulative effect or toxicity
   d. Drug displacement from protein binding sites

4. Which of these symptoms can be caused by adverse drug reaction?
   a. Confusion, unsteady gait
   b. Involuntary movements
   c. Weakness and fatigue
   d. All of the above

5. Drug review:
   a. Compares costs of drugs
   b. Need only be done once a year
   c. Includes evaluation of side effects
   d. Can only be done by physicians

6. The rate of noncompliance with a medication regimen in the elderly is:
   a. Lower than other age groups
   b. Higher than other age groups
   c. Same as other groups
   d. Unknown

7. Physiological changes of aging that greatly affect pharmacokinetics include all of the following except:

   a. Decrease in renal function
   b. Increase in lean body mass
   c. Decreased absorption in GI tract
   d. Increase in total body fat

8. The most accurate measure of renal function in the elderly is:

   a. Serum creatine
   b. Specific gravity
   c. Creatinine clearance
   d. Urine osmolarity

9. Patient assessment related to pharmacokinetics should include:

   a. State of hydration
   b. State of nutrition
   c. Cardiac output
   d. All of the above

10. Pharmacodynamics can be defined as:

    a. What drug does to your body
    b. What your body does to drugs
    c. Onset of action of drugs
    d. ''Steady state'' level of drug

11. Factors associated with noncompliance include all of the following except:

    a. Severity of illness
    b. Short illness
    c. Positive and rapid response to drug therapy
    d. Frequency of dosing

12. A measure that enhances compliance is:

    a. Limited information regarding drug side effects
    b. Child proof containers
    c. Multiple providers
    d. Use of blister packs, and medication dispensers

13. General prescribing principles for the elderly include:

    a. Use of new drugs whenever possible
    b. Giving verbal instructions carefully to patient
    c. Treating ALL conditions with drug therapy
    d. Start low, go slow

14. A thorough medication history includes questions about all of the following except:

    a. Storage of medications
    b. Alcohol use
    c. Family history
    d. Allergies

15. Over the counter (OTC) preparations:

    a. Cannot be efficacious
    b. Can cause serious adverse drug reactions
    c. Are not likely to be used by the elderly
    d. Are usually less expensive

16. Choose the most commonly prescribed cardiovascular drug:

    a. Thiazide diuretics
    b. Nitrates
    c. Digoxin
    d. Calcium channel blockers

17. Increased myocardial contractility and slowed heart rate are actions of:

    a. Calcium channel blockers
    b. Thiazide diuretics
    c. Nitrates
    d. Digoxin

18. Most common side effect of digoxin in the elderly is:

    a. Nausea and vomiting
    b. Visual disturbances
    c. Confusion
    d. Diarrhea

19. Which serum electrolyte should be monitored most carefully in the patient on digoxin?
    a. Sodium
    b. Potassium
    c. Chloride
    d. BUN

20. Nitrites and nitrates are used for:
    a. Prevention of myocardial infarction
    b. Management of HPTN
    c. Prevention and relief of anginal episodes
    d. Management of lipidemia

21. Which side effect is COMMON with nitrates?
    a. Orthostatic hypotension
    b. Flushing
    c. Constipation
    d. Photosensitivity

22. Alcohol can cause an adverse drug reaction with which class of drug?
    a. Anticoagulants
    b. NSAIDs
    c. Beta-blockers
    d. All of the above

23. When teaching the patient about sublingual nitrate use, after how many doses should patient contact health care provider if pain still persists?
    a. One dose
    b. Four doses
    c. Three doses
    d. Should call before taking ANY dose

24. The following dietary instruction would be given to a patient on thiazide diuretics:
    a. Eat foods high in fiber
    b. Eat foods high in sodium
    c. Avoid simple sugars
    d. Eat foods high in potassium

25. You would advise the patient on digoxin and hydrocholothiazide to contact the health care provider PROMPTLY for this condition:

    a. Cough
    b. Vomiting and diarrhea
    c. Altered taste sensation
    d. Headache

26. Ototoxicity is a side effect of which diuretic:

    a. Potassium sparing
    b. Thiazide
    c. Loop
    d. None of the above

27. A PREVENTABLE, reversible adverse effect of diuretic therapy is:

    a. Heart block
    b. Hypersensitivity
    c. Thrombocytopenia
    d. Urinary incontinence

28. Indications for calcium channel blockers include all of the following except:

    a. Coronary artery spasm
    b. Myocardial infarction
    c. Supraventricular arrhythmias
    d. Hypertension

29. Beta-blockers are contraindicated for patients with:

    a. Dementia
    b. Hypertension
    c. Glaucoma
    d. Diabetes mellitus

30. Hyperlipidemia and hyperglycemia are side effects of:

    a. Thiazide diuretics
    b. Beta-blockers
    c. Digoxin
    d. Calcium channel blockers

31. Patients receiving oral anticoagulant therapy should avoid:

    a. Bananas
    b. Cheese
    c. Licorice
    d. Legumes

32. An assessment of which of these skills should be completed before beginning to teach an elderly diabetic patient?

    a. Cognitive
    b. Visual
    c. Fine motor
    d. All of the above

33. Over the counter availability of this type of medication contributes to adverse drug interactions:

    a. Acetaminophen
    b. NSAIDs
    c. Psyllium
    d. 1/2% cortisone cream

34. Which anti-anxiolytic is most widely used by the elderly?

    a. MAO inhibitor
    b. Beta-blocker
    c. Benzodiazipine
    d. Alcohol

35. ''On an empty stomach'' means:

    a. One hour before or two hours after meals
    b. Two hours before or two hours after meals
    c. Two hours before or one hour after meals
    c. One half hour before or two hours after meals

36. What is the recommended length of treatment with H_2 blockers for gastric ulcer?

    a. Eight weeks
    b. Ten weeks
    c. Twelve weeks
    d. Nine weeks

37. Common side effects of benzodiazipines include all of the following except:
    a. Orthostatic hypotension
    b. Delirium
    c. Blurred vision
    d. Dementia

38. The MAJOR indication for use of antipsychotic drugs is:
    a. Depression
    b. Insomnia
    c. Schizophrenia
    d. Parkinson's disease

39. Akathisia is a side effect of:
    a. Antidiabetic drugs
    b. Digoxin
    c. Antidepressants
    d. Antipsychotics

40. Adjuvant therapy for pain control could include:
    a. Relaxation techniques
    b. NSAIDs
    c. Antidepressants
    d. All of the above

41. A new onset of symptoms in an elderly patient should always prompt:
    a. An EKG
    b. A urinalysis
    c. A drug review
    d. A mental status exam

Answers

1. c
2. b
3. a
4. d
5. c
6. b
7. c
8. c
9. d
10. a
11. b
12. d
13. d
14. c
15. b
16. c
17. d
18. c
19. b
20. c
21. b
22. d
23. c
24. d
25. b
26. c
27. d
28. b
29. d
30. a
31. c
32. d
33. b
34. d
35. a
36. c
37. d
38. c
39. d
40. d
41. c

Bibliography

Abrams, W., & Berkow, R. (1990). *The Merck manual of geriatrics.* Rahway, NJ: Merck, Sharp & Dohme Research Laboratories.

Acute pain management: Operative or medical procedures and trauma. Clinical practice guideline (1992) (AHCPR Pub.No. 92.0032). Rockville, MD: US Dept. of Health and Human Services. Agency for Health Care Policy and Research.

American Pain Society (1992). *Principles of analgesic use in the treatment of acute pain and cancer pain.* (3rd ed.). Skokie, IL: Author.

Bressler, R., & Katz, M. (1993). *Geriatric pharmacology.* New York: McGraw-Hill.

Hahn, K., & Wietor, G. (1992). Helpful tools for medication screenings. *Geriatric nursing.* 13(3) 160–66.

Kane, R., Ouslander, J., & Abrass, I. (1989). *Essentials of clinical geriatrics* (2nd ed.). New York: McGraw-Hill.

Malseed, R. & Harrigan, G. (1989). *Textbook of pharmacology nursing care.* Philadelphia: J. B. Lippincott.

McPherson, M. (1992, February). *Medication management issues of the geriatric client.* Presented at American Healthcare Institute Program on Drugs and the Elderly.

Punzi, H., & Flamenbaum, W. (1989). Hypertension. In H. Punzi & W. Flamenbaum (Eds.) *Clinical cardiovascular therapeutics,* Vol. 1. Mount Kiscoe, NY: Futura Publishing.

Skidmore-Roth, L. (1992). *Mosby's 1992 nursing drug reference.* St. Louis, MO: Mosby-Year Book.

Suddarth, D. (1991). Care of the older adult. In D. Suddarth (Ed.), *The Lippincott manual of nursing practice,* pp 118–125. Philadelphia: J. B. Lippincott.

ETHICAL AND LEGAL ISSUES

Deborah Francis

- Ethics can be defined as the moral rules that govern a society and assist us in determining what is right in a difficult situation. Health care or bioethics is the systematic process of applying fundamental moral rules or principles to a sensitive health care related problem in order to determine the best or right decision. Ethical dilemmas, in which there is clearly no best solution or in which decisions between equally unacceptable alternatives must be made, commonly and inevitably confront nurses working with the elderly. Applying basic ethical principles to guide the decision making process will ensure that these decisions are based on reason rather than on emotion.

  A. Ethical Principles:

     1. Autonomy: Every competent adult has the freedom to make and carry out his/her own decisions. Nurses must respect this right to self determination, which is considered more important than the values and beliefs of health care providers and what they perceive is most beneficial for the patient. Therefore, when ethical principles come into conflict, the autonomy of the competent patient must always take precedence.
     2. Beneficence/Nonmaleficence: This principle requires doing good or seeking alternatives for the patient that will provide the greatest good while preventing undo harm or nonmaleficence. The difficulty occurs in defining what is ''good'' for the patient, a concept that evokes different interpretations in different persons. When values come into conflict, it is important not to act paternalistically by doing what one perceives is best for the patient without respect for his/her personal autonomy.
     3. Justice: The principle of justice deals with treating individuals fairly and ensuring they get what they deserve. It is often referred to in discussions of distribution of services, especially regarding the differential treatment of some persons over others. Health care resources in this country tend to be rationed on the basis of age due in part to the escalating costs, stringent reimbursement criteria, and limited perceived benefit among the elderly. A person's functional status rather than chronological age needs to be considered when distributing scarce resources. Gerontological nurses must be prepared to advocate for their patients to receive new technologies and to promote the need

to expand services, such as home health care, currently restricted because of reimbursement restrictions.

4. Veracity/Confidentiality: The principle of veracity stipulates that all patients have the right to the truth and should not be deceived or misled by others. Nurses often struggle with the dilemma of how much information to disclose to a patient when the discomfort it may cause can potentially harm the patient. In such cases, the principles of beneficence and nonmaleficence come into conflict with veracity. Confidentiality is an important basic right that is guaranteed by the patients' bill of rights. A nurse has the responsibility to respect and protect the patient's confidentiality. Information may be disclosed only with the express permission of the patient or if required by law. Although the nurse must have access to confidential information necessary to provide competent patient care, she may not discuss it with anyone not directly involved in the patient's care.

B. Traditional Ethical Theories: Nurses should have an understanding of theoretical ethical approaches that can provide a basis to begin the ethical decision making process.

1. Utilitarian: The utilitarian approach focuses on what will provide the greatest good for the greatest number of people. This theory is often used to justify the termination of treatment for the elderly in an environment of scarce resources.

2. Deontology or Formalism: This theory suggests that the moral values of the nurse and the ethical principles or rules applied to the situation are more relevant to the decision than the consequences of the action. Decisions regarding death, suicide, euthanasia and prolongation of life are often based on this approach.

3. Egoism: Egoism suggests that the solution should be the one that will promote the greatest good for the decision maker regardless of the desires of the patient or family. Deciding not to disclose certain information because it may cause unnecessary discomfort to the patient is based on the egoist approach.

C. Ethical Decision Making Process: In addition to understanding basic ethical principles and theories, it has been suggested that in order to make sound ethical decisions, nurses should engage in values clarification, be aware of and adhere to the American Nurses Association Code of Ethics, collaborate with a multidisciplinary team and apply basic decision making models or frameworks.

1. Values Clarification: Before a nurse can systematically reason through an ethical dilemma, she must engage in the process of values clarification. All decisions are inherently dependent on personal values and belief systems. When confronted with a difficult ethical dilemma, examination and clarification of those values that are most significant to us is critical to the decision making process. Encouraging the patient and/or family to examine those values and beliefs considered most important in life is an important step to assisting them to make the best choice regarding medical care. This is especially important whenever advanced directives are being drawn up and when determining wishes for aggressiveness of care.

2. American Nurses Association (ANA) Code for Nurses: The ANA Code for Nurses with Interpretive Statements was first adopted by the ANA in 1950 and later updated in 1976 to guide the nurses' conduct and ethical decision making process. The code is a set of rules or guidelines that provides a standard of conduct by which all professional nurses are expected to practice. These standards may exceed those recognized by law, and the ANA has the right to reprimand, censure, suspend or expell any nurse found violating the code. Every nurse must be aware of and adhere to the code in her professional practice, as it is the recognized standard that guides ethically sound nursing conduct.

3. Ethics Committees: Most ethical dilemmas are best resolved through the collaborative effort of a team. When confronted with delicate ethical dilemmas, it is helpful to involve a multidisciplinary ethics committee designed to systematically examine the issues and make reasonable recommendations based on established ethical principles and theories. Besides consultation and review of cases, ethics committees are often responsible for ethics education, development of policies and procedures, and discussion of theological thought (Matteson & McConnell, 1988).

4. Ethical Decision Making Models: Various models or frameworks have been proposed to assist the nurse in working through an ethical dilemma. Although they vary in their approach, most consider the facts of the situation, the decision making questions and the underlying ethical theories (Aroskar, 1980). It has been suggested that it is not the specific model that is important, but the nurses' ability to apply a valid decision making model to an ethical dilemma.

- Informed Consent: Informed consent protects a person's autonomy by guaranteeing every competent adult the right to choose or to refuse medical interventions. A health care provider may not legally or morally touch or invade another person's body without explicit permission. To this end, except in cases of medical emergencies, competent adults must give voluntary written consent prior to all medical procedures or treatments or participation in a research project. Health care providers are legally responsible to provide patients with sufficient information in terms they can understand to allow them to make an informed choice. Valid informed consent must include the diagnosis or suspected diagnosis, nature and purpose of the proposed procedure or treatment and expected benefits, risks, consequences and/or side effects, probability of success, reasonable alternatives, and the probable consequences if patient refuses the proposed treatment. Informed consent is not possible if the patient is deemed incompetent or incapable to make a sound decision. In these situations, second party consent must always be obtained.
- Competence: The law presumes that all adults are competent to make their own decisions regarding medical care. Should the question of competence arise in a medical situation, only a court of law can declare a person legally incompetent. However, a health care professional has the ability to evaluate a person's mental capacity to determine whether he/she is competent to provide informed consent. Beauchamp & Childress (1983) suggest the theory of limited or intermittent competency. According to this concept, mental capacity is not an absolute attribute, but a variable one that depends on the gravity of the specific decision to be made and on the patient's mental condition at the time of the decision. A person may be competent to consent to a medical procedure, but may be incompetent to manage complicated financial matters.

Generally, persons who can demonstrate an understanding of their actions are considered competent. Specifically, competent adults must have sufficient language skills to communicate and understand, possess cognitive and conceptual abilities, be able to reason and deliberate and possess a sense of what is good or bad for their wellbeing in light of their personal goals (National Health Council, 1988). A cognitive examination is useful to determine competence and should include evaluation of the person's orientation to time, place and person, long and short-term memory, and the ability to reason abstractly about the consequences of conditions and actions. These factors all affect a person's judgment; however, impaired judgment alone does not deem a person incompetent. Mental capacity should be determined in the clinical setting prior to attempting to establish incompetency in a court of law.

A. Tests for Competence: Various tests for competency are used to obtain informed consent depending on the gravity of the situation. For a relatively benign procedure with few inherent risks, either evidence of choice by the patient who is able to say yes or no, or an acknowledgment that the choice the patient made is a reasonable one may be sufficient. The test of competence that is most consistent with the legal tenet of informed consent requires that the patient be able to understand the risks, benefits and alternatives to treatment. The fourth and highest level of competence measures the patient's actual understanding of the specifics of the situation (Chenitz, Stone & Salisbury, 1991).

B. Decisions on Behalf of Incompetent Patients:

   1. Surrogate Decision Maker: When the patient is deemed unable to make a decision due to a significant mental incapacity, consent for treatment should be obtained from the patient's surrogate decision maker. This is a person, usually a family member, appointed to plead a cause for another based on the patient's past wishes and values. Alternatives used to determine the best decision include the rational person, the substituted judgement approach and the durable statement of intent or advanced directive. The former considers what a rational person would do in the situation regardless of what the patient or health professional would choose. The substituted judgment approach attempts to determine what the patient would do in the situation if (s)he were competent to make the decision.

   2. Advanced directives are durable statements of intent based on a person's last expressed written wishes. In an effort to prevent confusion and disagreement regarding an incompetent patient's desires for medical care, the Patient Self Determination Act

(PSDA) was enacted in 1990 to encourage more adults to execute an advanced directive. This act mandates that all adult patients in any health care setting receiving federal funding have the right to control decisions and to plan ahead for their health care. In addition, it also encourages communicaton between patients, families and health care professionals as it clearly and specifically indicates a person's desires regarding agressiveness of care. Health care facilities must provide patients with written information about their legal rights to make decisions regarding their medical care, including the right to accept or refuse treatment and to formulate advance directives and must document whether an advance directive has been executed. If the patient does not have an advanced directive, information must be provided regarding the need for and process to complete one. These health care facilities must also educate their staff and inform the community of their policies on advance directives.

a. Living Will: A living will is a contract between a patient and a physician which specifies wishes concerning the end of life in case of terminal illness. Usually, a living will directs that if death is imminent, the process of dying should not be prolonged, but care necessary to maintain comfort and dignity will be provided while the illness takes its natural course. It is important to be aware of its legal status, because not all states recognize living wills, leaving health care providers legally liable for their actions in fulfilling the terms of the contract. The Natural Death Act was created in some states to legalize living wills and protect health professionals from any liability of abiding by the patient's wishes.

b. A Durable Power of Attorney for Health Care (DPAHC) authorizes another person or agent to make medical decisions on behalf of an individual if and when the patient becomes unable or unwilling to do so. It is a version of the power of attorney used in commercial transactions and transfers of properties. Whereby the power of attorney becomes invalid if and when the person becomes incapacitated, the DPAHC takes effect at precisely this time. Any competent adult over eighteen years of age may complete a DPAHC, which does not require an attorney to complete. The DPAHC has definite advantages over the living will and nurses should encourage interested patients to complete one. However, a nurse may not participate in any way in filling it out or witnessing it while practicing in a professional capacity. A DPAHC signed in or after 1992 is valid indefinitely; those signed prior to this are generally valid for seven years. It is recognized everywhere in the United States except in the District of Columbia, can be used to either prolong life or discontinue treatment, and may be revoked at any time. Unlike the living will, the DPAHC can be used to make decisions on behalf of individuals who are not terminally ill, but are incapable of making their own decisions.

3. Payee status: Individuals who are having difficulty managing personal finances may request that the Social Security Administration appoint a payee. All monies will be fowarded to the payee who will be entrusted to manage the funds for the older adult.
4. Legal guardianship or conservatorship is the legal appointment of a person, usually a family member, to make decisions on behalf of an adult legally deemed incapable or incompetent to make personal decisions or to provide for his/her own needs. To be declared incompetent, a person must suffer from a mental incapacity such as mental illness or a primary degenerative or alcohol related dementia, and the mental condition must adversely affect the person's ability to function. There are two basic types of guardianship. Guardianship of person is most restrictive and holds with it the potential for harm as the conservatee loses all constitutional rights and civil liberties, such as the right to vote, marry or make a will. Limited guardianship determines the specific areas that the individual is incapable of managing and assigns a guardian to act as the surrogate decision maker.

C. Do not resuscitate orders (DNR) are intended to prevent cardiopulmonary resuscitation (CPR) in the event of a cardiac arrest and are decided by the physician in consultation with the competent patient and/or family or the surrogate decision maker. Studies indicate that there is a general lack of awareness of the use of CPR among the public, and a reluctance among physicians to discuss the use of CPR with patients and family (Torian, Davidson, Fillit, Fulop & Sell, 1992; Stolman, Gregory, Dunn & Levine 1990). The lack of a DNR order in the medical record presumes that the patient desires full intervention, and holds the nurse legally responsible to initiate life sustaining treatment, regardless of whether the efforts may be futile and unnecessarily harmfull (Quill, 1992). Physicians must initiate discussions of life sustaining interventions and encourage the completion of advanced directives as early as possible. These discussions sould include not only the performance of CPR and use of a ventilator, but withholding of food, fluid and/or antibiotics in the case of an irreversible medical condition. Nurses need to assume an active role in educating patients and communicate to the physician any change of condition or need to clarify end of life treatment options. Health care institutions must consider developing guidelines for orders not to resuscitate (Davis & Aroskar, 1983).

Difficulties may arise when patients or families insist on resuscitation in cases considered to be medically futile or when the patient's wishes are not known and there is conflict among the family or health care providers. Faced with such ethical dilemmas, nurses have a variety of options:

1. Follow the DNR order
2. Refuse to carry out the DNR order
3. Contact the physician and/or family to request they reconsider the DNR option
4. Take the issue to the institution's ethics committee
5. Schedule a multidisciplinary team conference
6. Contact the local ombudsman program or adult protective services agency (Matteson & McConnell, 1988).

- Euthanasia: A highly controversial issue that addresses the active or passive act of hastening a person's death. Active euthanasia involves commiting an act that intentionally and directly leads to death. Passive euthanasia is an act of omission in which an intervention that would prolong life is witheld. Some argue that the need for euthanasia would be less if agreement over the issue of limiting care for persons in persistent vegetative states or with advanced dementia could be resolved or if medical technology could alleviate a person's suffering due to chronic pain. Opposition to euthanasia is grounded in arguments over morality and in the potential for indiscriminate use if it were to be legalized. However, there is a growing trend in this country to address its acceptance as evidenced by voters' recent consideration of the issue on state ballots.

- Restraints and Patient Rights: Physical and chemical restraint use in the elderly is common in this country. A physical restraint is any device that restricts the free movement of a person. A chemical restraint is any medication used for the sole purpose of controlling behavior or mood. The most common reasons to use restraints appear to be to protect a patient from harm and to prevent interference with medical treatment. The problem lies in the fact that restraints are commonly applied without the informed consent of the patient. All too often, the patient's right for autonomy is overlooked by the paternalistic act of the nurse who determines what is best for the patient on the grounds of beneficence. Before initiating restraints, it is essential to make every effort to determine the patient's abilty to understand the need for and the potential risk entailed in refusing restraints. When a patient cannot understand, the nurse should involve the patient's surrogate decision maker and ensure that the therapy is truly in the best interest of the patient by considering the risks and benefits of the restraints. The Omnibus Reconciliation Act (OBRA) of 1987 implemented new restrictions regarding restraint use in health care facilities. OBRA mandates that patients have the right to be free from any physical or chemical restraint imposed for purposes of discipline or convenience and not required to treat medical symptoms (Colorado Ombudsman Program, 1990). Restraints are allowed only to ensure the physical safety of the patient or other patients, and only upon the written order of the primary care provider that specifies the time and circumstances under which the restraints may be used.
- Research and the Elderly: It is generally accepted that much more research in the area of geriatrics and gerontological nursing is needed to promote our professional nursing practice. However, there are concerns that need to be addressed regarding the potential for exploiting the elderly as research subjects. This is particularly true when using institutionalized individuals who are particularly vulnerable. Prior to the initiation of any research with the elderly it is essential to assess the competence of the individual to completely understand the information and provide informed consent. It is also important to provide information about the research project in a manner that the elder can understand. Sometimes it is necessary to decide when verbal consent rather than written consent is

necessary. Finally, if the patient is unable to give informed consent, a type of proxy consent will have to be selected (Matteson & McConnell, 1988).

- Legal Issues

A. Malpractice and Negligence: The terms malpractice and negligence are commonly, but erroneously, used interchangeably. Negligence is the failure of an individual to do something that a reasonable person would do that results in injury to another. Malpractice is any negligent act performed within a professional capacity that causes harm to an individual by failing to act with the reason and skill expected of a professional. Examples of negligent acts within the scope of nursing practice that could result in malpractice suits include failure to properly administer medications, follow physicians orders, report patient changes, or follow established nursing procedure. An exception to this rule is the Good Samaritan Act which was enacted so that fear of malpractice suits would not prevent health care providers from assisting a victim in an emergency. In considering whether an act is negligent, it is necessary to determine whether the action was within the nurse's scope of practice and whether (s)he had the specific skills or knowledge to perform the activity. It is important for all professonal nurses to be covered by malpractice insurance in the event a malpractice suit is brought against him/her. According to common law, negligence involves four basic components (Klein, 1986):

1. Duty: A nurse's duty is defined by his/her scope of practice, and further outlined by the state's Nurse Practice Act, the job description and by judgments in previous court decisions.
2. Breach of Duty: Abandonment of professional duty, which can vary from failing to answer a patient's call light for several hours to inappropriate administration of medications.
3. Direct Causation and Damages: For malpractice to have occurred, an actual loss or damage must have occurred and direct causation between the breach of duty and the injury must be proved. Any negligent action performed by the nurse to or for the patient that results in actual damage to the patient can be considered malpractice. This could range from inappropriate restraint use to administering a lethal dose of medication.

B. Expert Testimony: Nurses with advanced education, expertise or knowledge are commonly requested to consult on or provide testimony on behalf of patients or health care facilities involved in a legal suit. Most commonly, these are malpractice suits. The expert witness is expected to examine the documented nursing practice in the case and/or testify regarding accepted standards of nursing care to assist in the determination of wrongful suit. The expert witness can expect to be compensated for her time as a nurse consultant.

- Elder Abuse: Elder abuse and neglect is the most recent and increasingly common form of domestic violence in which an elder or dependent adult is mistreated by another. Although the actual incidence is unknown, estimates suggest that between four and ten per cent of the elderly are abused. However, it is very common for the elder not to report the abuse or to deny its occurrence, suggesting the actual prevalence of the problem may be much higher.

A. Types of Abuse and Neglect:

1. Physical abuse: Nonaccidental use of physical force that results in bodily injury. This includes any physical beating or sexual assault.
2. Psychological or emotional abuse: Willful infliction of mental or emotional pain by verbal or nonverbal threat, intimidation, or humilitation.
3. Neglect: Failure of caregivers to fulfill their caretaking obligation.
4. Fiduciary or financial abuse: Unauthorized use of an elder's funds or resources.
5. Violation of rights: Denial of an elder's legal or unalienable rights.
6. Self Neglect/Self Abuse: Neglectful or abusive conduct toward oneself that threatens the older adult's safety or health.

B. Theories of Causation

1. Physical and Mental Impairments of the Elder: Functional and cognitive impairments render an elder dependent on others for assistance with basic activities of daily living. Such dependency needs over time can become overwhelming to even the most caring of caregivers.

2. Caregiver Stress: Most older adults live at home and are cared for by family members. The majority of caregivers are women and an increasing number are middle aged women with multiple demands of work, children at home and aging dependent parents. The stress can become overwhelming, particularly when there are so few community resources available to assist the caregiver.
3. Cycle of Learned Violence: There is an alarming trend of adults who were abused as children who are now caring for and abusing their parents.
4. Personality Traits of the Abuser: Drug and/or alcohol abuse or psychological problems of the caregiver commonly trigger an abusive situation.

C. Profile of the Victim: Victims tend to be female, over 75 years of age, who live with and are dependent on the abuser because of at least one physical or mental impairment that limits their activities of daily living. They may be socially isolated, frail, passive, and so afraid of change and/or loyal to the abuser that they deny or refuse to report the abuse.

D. Detection: Being aware of the risk factors and knowing what to look for is important in identifying abuse of the elderly. Elder abuse is often first identified in the hospital emergency room. In the community, home health and long term care nurses are in the position to not only intervene when abuse or neglect has occurred, but to detect high risk situations and prevent potential abuse.

1. Physical evidence: Bruises, burns, scratches, pinchmarks especially in unusual locations, injuries in various stages of healing, signs of untreated malnutrition or dehydration, evidence of misuse of medications, and unmet medical needs.
2. Suspicious indicators: Inconsistencies, such as any injury whose occurence is not consistent with the physical findings, history of similar injuries, pattern of seeking out different doctors or hospitals, elder brought to hospital by someone other than caregiver, or frequent use of emergency room.
3. Emotional indicators: Elder appears fearful, refuses to talk or establish or maintain eye contact, or cowers when touched as if in pain.

E. Intervention: The goals of intervention are to protect the patient and prevent any further injury. Most states have mandated elder and dependent adult abuse reporting laws. In California, for example, all health care providers are legally mandated to report suspected physical abuse. Additionally, they are encouraged to report other types of abuse and neglect. The state agency charged with protection of elders such as the Adult Protective Services agency should be notified of any suspected case of elder abuse, neglect, or any time an elderly person is being discharged into an unsafe or potentially harmful situation. Besides knowing when to report suspected abuse, nurses working with the elderly must be active in the education of public and professionals about the problem of elder abuse and support legislation and research to alleviate this problem. In addition, nurses need to advocate for the improvement of methods of detection and intervention, and incorporate a multidisciplinary approach in dealing with elder abuse.

Questions

Mrs. Jones is an 85 year old frail woman who lives alone in a run down mobile home with two dogs and multiple cats. She has no family and requires a walker to ambulate. She has been admitted to the hospital three times in the last six months for dehydration, falls and failure to thrive. Each time she is admitted she is confused, but she always clears enough prior to discharge to articulate how she can care for herself at home. Although you feel she requires more assistance at home and it would be in her best interest to be admitted to a nursing home, she insists on returning home and refuses a home health care referral.

1. In insisting on returning home with no assistance, Mrs. Jones is exercising her right to:
   a. Beneficence
   b. Justice
   c. Autonomy
   d. Fidelity

2. In encouraging Mrs. Jones to consider moving to a nursing home, the nurse is basing her intervention on the principle of:
   a. Beneficence
   b. Justice
   c. Autonomy
   d. Fidelity

3. Prior to sending Mrs. Jones home, it is important for the nurse to do all of the following except:
   a. File an elder abuse report with the local Adult Protective Services agency
   b. Document Mrs. Jones mental status and ability to understand the risks of returning home unassisted
   c. Attempt to locate a neighbor or other gatekeeper who can look in on her periodically
   d. Tell her you feel she would be better off in a nursing home and is doing the wrong thing by going home alone

4. The decision to transfer an elderly patient out of the ICU before he is medically stable because of a shortage of ICU beds is based on the ethical theory of:

   a. Formalism
   b. Nonmaleficence
   c. Utility
   d. Egoism

5. In order to assist the nurse to make the best decision in a situation that poses a difficult ethical dilemma, it is important to possess a basic understanding of all of the following except:

   a. Ethical principles and theories
   b. ANA Code of Nurses with Interpretive Statements
   c. The patient's last expressed wishes and values
   d. The family's feelings regarding what a competent patient should do

6. Values clarification is an important step in the process of:

   a. Assisting the patient to determine the specific type and content of advanced directive
   b. Discussing specifics regarding do not resuscitate orders
   c. Determining the best possible choice in a difficult decision in which no alternative appears acceptable
   d. All of the above

7. Nurses need to be aware of the ANA Code for Nurses with Interpretive Statements because of all of the following except:

   a. Nurses are held legally liable to follow the code
   b. It sets the standard for professional practice
   c. Failure to do so can result in loss of licensure or reprimand
   d. It serves to guide the ethical conduct of the nurse

8. According to the law of informed consent, in order for a patient to consent to a medical procedure, he/she must:

   a. Be judged competent in a court of law
   b. Demonstrate the procedure that will be performed
   c. Be declared competent by a psychiatrist
   d. Understand the risks and benefits of the procedure

9. All of the following is true regarding informed consent except that it:
   a. Protects a person's autonomy by protecting his right to choose
   b. Is necessary prior to any medical intervention or participation in a research project
   c. Must be obtained even if the patient's competence is in question
   d. Requires health care providers to provide patients with information in terms they can understand

10. The law presumes that all adults:
    a. Have expressed their wishes regarding medical care to a surrogate decision maker
    b. Are competent to make their own medical decisions
    c. Need an evaluation by a psychiatrist before being declared incompetent
    d. Require an evaluation of their mental status prior to obtaining informed consent

11. The concept of limited competence refers to the fact that:
    a. Competence is not absolute and a person can be competent in one area and incompetent in another
    b. Incompetence can be determined by only a limited number of health care providers
    c. Incompetence depends on an evaluation of limited mental capacity
    d. A person can be declared incompetent only by a court of law

12. The law of informed consent is based upon the fact that:
    a. The patient is able to make a reasonable choice
    b. The patient fully understands every detail about the medical procedure involved
    c. The patient appears to understand the risks and benefits of and alternatives to the intervention
    d. The patient is able to make a choice

13. The person identified to make a decision for a patient whose mental capacity renders him incapable of giving informed consent is called a(n):
    a. Advanced directive
    b. Substituted judge
    c. Surrogate decision maker
    d. Rational person

14. Advance directives provide an individual with the opportunity to express his/her wishes regarding:

    a. Burial
    b. Where they would like to die
    c. Specifically how they would like to die
    d. Life prolonging measures

15. The Patient Self Determinaton Act applies to all of the following settings except:

    a. Acute care hospitals
    b. Skilled nursing facilities
    c. Senior centers
    d. Hospice

16. The Patient Self Determination Act provides the following:

    a. Older adults are required to have durable powers of attorney in the event they become incapacitated.
    b. The primary care provider is responsible for determining what the appropriate advanced directive should be for each of their patients.
    c. The health care institution is required to ask each person admitted if they have an advanced directive and if they do not, provide them with information on how to execute one.
    d. None of the above

17. A living will goes into effect:

    a. With all types of illness
    b. When a person cannot verbally express his wishes
    c. When the family of the patient requests it
    d. When the patient has a terminal illness

18. All of the following is true regarding a Durable Power of Attorney for Health Care except:

    a. It is recognized in all fifty states
    b. It goes into effect when the patient is no longer able or unwilling to make decisions for self
    c. A nurse should encourage all patients to complete one and can witness it for the patient
    d. It designates another person to make specific decisions for the patient

19. Guardianship of person:

    a. Does not require the involvement of an attorney
    b. Designates another person to make all decisions for the patient
    c. Allows the patient's right to vote and to marry
    d. Can be obtained for a person who can no longer function independently, but is cognitively intact

20. OBRA mandates that nurses may use physical and chemical restraints only:

    a. To ensure the physical safety of the patient or other patients
    b. With permission from the family
    c. When there is a standing order from the physician for their use
    d. To avoid a malpractice suit in case a patient falls

21. The group of older adults most vulnerable for exploitation as research subjects tends to be those:

    a. Acutely ill hospitalized elders
    b. Persons living in skilled nursing facilities
    c. Community dwelling elders
    d. Who have no primary care provider

22. For an action to be considered malpractice, all of the following must have occurred except:

    a. An injury occurred as a direct result of an act by the nurse
    b. The nurse clearly possesses the skill to perform the act
    c. The injury occurred in response to a medical emergency while off duty
    d. The act was within the nurse's scope of practice

23. According to law, negligence involves all the following except:

    a. Duty
    b. Injury
    c. Justice
    d. Direct causation

24. Situations that are suspected to be elder abuse and should be reported to the proper authorities include:

    a. Verbal threats to place in a nursing home
    b. Administering medications for the sole purpose of controlling behavior
    c. Sexual assault of an elder
    d. All of the above

25. Nurses working with the elderly are responsible for all of the following except:

    a. Knowing what the state mandated elder abuse requirements are
    b. Notifying the family when suspected abuse has occurred
    c. Being able to identify physical or suspicious indicators of abuse
    d. Knowing when and to whom to report suspected elder abuse

26. All of the following are considered causes of elder abuse except:

    a. Caregiver burden
    b. Alcohol abuse
    c. Learned violence
    d. Lack of education

27. An 85 year-old resident of a skilled nursing facility has advanced Alzheimer's disease and is functionally dependent in all of the ADLs. His wife's wishes for life sustaining treatment are not known and the family have expressed a desire for full intervention in the event of a cardiac arrest. There is no DNR order in the medical record and the nursing staff feel uncomfortable about initiating CPR on this patient. Their options include all of the following except:

    a. Contact the physician to request that he reconsider the no DNR order.
    b. Convene a multidisciplinary team conference to express feelings and consider alternatives.
    c. Contact the family to tell them you will not perform CPR.
    d. Contact the institution's ethics committee.

28. A nurse's responsibility in ensuring that patient's end of life options are honored include all except:

    a. Educating patients and families regarding the risks and benefits of life sustaining treatment.
    b. Communicating any change of condition to the physician that may warrant reconsidering DNR order.
    c. Communicating to physician a change in the patient's wishes.
    d. Documenting physician/patient discussions regarding treatment options.

Answers

1. c
2. a
3. d
4. c
5. d
6. d
7. a
8. d
9. c
10. b
11. a
12. c
13. c
14. d
15. c
16. c
17. d
18. c
19. b
20. a
21. b
22. c
23. c
24. d
25. b
26. d
27. c
28. d

Bibliography

American Association of Retired Persons. (1991). Long term care ombudsman program. *Fact sheet on nursing homes.* American Association of Retired Persons: Washington, DC.

American Nurses Association. (1987). *Standards and scope of gerontological nursing practice.* Kansas City, MO: American Nurses Association.

Aroskar, M. (1980). Anatomy of an ethical dilemma theory and practice. *American Journal of Nursing. 4,* 658–663.

Beauchamp, T. L. & Childress, J. F. (1982). *Principles of biomedical ethics* (2nd ed.). New York: Oxford University Press.

Catholic Health Care Association. (1991). *The Patient self determination act health care decisions in advance.* St. Louis, MO: The Catholic Health Care Association.

Chenitz, W. C., Stone, J. T., & Salisbury, S. A. (1991). *Clinical gerontological nursing: A guide to advanced practice.* Philadelphia: W. B. Saunders Company.

Colorado Ombudsman Program. (1990). The use of restraints in nursing homes. *Here's help from the Colorado ombudsman program.* Denver: The Colorado Ombudsman Program.

Davis, A. J., & Aroskar, M. A. (1983). *Ethical dilemmas and nursing practice.* East Norwalk, CT: Appleton-Century-Crofts.

Johnson, R., & Justin, R. (1988). Documenting patients' end-of-life decisions. *Nurse Practitioner. 13*(6), 41–52.

Klein, C. (1986). Scope of practice. *Nurse Practitioner, 11*(11), 67–72.

Miller, C. (1990). *Nursing care of older adults: Theory and practice.* Glenview, IL: Scott Foresman/Little Brown Higher Education.

Miskin, B. (1986). *A Matter of choice: Planning ahead for health care decisions.* Washington, D.C: American Association of Retired Persons.

Moore, V. (1992). Self determined advance directives: New issues in primary care. *Nurse Practitioner Forum. 3*(1), 10–30.

National Health Council, Inc. (1988). *Whose choice is it anyway? Autonomous decision making at the end of life.* New York, N.Y: National Health Council Inc.

Office of the Inspector General Department of Health and Human Services. (1990). *Resident abuse in nursing homes: Understanding and preventing abuse.* Washington, DC: Department of Health and Human Services.

Quill, T. E., & Bannett, N. M. (1992). The effects of a hospital policy and state legislation on resuscitation orders for geriatric patients. *Archives of Internal Medicine, 152,* 569–572.

Stolman, C. J., Gregory, J. J., Dunn, D., & Levine, J. L. (1990). Evaluation of patient, physician, nurse, and family attitudes toward do not resuscitate orders. *Archives of Internal Medicine, 150,* 653–658.

Torain, L. V., Davidson, E. J., Fillit, H. M., Fulop, G., & Sell, L. L. (1992). Decisions for and against resuscitation in an acute geriatric medicine unit serving the frail elderly. *Archives of Internal Medicine, 150,* 561–565.

Professional Issues, Role Functions, and Health Policy

Pamela Cacchione

Theoretical Foundations

The advanced practice nurse in gerontology as well as the generalist nurse in gerontology is confronted by professional role development, the ability to promote change and resolve conflict, and the acquisition of decision making strategies. Models used to support the nurse in these areas include:

- Role Theory: Ralph Linton (1936) studied role in relation to culturally and socially determined occurrences. Role was defined as an ''external constraint'' and status as a collection of rights and duties. In Linton's theory, the inherent changes in a nurse's role have occurred partly as a result of culturally and socially determined external limits that have necessitated changes in the traditional role so as to provide for new positions with increased status. Role making and role modification were added to the concept of role by Mead (1967) and Moreno (1962). Role modification occurs when a disequilibrium of previously established roles and relationships are inadequate to meet current health care delivery needs. The roles of Clinical Nurse Specialist (CNS) and Nurse Practitioners (NP) grew out of this disequilibrium of the health care delivery system.
- Change Theory: There are several theories and models of change.
    1. Lewin's theory of change: Lewin's (1951) theory has three steps: unfreezing, moving to a new level, and refreezing. Unfreezing involves motivating participants in the direction of change. Moving to a new level occurs when participants have gathered enough information to recognize the need to alter their behavior, and refreezing occurs when participants have integrated the change into their participants' personalities (Lancaster & Lancaster, 1982).
    2. Chinn has described three models of change:
        a. The systems model: Uses assessment of the scope of the problem by defining the variables, stress, tension, and conflict surrounding the problem. The nurse then involves people who are ready, and those who are resistant to change in the planning. Then a pilot program is run and revised as needed (Menard, 1987).
        b. The developmental model: Involves diagnosing the transitional or critical areas and deciding what is inhibiting change from occurring. Personal factors which have been identified to inhibit change include: insecurity about a new role, self-doubt of

performance in a new situation, old role as a habit, poor coping methods regarding change, fear of loss of current job satisfaction and ignorance of implications of the planned change (Menard, 1987). Social factors which have been identified to inhibit change include: insufficient time for accomplishment, lack of employee input, inflexible plans, lack of money and lack of consideration of local or community conditions. Change may also be inhibited if there is a perceived threat to employee's economic interests, ethics, culture or religious or moral interests (Menard, 1987).

c. The ''model for change'': Includes elements of the developmental model, the systems model and is supported by Lewin's theory. In this case the change agent is an insider and active participant in the change. When the situation is unfrozen this breaks a habit and creates disequilibrium. The direction that will be taken is the responsibility of those involved and is arrived at in a collaborative manner. When the situation becomes comfortable, stable refreezing takes place (Menard,1987).

- Conflict Resolution: Conflict is often inevitable. Therefore effective conflict resolution is an essential part of nursing. There are three ways of dealing with conflict: avoidance, defusing or cooling down, and confrontation (Marriner-Tomey, 1992). Avoidance and defusing are passive methods of conflict resolution and usually not very successful; therefore confrontation will be discussed. Confrontation involves three stages: assessment, direct confrontation, and resettlement. Assessment includes determining what the problem is and how it is affecting you and others. A thorough assessment is essential in order to eliminate getting side tracked by peripheral issues. The second stage of direct confrontation is based on good communication skills. Guidelines for this stage include sticking to the facts, handling one subject at a time, and avoiding interrupting others. Everyone should have the chance to provide feedback after everyone has spoken (Marriner-Tomey, 1992). The final stage is resettlement which includes agreeing that a problem exists and jointly devising a strategy for resolution. This involves agreeing on what the key issues are and what steps need to be taken to resolve the conflict. Goals should be developed and the steps to meet these goals should be prioritized. A method for follow-up and reevaluation should be part of the plans for resolution. This is an effective process for conflict resolution.

- Decision-making models include the normative model of decision making and the descriptive model of decision making.
    1. The normative model is founded on two fundamental assumptions:
        a. All decisions are made with the objective of maximizing some predetermined goal or desired value
        b. All decisions are made to seek pleasure and avoid pain.
        c. Based on these assumptions decisions should be approached in the following manner:
            (1) The problem is defined and analyzed
            (2) All alternatives are identified
            (3) Each alternative is evaluated on its benefits and disadvantages
            (4) Alternatives are ranked and the alternative that maximizes the desired goal is selected, implemented, and reviewed (Lancaster & Lancaster, 1982).
    2. The descriptive model of decision making is based on the fact that people do not have all the information in order to utilize the normative model. Therefore the descriptive model characterizes people as being subjectively rational i.e., they make decisions on the basis of incomplete information and they seek satisfactory rather than optimal solutions to their problems (Lancaster & Lancaster, 1982). The descriptive model of decision making involves the individual subjectively defining a problem and identifying acceptable alternatives. Once alternatives are identified they are evaluated, one or two are chosen, and then the alternatives are implemented and evaluated (Lancaster & Lancaster, 1982).

Professional Issues

- Credentialing: A profession's efforts to acknowledge and recognize those who have achieved a level of skill and knowledge. This is also a method of self regulation; a means of demonstrating to and assuring the public of the profession's commitment to fulfilling its responsibility and thereby ensuring society's trust (Cary, 1989). There are basically four types of credentialing.
    1. Accreditation: Process by which a voluntary, nongovernmental agency or organization appraises and grants accreditation status to

institutions and or programs or services which meet predetermined structure process and outcome criteria (Geolot, 1986). Nursing schools are accredited by the National League for Nursing. The Joint Commission on Healthcare Organizations accredits hospitals and other health care organizations and agencies.

2. Licensure: Process by which an agency of state government grants permission to individuals accountable for the practice of a profession to engage in the practice of that profession and prohibits all others from legally doing so. It permits use of a particular title. Its purpose is to protect the public by ensuring a minimum level of professional competence (Geolot, 1986). Registered Nurses are licensed.
3. Certification: Process by which a non-governmental agency or association certifies that a licensed individual has met certain predetermined standards specified by a profession for specialty practice. Its purpose is to assure various publics that an individual has mastered a body of knowledge and acquired skills in a particular specialty (Geolot, 1986). Gerontology generalists, Gerontological Clinical Nurse Specialists and Gerontological Nurse Practitioners can be certified by the American Nurses' Credentialing Center if they meet certain criteria and receive a passing score on certification examinations. Certification must be renewed periodically by fulfilling the requirements for renewal.
4. Endorsement: An individual state's acknowledgement and acceptance of another state's Registered Nurse licensure. This has been made available because of the national licensure examination. The candidate must have attained a passing score on the national examination.

- Academic degrees: A reflection of the level of educational preparation a nurse has accomplished. Currently, there are nurses practicing with preparation in diploma programs which are usually conducted within a hospital setting. This type of basic education for nurses is being replaced with nurses prepared in academic programs where associate, baccalaureate, and master's degree are awarded upon successful completion of the programs. Many nurses receive their basic nursing preparation in either associate degree or baccalaureate degree programs and some continue their education and receive Master's degrees. They may also continue their education and receive doctoral degrees in nursing or other disciplines.

- Continuing Education: A more informal method of gaining or maintaining knowledge in a particular area of interest. Continuing education is essential for nurses to practice safely. Continuing Education Credits or contact hours are granted for self or independent study and attendance at lectures, symposia, and conferences which meet specified criteria. These credits are helpful in maintaining the level of certification one has reached.

- Standards of Gerontological Nursing: As the official organization of professional nursing, the American Nurses' Association has defined the standards and scope of gerontological nursing practice.

Standard I. Organization of Gerontological Nursing Services.

All gerontological nursing services are planned, organized, and directed by a nurse executive. The nurse executive has baccalaureate or master's preparation and has experience in gerontological nursing and administration of long-term care services or acute care services for older clients.

Standard II. Theory

The nurse participates in the generation and testing of theory as a basis for clinical decisions. The nurse uses theoretical concepts to guide the effective practice of gerontological nursing.

Standard III. Data Collection

The health status of the older person is regularly assessed in a comprehensive, accurate, and systematic manner. The information obtained during the health assessment is accessible to and shared with appropriate members of the interdisciplinary health care team, including the older person and the family.

Standard IV. Nursing Diagnosis

The nurse uses health assessment data to determine nursing diagnoses.

Standard V. Planning and Continuity of Care

The nurse develops the plan of care in conjunction with the older person and appropriate others. Mutual goals, priorities, nursing approaches, and measures in the care plan address the therapeutic, preventive, restorative, and rehabilitative needs of the older person. The care plan helps the older person attain and maintain the highest level of health, well-being, and quality of life achievable, as well as a peaceful death. The plan of care facilitates continuity of care over time as the client moves to various care settings, and is revised as necessary.

Standard VI. Intervention

The nurse guided by the plan of care, intervenes to provide care to restore the older person's functional capabilities and to prevent complications and excess disability. Nursing interventions are derived from nursing diagnosis and are based on gerontological nursing theory.

Standard VII. Evaluation

The nurse continually evaluates the client's and family's responses to interventions in order to determine progress toward goal attainment and to revise the data base, nursing diagnoses, and plan of care.

Standard VIII. Interdisciplinary Collaboration

The nurse collaborates with other members of the health care team in the various settings in which care is given to the older person. The team meets regularly to evaluate the effectiveness of the care plan for the client and family and to adjust the plan of care to accommodate changing needs.

Standard IX. Research

The nurse participates in research designed to generate an organized body of gerontological nursing knowledge, disseminates research findings, and uses them in practice.

Standard X. Ethics

The nurse uses the Code for Nurses established by the American Nurses' Association as a guide for ethical decision making in practice.

Standard XI. Professional Development

The nurse assumes responsibility for professional development and contributes to the professional growth of interdisciplinary team members. The nurse participates in peer review and other means of evaluation to assure the quality of nursing practice.

Note. From American Nurses' Association.(1987). *Standards and Scope of Gerontological Nursing Practice* (pp 1– 27). Kansas City, MO: Author. Reprinted with permission.

- Scope of Practice: Is defined by a state's nurse practice act, the rules and regulations of the nurse practice act, previous court decisions, the community's standard of care, and the nurse's job description. The nurse practice act varies from state to state and is available from each state's Board of Nursing. Ultimately each nurse is responsible for their own scope of practice and level of competence.

- Clinical Privileges: Are available to advanced practice nurses through contractual agreements with different facilities. The advanced practice nurse can gain admitting privileges to hospitals through the administration in the hospital setting. Geropsychiatric clinical nurse specialists, in some areas, have been able to get admitting privileges to mental health facilities. Gerontological nurse practitioners may have admission privileges in hospitals and long term care facilities.
- Protocol Development: Nurse Practitioners in many states are required to practice in collaboration with a physician utilizing protocols (or standing orders) for treatments of common conditions. These protocols are developed collaboratively by the nurse practitioner and the physician. Regulations regarding direct and indirect supervision of the nurse practitioner differ depending upon the state and area of practice.
- Professional Organizations: Have multiple purposes such as working to maintain a high standard of service to the community, working for the welfare of their members, and organizing their members collectively. Legislative and regulatory changes through political action are done through professional organizations. This method is resource-intensive and requires coordination with local, state, and national nursing associations (Sullivan, 1992).
    1. The American Nurses' Association (ANA): A national organization of professional nurses that focuses on standards of health care, nurses' professional development, and economic and general welfare of nurses. The ANA, comprised of individual state nurses associations, is the largest lobbying group for nurses.
    2. National League for Nursing (NLN): A national organization of nurses and lay people concerned with improving nursing education, nursing service, and the delivery of health care. The NLN is the official accrediting agency for nursing schools.
    3. Specialty Organizations: There are several specialty organizations which focus primarily on servicing their members through education and lobbying efforts.
        a. National Gerontological Nurses Association (NGNA) is a non-profit association created specifically for nurses specializing in

the delivery of health care to the elderly. The membership includes RNs, LPNs and other associate members interested in nursing care of the elderly (Meyers, 1993).

b. Gerontological Society of America (GSA) is a society founded to promote the scientific study of aging and to encourage exchanges among researchers and practitioners from the various disciplines related to gerontology. The GSA's members include: gerontological researchers, educators, and practitioners in biological, medical, behavioral, social sciences and humanities.

c. American Association of Retired Persons (AARP) is a lay persons' association which provides multiple services to the elderly and those interested in elder care. The AARP's members are seniors age 55 and older. The AARP has a very active legislative division which has tremendous grass roots support among its members making it a very strong force in Washington, D.C.

- Reimbursement: Essential in maintaining the viability of nurses in advanced practice. Direct reimbursement does the following for nurse practitioners and clinical specialists: Increases the availability and improves accessibility of health care to the elderly consumer; increases consumer choice of health care providers; provides for comprehensive health care for the elderly consumer; provides for cost-effective health care through improved utilization by nurse practitioners; legitimizes the nurse practitioner role; and decreases restrictions on practice imposed by limited reimbursement mechanisms (Bodenhorn, Celentano, Hardy-Havens, Millonig, 1991). There are two methods of gaining direct reimbursement.

  1. Agreements with individual insurance carriers: these agreements are negotiated on an individual level and are the suggested method for seeking direct reimbursement. A number of states have legislation to authorize reimbursement to the nurse practitioner from private and commercial insurers (Sullivan, 1992).

  2. Governmental systems for direct reimbursement include:

     a. Medicare: A government health insurance system which covers the elderly and the disabled. This program covers hospital services, physician services and other medical services. Medicare includes two parts: Part A Hospital insurance and Part B Supplementary insurance (Bodenhorn et al. 1991). Part A of medicare covers inpatient hospital care, short term skilled nursing facility care following a hospital stay, limited home health care visits and hospice care (Bodenhorn et al. 1991). Part B of Medicare covers any person entitled to Part A and all persons over the age of 65 if they enroll. This is a voluntary program and individuals must pay a premium to receive benefits. The program covers physician services, and some non-physician providers e. g., physical therapists, outpatient hospital care, laboratory and x-ray services and other related medical services and supplies (Bodenhorn et al. 1991). Some durable medical equipment is covered under Medicare Part B. The following legislation has provided for reimbursement for Nurse Practitioners and in some cases Clinical Nurse Specialists.

(1) Rural Nursing Incentive Act of 1991: Grants direct reimbursement from Medicare to all nurse practitioners and clinical nurse specialists practicing in designated rural areas (Mittelstadt, 1993).

(2) Indirect reimbursement from Medicare: Regulatory changes were enacted by the Health Care Financing Administration in 1990 which allows employers of nurse practitioners to receive direct payment from Medicare for services provided in a nursing facility (Sullivan, 1992).

(3) Omnibus Budget Reconciliation Act (OBRA): Authorizes payment of services of nurse practitioners under Medicare in nursing homes. This is indirect reimbursement through a nurse practitioner's employer whether a physician, nursing home or hospital (Mittelstadt, 1993). OBRA also allows nurse practitioners or clinical nurse specialists to certify and recertify the medical necessity for skilled nursing facility services under Medicare; the advanced practice nurse can not be employed by the facility caring for the patient for whom the certification is declared (Bodenhorn et al, 1991).

b. Medicaid: A combined state and federal government insurance program for persons of very low income. Nationally, the average income eligibility requirement for medicaid is less than half of 1990 federal poverty level. At least 42 states currently authorize direct reimbursement to nurse practitioners with varying restrictions (Pearson, 1993).

- Prescriptive Authority: Prescribing of drugs is an act essential to the assessment, diagnosis and treatment in the provision of primary care (Harkless, 1989). Prescribing privileges, which vary from state to state, are granted from state legislation, frequently under the provision of pharmacy bills. These bills frequently cover the prescribing privileges of nurse practitioners, nurse midwives, and clinical nurse specialists. Prescriptive authority is limited by formulary or protocols/practice agreements (Harkless, 1989).
- Interdisciplinary Practice: Is essential in the care of the elderly client. Nurses are expected to be active members of the interdisciplinary team. This team may include the patient, patient's family, nurses from the setting, possibly home care nurses, physical therapists, occupational therapists, speech therapists, social workers, chaplains, ethicists, a psychiatrist, and possibly a physician. The advanced practice nurse should be aware of the various roles and knowledgeable about who to refer to and collaborate with in patient care, staff education, or research

Practice Role Functions

- Clinician: The clinician role is the basis for the generalist's nursing practice. CNSs and NPs also have strong clinician roles. The clinical care of the elderly by advanced practice nurses includes providing direct patient care as well as developing advanced nursing interventions for the elderly clients.
- Educator: Being an educator is a large portion of the generalist, CNS and NP roles. This includes education of patients, their families, community groups and colleagues.
    1. Important teaching learning principles to remember are:
        a. Physical and mental readiness are necessary for learning. Obviously this varies from individual to individual therefore an assessment of readiness should be conducted prior to teaching whenever possible.
        b. An individual must be motivated to learn. The nurse should target the chief concern for that individual first, and focus the

teaching in this area. The nurse can offer incentives for learning, set realistic objectives, and organize the material to facilitate learning.

c. Learning can occur through imitation. Role modeling is an excellent teaching technique.

d. Effective learning requires active participation. Material learned through active involvement which incorporates several of the senses, has the highest level of retention.

e. Reinforcement strengthens learning. Rewards for appropriate learned behavior strengthen the newly gained knowledge (Menard, 1987).

f. Special guidelines for teaching elderly clients include:

   (1) Utilize a method that is self-paced rather than externally paced.

   (2) Emphasize the integration and application of knowledge and experience, rather than the acquisition of large amounts of new knowledge.

   (3) Use visual methods that are meaningful and lend themselves to thoughtful analysis.

   (4) Use auditory methods, alone or in combination with visual ones, for information that is factual and straightforward.

   (5) Provide advance organizers, such as outlines, written cues, and introductory overviews (Miller, 1990).

   (6) Make certain all sensory aids are in place, e.g., hearing aids, glasses.

   (7) Provide material in large print and on non-glare paper.

g. Group instruction is economical, efficient and it provides peer support, reinforcement and social pressure. Group instructions increase opportunities for self-rewards and decrease feelings of isolation (Menard, 1987).

2. Staff Development: A broad term used to describe the presentation of orientation, inservice education, and continuing education. It is the process by which formal and informal learning opportunities are

provided so that nurses may fulfill job expectations within a given agency or organization (Schweiger, 1986).

3. Selected nursing models relevant to gerontology which are important in educational efforts include:

    a. Adaptation Theory (Andrews & Roy, 1991): Views client as an adaptive system. The goal of nursing is to help the person adapt to changes in physiological needs, self concept, role function, and interdependent relations during health and illness. The need for nursing care arises when the client cannot adapt to environmental demands.

    b. Self-Care Theory (Orem, 1991): Views individuals as having to meet certain needs or life demands including air, food, water, excretion, activity, rest, solitude, social interaction, avoidance of hazards to life, and well being. Each individual has unique capacities and limitations regarding the ability to fulfill these demands. Self care capacity exists when individuals are able to be independent and take responsibility for meeting these needs. A self care limitation exists when an individual's ability to fulfill a demand is partially or totally restricted. Nursing actions focus on promoting capacity and reducing limitations of the individual so that care can be provided for self as independently as possible.

    c. Unitary Man (Rogers, 1979): Views man as an energy field coexisting within the universe who is in continuous interaction with his environment. Rogers describes man as a four dimensional energy field identified by pattern and manifesting characteristics which are specific to the whole and can not be determined from knowledge of the parts. Rogers utilizes the four dimensions to derive principles about how human beings develop.

- Consultant: Consultation has been described as a process of interaction between two professional persons: the consultant, who can be the CNS or NP, and the consultee, who invokes the consultant's help in regard to a current work problem. This problem must be identified within other's area of expertise. The process of consultation (Caplan, 1970) involves assessment of the consultation problem following the consultation request, developing a consultation report, implementation of the consultant's recommendations, and follow-up (Caplan, 1970).

1. Communication techniques: Communication is a major avenue for the advanced practice nurse to enhance their image during consultation. Communication occurs through structure and process. Structure includes regular meetings and documentation, while the process includes establishing paths of decision-making, and methods of conflict resolution.

2. Problem-solving skills: Problem solving skills are essential at all levels of nursing. These skills are developed through expanding ones clinical knowledge base and the use of the nursing process. Assessment is the first step toward solving the problem; development of a plan that can be either interdisciplinary or for the sole practitioner is the next step, which is followed by implementation of the plan. Unfortunately, in the role of the consultant, the plan may never be implemented because the consultee has the final decision on the plan of action. In an attempt to have the plan implemented, it is beneficial to communicate directly to whomever requested the service. Evaluation and revisions of the plan is the final step. This evaluation and follow-up process is very valuable and should not be underestimated; it is essential for continuity of care for the elder adult.

3. Networking: The process of developing contacts and professional acquaintances with people who have similar professional interests. The ongoing development of a professional network is extremely beneficial for the advanced practice nurse. It can lead to further consulting possibilities, new job opportunities, research opportunities (individual and collaborative), and further professional development.

- Researcher: Participation in research is an expected role of a master's degree prepared nurse. It requires that the nurse:

  1. Maintain a current scientific base of practice. It is the responsibility of the advanced practice nurse to know the latest research findings.

  2. Identify gerontological nursing problems to research in the setting in which (s)he is employed. This includes encouraging and supporting other nurses in pursuing research problems in the elderly.

  3. Have a knowledge of the rights of human subjects. which include informed consent, protection from physical or emotional harm, privacy and confidentiality. To safeguard these rights institutions have internal review boards to approve research proposals prior to their implementation (Waltz, Strickland & Lenz, 1991).

4. Have a knowledge of the institutional, human and material resources available to nurse researchers and access to these resources. This usually entails collaboration with the other individuals.
5. Be prepared to evaluate, interpret, and disseminate research findings to colleagues which can be done through informal communication, formal consultations, publications and continuing staff education.

- Administrator: Strong clinical skills can enhance the administrative role, if and when a CNS or NP pursue an administrative position. The administrator is part of a management team which utilizes a management process that includes: planning, organizing, staffing, directing, and controlling (Marriner-Tomey, 1992). Although administration is separate from leadership, effectiveness is related to leadership, and requires vision, and judgement (Marriner-Tomey, 1992). The following are activities which are part of the nurse administrator's role:
    1. Peer review: This is the critical evaluation of one's work by a colleague equal in qualifications, expertise, and position. It is thought that this is the best type of evaluation, when accompanied by self-evaluation, to meet the needs of advanced practice nurses (Menard, 1987). Administrators may be responsible for developing a peer review system. The guidelines for such a system include: first, the evaluation should be based on the advanced practice nurse's role functions, second the criteria should be developed to measure these role functions and third, the advanced practice nurse is given the opportunity to hear his/her peer review in order to take action (Menard, 1987).
    2. Interdisciplinary team building and development: The interdisciplinary team's purpose is to discuss, plan, implement, and review the ongoing care of particular patients. There is also a large educational component to interdisciplinary teams. These interdisciplinary teams can be developed wherever there are multiple disciplines working together for the benefit of patients: acute care, long term care, adult day care, psychiatric settings and primary care. Advanced practice nurses can influence interdisciplinary team building either in the role of clinician or administrator.
    3. Continuous quality improvement: The emphasis has recently shifted from quality assurance to that of continuous quality improvement. Continuous quality improvement is based on two fundamental concepts: overall systemic improvement, and the inclusion of customers in the process (Dienemann, 1992). Continuous quality improvement

requires the rejection of dualistic thinking as a way of assigning blame and correction of negative quality outcomes. Quality is a joint venture between caregiver and care receiver, between provider and payer, between education and practice and research (Mitty, 1992). This is the current approach to quality improvement for the elderly in acute and long term care settings.

In a successful continuous quality improvement program a team approach is most frequently utilized which includes the following steps:

a. Find a process to improve.
b. Organize a team that knows the process.
c. Clarify current knowledge of the process.
d. Understand causes of process variation.
e. Select the process improvement.
f. Plan the improvement.
g. Do data collection, data analysis, and improvement.
h. Check data for process improvement and customer outcome.
i. Act to maintain and continue improvement (Street & Alvis, 1992).

- Case Manager: Case managers coordinate services for the elderly, and can follow patients from primary care through the health care maze to help the patient receive the best care possible; in addition, case managers can assess the health care system to provide the most appropriate care possible. The important goals and outcomes of nursing case management are to optimize and increase the client's self care abilities, enhance quality of life and adjustment to altered health states, prevent inappropriate hospitalizations and decrease recidivism, provide quality health care with decreased fragmentation of care across settings and to promote health care cost containment (Papenhausen, 1990).
- Client Advocacy: An advocate supports, defends, and maintains the cause of someone or something. Advocacy has been called that part of the person's nature known as ''selfish benevolence'' (Kerschner, 1976). The advocate works to change the power structure so that the situation of his or her client may be socially, politically, or economically improved. This is done through ones own caring efforts to educate and support the client (Kohnke, 1982).

Settings for Practice

- Institutional living: The most common form, but not the only form of institutional living for the elderly is nursing home care. Other examples of institutional living include: chronic and rehabilitation hospitals, domiciliary care facilities, caretaker environments, congregate housing, and life care retirement communities. Some of these will be discussed. Nursing homes have three levels of care: skilled, intermediate, and residential.
    1. Skilled nursing facilities: Defined by federal regulations, which require 24 hour skilled nursing care under the supervision of a physician.
    2. Intermediate care facilities: Provide health care and services to individuals who do not require the care and treatment which a hospital or skilled nursing facility provides.
    3. Residential care facilities: Provide a lower level of care with room, board and some degree of supervision. There are no federal licensure categories for these types of facilities.
    4. Life care communities: Provide housing and services, including health care, in an independent residential setting. The communities guarantee shelter and various health care services for life, for a large one-time entry fee and an additional monthly fee.
- Community-based services: Community based services are many and their availability and accessibility is variable depending upon location, funding and community coordination. These include home care agencies, public health agencies, area agencies on aging, social service and adult protective service agencies, adult day care, and rehabilitative and medical services.
- Community living: Over 80% of the elderly live in the community. Some of these elderly require very little support and some require 24 hour custodial care. The majority of elderly, as well as their families, support remaining in the community as long as possible.
- Hospital care: Hospital care is inevitable for almost all elderly. Hospital care is necessary when an illness, physical or mental, can not be managed in any other setting. The degree of illness creates the need for acute medical or psychological care. The length of stay in a hospital setting is determined by the individual's illness and the Diagnostic Related Grouping (DRG) reimbursement system. This system impacts length of stay for

the elderly by predetermining the number of days a patient's care can be paid for. The elderly often require longer to recuperate from procedures and illnesses, however, there is not an adjustment made for this by the DRGs. Hospitalizations of the elderly often result in placement in long term care, either due to failure to recuperate in the time allotted, or the need for short term rehabilitation.

- Hospice care: Hospice care is the end of the continuum of long term care and often occurs in the community where the continuum begins. This is ideal when a terminal event can occur in a familiar setting where the individual is surrounded by family and friends. Hospice care is comprehensive comfort care for patients with terminal illnesses such as cancer and Alzheimer's disease. The hospice care includes family and friends of the patient and assists them with their bereavement. Hospice care can be either in the patient's home or in a community or hospital based setting.

Organizational Issues

- Long-term care continuum: A range of services that addresses the health, personal care, and social needs of individuals who lack some capacity for self-care. Services may be continuous or intermittent, but are delivered for sustained periods to individuals who have a documented need, usually measured by some index of functional incapacity (Kane, Ouslander & Abrass, 1984). Long-term care is not just provided in a nursing home; it is most often provided by families. There are a number of factors which affect the long- term care continuum

    1. Demographics: The United States Census Bureau predicts between 1984 and 1999 a 58% increase in the number of people aged 75 to 84. Elderly above 85 are projected to increase 132% during this same period. Thus the numbers of frail elderly continues to increase (Caudill, 1993).

    2. Demand for professionals and paraprofessionals: Nursing homes are expected to need more than one million nurses by the year 2000 which is double that in 1990 (Caudill, 1993).

    3. Increasing costs for health care coupled with a reduction in reimbursement for health care services: In 1984 the national health expenditures were approximately 10.6% of the gross national product (GNP); the percentage is expected to be 15.3% of the GNP by 1993. As this increase continues there is a federal policy for cost containment and cutbacks in funding.

4. Growth in consumer education: Consumers are learning that they have choices in health care and a right to participate in health care decisions.

- Continuous quality improvement: Continuous quality improvement is a concept which includes: quality assurance, problem resolution and quality improvement. Quality assurance involves the provisions of services that meet an appropriate standard. Problem resolution involves including all departments involved in the issue at hand. Quality improvement is the continuous process involving all levels of the organization working together across departmental lines to produce better services for health care clients (Moran & Johnson, 1992).

- Quality Assurance: Quality assurance programs are still present in the health care field while the transition is made to continuous quality improvement. The purpose of a quality assurance program is to ensure excellent physical and psychosocial care and improve the quality of life of the patients and residents. A facility's most valuable resource is a knowledgeable staff that has the ability to assess health problems and the environment of the residents and develop individualized goals and service plans (Stillwell, 1990). In a successful quality assurance program, the talents and expertise of the staff would be used to build an individualized program or to modify prepackaged programs to individual agency objectives (Stillwell, 1990).

Health Policy Issues

- Health care financing: Health care financing comes in many shapes and sizes from basic packages from the government to prepaid private insurance. The different types of health care financing will be summarized below.

1. Medicare: A federal government health insurance program for persons who age are 65 years and older and for some disabled persons. There are two parts to Medicare: Part A and Part B. Part A is the hospital insurance portion which covers inpatient hospital care, skilled nursing facility care, home health care and hospice care. Medicare Part A is financed primarily through a payroll tax. (Federal Register, 1992) Part B is the medical insurance portion of medicare which covers physicians' services, other out patient hospital services and cost of durable medical equipment. It is financed through monthly premiums and is voluntary. Individuals must enroll and pay a premium to receive benefits. Medicare generally pays 80% of

the reasonable charges for covered services, after the beneficiary has met the annual deductible (Sec. 4302, Public Law, 1990). One of the major limitations of Medicare is the lack of coverage for preventive services. Nor are medications, dental, vision care, or nonskilled long-term care covered.

Medicare is administered by the Health Care Financing Administration (HCFA) in the Department of Health and Human Services (HHS). These organizations utilize intermediaries for Part A and carriers for Part B to perform the day to day operations such as reviewing and paying claims. Private insurers such as Blue Cross/ Blue Shield act as these intermediaries or carriers (Bodenhorn et al. 1991).

2. Medicaid: Medicaid is a combined federal/state program that is administered by the individual states. Low income individuals qualify for Medicaid if they are blind, disabled, or members of families with children. In 1973, Medicaid was extended to all adults who met the criteria for Supplemental Security Income, including people who required long-term care (Miller, 1990).
3. Supplemental Insurance, otherwise known as Medigap insurance is a response to the limitations of Medicare coverage. About two-thirds of older adults purchase Medigap insurance. These insurance programs cover the copayment and deductibles for services covered by Medicare (Miller, 1990). There has been a lot of fraud in the area of Medigap insurance. It is essential for the elderly to be well informed regarding amount and kind of coverage.
4. Civilian Health and Medical Program of the Uniformed Services (CHAMPUS): This is a federal health plan that provides coverage to military personnel and their families. The program coverage extends to active duty personnel and their dependents, retirees, dependents and surviving dependents of service members. (Bodenhorn et al. 1991). Nurse practitioners are an integral part of primary care for the CHAMPUS program.
5. Health Maintenance Organizations (HMO): Prepaid health care organization that combines health care financing and health care delivery, emphasizing health promotion and health maintenance. Individual's choice of health care provider and agencies and hospitals are prescribed by the plan.

6. Preferred Provider Organizations (PPO): Formal arrangements where services of a panel of health care providers is marketed to purchasers for which payment is on a prospectively negotiated fee. Subscribers have an economic incentive to use the select panel.

- Allocation of Resources: The allocation of health resources to provide the maximum healthcare benefit to patients; this includes financial resources as well as health services and health personnel. As the aging population continues to grow additional strains are placed on the health care system to provide services to these individuals. This leads to disparities in distribution of services. A person's functional status rather than chronological age needs to be considered when distributing scarce resources. Gerontological nurses will be forced to become advocates for their patients to ensure ethical distribution of these resources.
- Access to care: Limited for those who do not have health insurance or have very limited insurance. This is a major impediment to health maintenance and health promotion. The elderly may have limited access to care due to disabilities as well as financing. It is often very difficult for the elderly to get to their primary care provider.
- Availability of Care: More and more hospitals have moved away from the inner cities to the suburbs. This has left many urban elderly without available health care. Rural areas also have tremendous problems with available health care. A large number of small rural hospitals have closed or converted to long term care facilities. This has dramatically limited the availability of health care for rural areas.

Political Activity

- Knowledge of the legislative process

   1. Congress: Congress is made up of two houses: the House of Representatives and the Senate. Members of the House of Representatives are elected for two-year terms by the residents of a district within a state. There are 435 members of the House of Representatives. The senate is made up of two senators from each state who are elected to six-year terms. Each representative and senator serves on a number of committees and subcommittees. Committee assignments are based on a number of factors: seniority, the member's interests and issues, and industries relevant to the constituent base.

2. The process of a Bill Becoming Law: Few pieces of legislation introduced in Congress actually become laws; most die in committee. The following is a brief outline of how a bill becomes law

   a. A senator or representative may request that a bill be prepared. Outside organizations often assist in its writing.

   b. A bill is introduced by a senator or representative in their respective House of Congress. The clerk of the respective House assigns a number and title to the bill, and the information is published in the *Congressional Record*

   c. The bill is then assigned to the committee or committees responsible for the particular area or issue. The chairman of the committee then assigns the bill to a subcommittee

   d. The subcommittee may hold hearings on the bill and invite testimony from public and private witnesses. Individuals may make their views known by testifying before the subcommittee, by providing a written statement or by allowing interest groups to represent their views.

   e. Once the hearings are completed, the subcommittee may meet to "mark up" the bill to consider amendments. It then votes on whether to report the bill favorably to the full committee. If not favorably reported, the bill dies.

   f. The full committee may repeat any or all the subcommittee's actions: hearings, mark up and vote. If the committee votes favorably on the bill, it is ordered reported to the respective side of Congress either the House of Representatives of the Senate.

   g. When the bill reaches the floor of the House or Senate, the membership of the entire body can debate it. At this stage, the bill may be further amended, voted up or down, referred back to committee or tabled. Should either of the two latter happen, the bill typically dies.

   h. If the bill is passed by the House or Senate, it then is referred to the other body for consideration. A House-passed bill may be placed directly on the Senate Calendar, bypassing the subcommittee and committee reviews. Usually, however, the subcommittees and committees in both bodies have an opportunity to hold hearings, debate and amend legislative proposals. Related or identical legislation often proceeds through the House and Senate simultaneously and is combined at some point in the process.

i. If there are significant differences between the House and Senate versions of the bill, an ad hoc "conference committee" is appointed by the President of the Senate and the Speaker of the House to resolve the differences. Conference committees are often composed of senators and representatives on the committees which originally considered the legislation.

j. If the conferees are unable to reach agreement, the legislation dies. If they do reach agreement, the bill is sent back to both houses where both must then approve the conference committee bill.

k. The bill then goes to the President for his signature. He may have four options:

(1) He can sign the bill and it becomes law

(2) He can take no action and the bill becomes law in 10 congressional days.

(3) He can take no action while Congress is adjourned at the end of the second session, the bill is "pocket vetoed" and the bill dies.

(4) Or the president may veto the bill.

Note. From *Advocacy Handbook: How to Lobby* by Daughters of Charity National Health Care System (1991). Adapted by permission.

- Advocacy for the development and implementation of public policy.

1. Nine steps to lobbying your legislators are listed below.

a. Establish contact with your state's congressional delegation, whether or not your senator and representatives sit on key authorizing or budget committees. Turn these contacts into relationships. Do not wait until you are angry to let them hear from you. Your job is to educate.

b. Determine which members of the staff handle health care issues in each office of your delegation.

c. Write to the appropriate staff; introduce yourself; explain your business and the services you provide, and let them know what a vital role you play in your community

d. Follow up with a phone call to make sure that the health care staff received your letter and to answer any questions they might have.

e. Make an appointment to meet with staff, either in Washington, D.C., or your home district.

f. "Prepare, prepare, prepare" for the meeting. If you plan to discuss a particular piece of legislation, learn the vocabulary of the legislation and where it stands in committee. You will also need to educate the staff about your practice and its importance and concerns.

g. Prepare some brief written materials, written in lay language to distribute at you meeting.

h. After your visit, be sure to send a thank you note summarizing the key points of your visit. Keep in touch with the office on a regular basis at least once a month.

i. Arrange for either the staff or your legislator to visit your practice setting for a "hands on tour". During this visit explain the high cost of delivering care and the types of community and charity care delivered. (Daughters of Charity National Health Care System, 1991).

2. The American Nurses' Association—One of nursing's major lobbying organizations. One of the purposes of the ANA is to prepare the members for political action through formal conferences and through their mailings about legislative issues. As nurses become more involved in political activities through networks, coalitions, political action committees, they gain recognition and power in the political arena. This involvement can facilitate the development of partnership relationships between nurse and their clients in working toward shared goals, which promote health, self-reliance and competence (Flynn & Martin, 1989).

Questions

1. Certification is intended to provide the following for nurses
    a. License them as advanced practice nurses
    b. Recognize their expertise in a given specialty area
    c. Increase their pay
    d. None of the above

2. According to role theory the CNS and NP movement grew out of:
    a. The disequilibrium of the health care system
    b. Nurses' desire to be more like physicians
    c. The need for nurses to be recognized as expert clinicians
    d. The surplus of physicians in rural areas

3. Conflict resolution is best resolved using which of the following methods:
    a. Avoidance
    b. Diffusion
    c. Cooling down
    d. Confrontation

4. Decision making models come in two styles, which are the two styles?
    a. Active and passive
    b. Normative and descriptive
    c. Collegial and interdisciplinary
    d. Individual and group

5. Continuing education is important for nursing as a profession because:
    a. It provides a method for all nurses to remain current
    b. It is necessary for licensure in all states
    c. It provides revenue for management
    d. All of the above

6. Protocol development:
    a. Is required in some states for NPs in collaborative practice with physicians
    b. Is the least restrictive form of NP prescription privileges
    c. Can prevent malpractice cases
    d. Is a very new phenomenon in nursing

7. Reimbursement for NPs and CNSs is
   a. Not available
   b. Available only in rural areas
   c. Available in some states directly and indirectly through private insurance, medicare and medicaid
   d. None of the above

8. Reimbursement is essential to advanced practice nurses because:
   a. It increases access to care for the elderly
   b. It is more cost effective
   c. It legitimizes the advance practice roles
   d. All of the above

9. Prescription authority for nurses:
   a. Is available in all 50 states
   b. Varies from state to state
   c. Is doomed due to the over surplus of physicians
   d. Is only available via the use of protocols

10. Education of the elderly should always:
    a. Be done in a loud tone in a bright room
    b. Be adapted to the elderly persons limitations
    c. Be done individually, never in a group
    d. Be externally paced

11. Which of the following is not always a part of the consultation?
    a. The consultation report
    b. The assessment of the problem
    c. Follow up on the recommendations made
    d. The consultant's recommendations are followed

12. Research in nursing:
    a. Is limited to doctorally prepared nurses
    b. Can be done in any setting except the nursing home due to OBRA regulations
    c. Is a role for all nurses, especially masters and doctorally prepared nurses
    d. All of the above

13. The rights of human subjects include all except:
    a. The right to be paid $20.00 an hour for being a research subject
    b. The right to know the benefits and risks of participating in a research project
    c. The right to know what alternative treatments are available other than being involved in a research project
    d. Informed consent

14. Advanced practice nurses should:
    a. Evaluate, interpret, and disseminate research findings
    b. Be involved in at least one research study at all times
    c. All have administrative positions
    d. Only work in underserved areas to improve access to health care

15. Which health care delivery system allows the greatest choice of primary care provider?
    a. Preferred Provider Organizations
    b. Health Maintenance Organizations
    c. Private Providers
    d. Medicare Part B

16. The steps that a continuous quality improvement team follow include all except the following:
    a. Clarify current knowledge of the process
    b. Organize a team that is not knowledgeable about the process so they will not be biased
    c. Do data collection, analysis and improvement
    d. Understand the causes of variation of the process

17. Case managers are utilized in all of the following except:
    a. Long term care facilities
    b. Acute care facilities
    c. Senior centers
    d. The community setting

18. Interdisciplinary care is useful:
    a. Only in the acute care and long term care setting
    b. For the family but not the patient

c. For all geriatric patients
d. All of the above

19. Chinn described 3 models of change. Which of the following is not one of Chinn's models for change?

    a. The systems model
    b. The development model
    c. The model for change
    d. The collaboration model

20. Which of the following is not a goal of case management:

    a. Monitor inappropriate hospitalizations
    b. Optimize client's self care abilities
    c. Enhance quality of life for client
    d. Decrease the fragmentation of care across settings

21. Peer review is:

    a. When a higher level colleague provides the nurse with a critical evaluation
    b. A method for management to avoid doing reviews
    c. Based on the nurse's role functions
    d. Thought to be of limited use for advance practice nurses

22. Networking is thought to be beneficial for all nurses because it:

    a. Helps nurses develop contact with other professional with similar interests
    b. May open up new job opportunities
    c. May open up research opportunities
    d. All of the above

23. The National League of Nursing:

    a. Provides certification for advanced practice nurses
    b. Is made up of nurses and lay persons interested in nursing education
    c. Provides continuing education credits.
    d. All of the above

24. Which of the following is not a standard of gerontological nursing practice?

    a. Nursing diagnosis
    b. Professional development

c. Intervention
d. Cost containment

25. Your 83 year old female community patient has a diagnosis of Alzheimer's disease. Her family wants to participate in her terminal care what would you suggest?

    a. That they should hospitalize her and the family should be present 24 hours a day.
    b. They should place her in a nursing home with a private duty nurse
    c. They should utilize respite care
    d. They should enroll her in hospice care

26. Continuous quality improvement includes all of the following except:

    a. Quality assurance
    b. Problem resolution
    c. Individual responsibility
    d. Quality improvement

27. Which health care financing measure is a supplemental federal government program that elderly people enroll in?

    a. Medicaid
    b. Medicare Part B
    c. Medigap
    d. Medicare Part A

28. What factors have affected availability of care to the elderly?

    a. Lack of insurance coverage beyond Medicare
    b. The move of the urban hospitals to the suburbs
    c. The rural hospitals converting to nursing homes
    d. All of the above

29. Which of the following facilities does not have federal licensure requirements?

    a. Chronic care facilities
    b. Skilled nursing facilities
    c. Intermediate care facilities
    d. Residential care facilities

30. The purpose of a quality assurance includes all of the following except:
    a. Improve quality of life of patients
    b. Ensure excellent physical care
    c. Improve the cost effectiveness of nursing care
    d. Ensure excellent psychosocial care

31. Civilian Health and Medical Program of the Uniformed Services (Champus) is a health plan that covers:
    a. Only the enlisted person and their dependents
    b. Military personnel and their families, including retired and active duty
    c. Only the retired military personnel and their dependents
    d. None of the above

32. Which of the following is not a step in lobbying your legislator?
    a. Your legislator is very busy so only educate your legislator when there is a bill currently being addressed that you are interested in.
    b. Determine which members of the legislator's staff handle health care issues.
    c. Communicate with the health care staff in writing, by phone, and in person when you are able.
    d. After meeting with the health care staff, write a thank you note, reviewing the key points of your meeting.

Answers

1. b
2. a
3. d
4. b
5. a
6. a
7. c
8. d
9. b
10. b
11. d
12. c
13. a
14. a
15. c
16. b
17. c
18. c
19. d
20. a
21. c
22. d
23. b
24. d
25. d
26. c
27. b
28. d
29. d
30. c
31. b
32. a

Bibliography

American Nurses' Association (1987). *Standards and scope of gerontological nursing practice.* Kansas City: American Nurses' Association.

American Nurses' Association (1980). *Nursing a social policy statement.* Kansas City: American Nurses' Association.

Andrews, H., & Roy, C. (1991). *Essentials of the Roy adaptation model.* Norwalk, CT: Appleton and Lange.

Barresi, C., & Stull, D. (1993). *Ethnic elderly & long-term care.* New York: Springer Publishing.

Bodenhorn, K., Celentano, D., Hardy-Havens, D., & Millonig, V. (1991). Health policy issues. In V. Millonig (Ed.), *The adult nurse practitioner certification review guide* (pp. 199-232). Potomac, MD: Health Leadership Associates.

Caplan, G. (1970). *The theory and practice of mental health consultation.* New York: Basic Books.

Carey, A. (1989). Credentialing: Opportunities and responsibilities in nursing. In C. Lambert & V. Lambert (Eds). *Perspectives in nursing: The impacts on the nurse, the consumer, and society* (pp. 33-52). Norwalk: Appleton & Lange.

Caudill, M. (1993). Governmental policies affecting the elderly and acquired immunodeficiency syndrome. In D. Carneval & M. Patrick (Eds.). *Nursing management for the elderly.* Philadelphia: J. B. Lippincott.

Dempster, J. (1991) The nurse practitioner and autonomy: Contributions to the professional maturity of nursing. *Journal of the american academy of nurse practitioners, 3*(2), 75-78.

Daughters of Charity National Health System (1991). *Advocacy handbook: How to lobby.* St. Louis: The Daughters of Charity National Health System.

Dienemann, J. (1992). *Continuous quality improvement in nursing.* Washington, D.C.: American Nurses Publishing

Edwards, J. (1991). What's holding back the nurse practitioner movement? *Imprint, 38*(4), 65-66.

Eliopoulus, C. (1990). *Health assessment of the older adult.* Reading: Addison Wesley.

Fawcett, J. (1989). *Analysis and evaluation of conceptual models in nursing* (2nd ed.). Philadelphia: F. A. Davis.

Federal Register (1992). *Medicare program inpatient hospital deductible and hospital and extended care services coinsurance amounts for 1993.* 57 FR # 229, November 27, 1992 at 56345

Flynn, B. C., & Martin, J. (1989). Demystifying political involvement. In C. Lambert & V. Lambert (Eds). *Perspectives in nursing: The impacts on the nurse, the consumer, and society* (pp. 453-475). Norwalk, CT: Appleton & Lange.

Geolot, D. H. (1986). The relationship between certification and practice. *Nurse practitioner, 11*(3), 55-58.

Hamric, A. B. & Spross, J. A. (1989). *The clinical nurse specialist in theory and practice* (2nd ed.). Philadelphia: W. B. Saunders.

Harkles, G. E. (1989). Prescriptive authority:Debunking common assumptions. *Nurse practitioner, 14*(8),57-61.

Heine, C. (1988). The gerontological nurse specialist: Examination of the role. *Clinical Nurse Specialist, 2*(1), 6-11.

Hooyman, N., & Kiyak, H. (1991). *Social gerontology a multidisciplinary perspective.* Boston: Allyn and Bacon.

Kane, R., Ouslander, J., & Abrass, I. (1984). *Essential of clinical geriatrics.* New York: McGraw Hill.

Kane, R., Garrard, J., Buchanan, J. L., Rosenfeld, A., & Skay, C. (1991). Improving primary care in nursing homes. *Journal of the American Geriatrics Society, 39*(4). 359-367.

Kerschner, P. A. (Ed.). 1976. *Advocacy and age.* Los Angeles: Andrus Gerontology Center.

Kohnke, M. F. (1982). *Advocacy: Risk and reality.* St. Louis: C. V. Mosby.

Labar, C. (1990). The issue of third party reimbursement—Advice for nurse practitioners from national expert. *Nurse Practitioner, 15*(3), 46-47.

Lancaster, J., & Lancaster, W. (1982). *Concepts for advanced nursing practice: The nurse as a change agent.* St. Louis: C.V. Mosby.

Linton, R. (1936). *Study of man.* New York: Appleton, Century, Crofts.

Marriner-Tomey, A. (1992). *Guide to nursing management* (4th ed.). St. Louis: Mosby Year Book

Mead, J. (1967). *Mind self and society* (2nd ed.). Chicago: University of Chicago Press.

Menard, S. W. (1987). *The clinical nurse specialist perspectives on practice.* New York: Wiley Medical Publication.

Meyers, D. (1993). Gerontological nursing and the national gerontological nursing association. *Geriatric Nursing, 14*(2), 101-103.

Miller, C. (1990). *Nursing care of older adults: Theory and practice* Glenview: Scott Foresman/Little Brown Higher Education.

Miller, T. V., & Rantz, M. (1989). Quality assurance: Guaranteeing a high level of care. *Journal of Gerontological Nursing, 15*(11), 10-15.

Mittelstadt, P. C. (1993). Federal reimbursement of advanced practice nurses' services empowers the profession. *Nurse Practitioner, 18*(1), 43-49.

Mitty, E. (1992). *Quality imperatives in long term care. The elusive agenda.* New York: National League for Nursing Press.

Montz, D., & Ostfeld, A. (1990). The epidemiology and demography of aging. *Principles of geriatric medicine and gerontology.* New York: McGraw Hill Information Systems.

Moran, M. J., & Johnson, J. E. (1992). Quality improvement: The nurse's role. In J. Dienemann (Ed.), *Continuous quality improvement in nursing.* Washington, D.C.: American Nurses Publishing.

Moreno, J. L. (1962). Role theory and emergence of self. *Group Psychotherapy, 15,* 114-117.

Orem, D. (1991). *Nursing concepts of practice* (4th ed.). St. Louis: Mosby Year Book.

Papenhausen, J. L. (1990). Case management:A model of advanced practice? *Clinical Nurse Specialist, 4*(4), 169-170.

Pearson, L. (1993). 1992-93 Update: How each state stands on legislative issues affecting advanced nursing practice. *Nurse Practitioner, 18*(1), 23-38.

Pawlson, L. G. (1990). Health care implications of an aging population. In W. R. Hazzard, R. Andres, E. L. Bierman & J. P. Blass (Eds.) *Principles of geriatric medicine and gerontology* (2nd ed.). New York: McGraw-Hill Information Services.

Public Law (1990). *Provisions relating to medicare part B premium and deductible.* Section 4302, Pub. L. 508, 101st Congress, Second Session.

Rogers, M. E. (1979). *An introduction to the theoretical basis of nursing.* Philadelphia: F. A. Davis.

Roy, C. (1986). The Roy adaptation model. In J. P. Riehl, & C. Roy (Ed.). *Conceptual models for nursing practice.* New York: Appelton-Century-Crofts.

Schroer, K. (1991). Case management: Clinical nurse specialist and nurse practitioner, converging roles. *Clinical Nurse Specialist, 5*(4), 189-194.

Schweiger, J. L. (1986). *Handbook for first-line nurse managers.* New York: John Wiley and Sons.

Severance, D. (1991) Prescriptive authority. *Frontier Nursing Service Quarterly Bulletin, 66*(4), 1-4.

Somers, A. R., & Spears, N. L. (1992). *The continuing care retirement community.* New York: Springer Publishing.

Stillwell, E. (1990). Assuring quality of care. *Journal of gerontological nursing, 16*(7), 3.

Street, E., & Alvis, D. (1992). A quality improvement process team. In J. Dienemann (Ed.), *Continuous quality improvement in nursing.* Washington, D.C.: American Nurses Publishing.

Sullivan, E.M. (1992). Nurse practitioners & reimbursement. *Nursing and Health Care, 13*(5), 236-241.

Trocchio, J., & Holloway, K. (1990). Quest for quality:Here's a program to help you grade your facility. *Geriatric Nursing, 11*(2), 34-36.

Waltz, C. F., Strictland, O. L., & Lenz, E. R. (1991). *Measurement in nursing research* (2nd ed.). Philadelphia: F. A. Davis.

INDEX

Certification Review Courses

A variety of Certification Review Courses are offered annually in the Washington, D.C. area.

■ **ANA APPROVED COURSES** ■

■ **95% TO 98% PASS RATE** ■

■ **ALL FACULTY CERTIFIED** ■

For information regarding these courses contact:

Health Leadership Associates, Inc.
P.O. Box 59153
Potomac, MD 20859

(301) 983-2405

AUDIO CASSETTES
Of Certification Review Courses

Live unedited audio recordings are available for those who are unable to attend our certification review courses which are offered annually. The audio recordings are an invaluable aid when studying for certification examination. If you cannot attend the courses, these cassettes are the next best thing to being there! Audio recordings are available for the following nursing specialties.

- *• Generalist Pediatric Nurse
- *• Generalist Gerontological Nurse
- • Generalist Medical-Surgical Nurse
- • Rehabilitation Nurse
- • Generalist Psychiatric and Mental Health Nurse
- *• Gerontological Nurse Practitioner
- • Clinical Specialist in Adult Psychiatric and Mental Health Nursing
- †*• Adult Nurse Practitioner
- †*• Pediatric Nurse Practitioner
- • Test Taking Strategies and Techniques
- †*• Childbearing Management
- • Ambulatory Women's Health Nurse
- • Community Health Nurse
- *• Ob-Gyn Nurse Practitioner
- • Nursing Administration

* These audio cassettes are available with corresponding Review Guides.

† These courses are the components of the FNP Certification Review Course.

For additional information contact:

Health Leadership Associates, Inc.
P.O. Box 59153
Potomac, MD 20859
(301) 983-2405

FORTHCOMING PUBLICATIONS

Published by Health Leadership Associates, Inc.

Psychiatric Certification Review Guide for the Generalist and Clinical Specialist in Adult Psychiatric and Mental Health Nursing

(Available Spring 1994)

Medical Surgical Nursing Certification Review Guide for the Generalist and Clinical Specialist

(Available Winter 1995)

Before and After Menopause

A "must" book

For clients, patients, colleagues, friends, relatives and you.

(Available Fall 1994)

The most current up to date information on the climacteric, menopause and postmenopause. Provides an explanation of the changes that occur during these periods in a woman's life and provides a summary of the research and latest up to date recommendation regarding treatment. Educates the reader so they can play a major part in collaboration with their health professional in their individualized management program.

For additional information contact:

Health Leadership Associates, Inc.
P.O. Box 59153
Potomac, MD 20859
(301) 983-2405

Additional Certification Review Guides

by Health Leadership Associates, Inc.

(Certification Review Specialists)

• The Review Guides Specifically Designed To Help You Prepare For Certification •

Review Guide Order Form

QTY	BOOK TITLE		AMOUNT
_____	Generalist Pediatric Nurse Certification Review Guide (2nd Edition)	43.95	_____
_____	Pediatric Nurse Practitioner Certification Review Guide (2nd Edition)	43.95	_____
_____	Adult Nurse Practitioner Certification Review Guide (2nd Edition)	43.95	_____
_____	Ob-Gyn Nurse Practitioner Certification Review Guide	43.95	_____
_____	Family Nurse Practitioner Package (Includes 3 Guides: ANP, PNP, & Ob-Gyn)	112.00	_____
_____	Gerontological Nursing Certification Review Guide for the Generalist, Clinical Specialist and Nurse Practitioner	43.95	_____
		SUB TOTAL	_____
		Maryland Residents add 5% sales tax	_____
		Shipping & handling $4.95 one book, Add $2.00 for each additional book	_____
		TOTAL	_____

For orders of 10 or greater, call 1-800-435-4775. International shipping fees additional, please inquire.
All prices subject to change without notice.

Name ______________________________

Address ______________________________

City ____________________ State __________ ZIP __________

Telephone Home: (   ) ______________ Work: (   ) ______________

☐ Check or Money Order (U.S. funds payable to Health Leadership Associates, Inc.)

☐ Purchase Order is attached P.O. # ______________________________

☐ MasterCard ☐ VISA Credit Card # ______________________________

Signature ______________________________ Exp. Date __________

Return Mail Order to: Health Leadership Associates, Inc.
P.O. Box 59153 • Potomac, MD 20859
(301) 983-2405

For MasterCard and VISA orders only: Call Toll Free 1-800-435-4775

How did you hear about H.L.A.? ______________________________

____